P9-BYT-081

# Chronic Fatigue, Fibromyalgia & Lyme Disease

SECOND EDITION

*Burton Goldberg*
*Larry Trivieri, Jr.*

Celestial Arts
Berkeley · Toronto

# CREDITS FOR THE SECOND EDITION

President: Burton Goldberg
Editor: Larry Trivieri, Jr.
Writer: Larry Trivieri, Jr.
Contributors: Kristen Bole, D.J. Fletcher, Tom Klaber,
 Richard Leviton, Stephanie Marohn

Portions of this book were previously published, in a different form, in
*Alternative Medicine: The Definitive Guide* and *Alternative Medicine Digest*

Celestial Arts
P.O. Box 7123
Berkeley, CA 94707
www.tenspeed.com

Distributed in Australia by Simon & Schuster Australia, in Canada by Ten
Speed Press Canada, in New Zealand by Southern Publishers Group, in
South Africa by Real Books, and in the United Kingdom and Europe by
Airlift Book Company.

Cover design by Betsy Stromberg

LIBARY OF CONGRESS CATALOGING-IN-PUBLICATION DATA
Goldberg, Burton, 1926-
    Chronic fatigue, fibromyalgia, & Lyme disease : an alternative
medicine definitive guide / by Burton Goldberg and Larry Trivieri, Jr.—
2nd ed.
        p.   cm.
First ed. published in 1998 under title: Alternative medicine guide to
chronic fatigue, fibromyalgia & environmental illness.
    ISBN 1-58761-191-0
    1. Chronic fatigue syndrome — Alternative treatment.
2. Fibromyalgia — Alternative treatment.   3. Environmentally
induced diseases — Alternative treatment.   4. Lyme disease —
Alternative treatment. I. Trivieri, Larry, 1956– .  II. Goldberg,
Burton, 1926– .  Alternative medicine guide to chronic fatigue,
fibromyalgia & environmental illness.   III. Title.
RB150.F37G643   2004
616'.0478 — dc22                                    2003025247


    2   3   4   5   —   08   07   06   05   04
Printed in the United States

# Important Information

This book was written as an educational tool to enable you to better understand, assess, and choose the best course of treatment when chronic fatigue, fibromyalgia, environmental illness, or Lyme disease strikes. It will also show you how to prevent these conditions from striking in the first place. It could save your life.

In reading this book, please remember that it is not another catalog of mainstream medicine's conventional treatments and drugs that are used to treat these diseases. It is about effective *alternative* approaches to these conditions—approaches generally not understood and, at this time, not endorsed by the medical establishment. Therefore, we urge you to discuss the treatments described herein with your doctor. If your doctor is open-minded, you may actually educate him or her. We are gratified to know that many of our readers have found their physicians to be open to new ideas.

Use this book wisely. Because many of the treatments it describes are, by definition, alternative, they have not been investigated, approved, or endorsed by any government or regulatory agency. National, state, and local laws may vary regarding the use and application of many of the treatments that are discussed. Accordingly, this book should not be substituted for the advice and care of a physician or other licensed healthcare professional. Pregnant women, in particular, are urged to consult with a physician before commencing any therapy. Ultimately, you, the reader, must take responsibility for your health and how you use the information in this book.

Neither AlternativeMedicine.com, Burton Goldberg, nor Larry Trivieri, Jr. have a financial interest in any of the products or services discussed in this book, other than the citations to AlternativeMedicine.com's other publications. All of the factual information in this book has been drawn from the scientific literature.

# Contents

# You Don't Have to Endure Chronic Fatigue

If you have chronic fatigue syndrome or one of its close relatives—fibromyalgia, environmental illness, and Lyme disease—you most likely have experienced years of frustration trying to find relief from your puzzling assortment of symptoms. You may have spent years just trying to find a doctor who could find out what was wrong with you. In the process, you probably encountered many medical professionals who dismissed your complaints as neurotic imaginings.

If you were fortunate enough to find a physician who acknowledged your problem by giving it a name, a name was likely all you got. Conventional medicine is usually baffled by these disorders and can only offer drugs to temporarily ease some of the symptoms: painkillers for the muscle pain of CFS and fibromyalgia; antihistamines for the allergies of CFS and environmental illness; antibiotics for Lyme disease; antidepressants for the mood disorders of all four. But such conventional drugs produce their temporary relief only at the cost of considerable side effects and toxicity.

It is not only conventional physicians who have failed you. It is the whole conventional medical establishment, which has for more than a decade debated whether CFS even exists and, if it does, arguing over the number and nature of symptoms that qualify a person for the distinction of having CFS. This has been the pursuit of the U.S. government's Centers for Disease Control—whose accomplishments, after more than ten years of investigating CFS, consist of the development of formal diagnosis criteria.

But they are no closer to discovering what causes CFS (or how to treat it) than they were in the mid-1980s, when the outbreak in Incline Village, Nevada, first drew their attention to what would become an epidemic. Conventional medical research seems, as it is with most illnesses, capable only of focusing on the search for that single cause that will then yield the mythical "magic bullet" cure. That is not the way alternative medicine goes about dealing with a complex illness like chronic fatigue.

The good news is that you don't have to wait for the magic bullet (which will never arrive). Alternative medicine has practical solutions for you now. Physicians of alternative medicine know that illness is multifactorial. Particularly in the case of such complex disorders as CFS, fibromyalgia, and environmental illness, no one cause is responsible. Multiple imbalances and deficiencies combine to produce the breakdown of the body. And all three of these disorders can be severely complicated by Lyme disease, a condition that has become pandemic in this country and still, for the most part, goes undetected, because its many symptoms are often mistakenly identified as other illnesses.

Knowing this, alternative medicine physicians have set about to systematically identify these factors—from viruses and yeast overgrowth to heavy metal toxicity and nutritional deficits—through precisely targeted, nontoxic tests. Once the underlying factors have been pinpointed, a treatment plan can be designed to address each one. Instead of treating symptoms, which can only produce temporary relief at best, alternative medicine goes to the root causes and so can provide a real and lasting solution to your health problems.

In addition, alternative physicians know that if you want good results, you must always consider the body as a whole. For example, prescribing supplements for patients with severe nutritional deficiencies without first addressing their digestive problems will yield little or no results—because until the patient's faulty digestion is addressed and resolved, nutrients cannot be properly absorbed. All the systems of the body are interrelated; that is why holistic medical treatment is such an effective model. Holistic medicine also knows that no two people, even with the same illness, will require the same treatment. "Cookbook prescriptions" have no place in the world of alternative medicine.

In this book you will learn how over 50 alternative medicine physicians reverse CFS, environmental illness, fibromyalgia, and Lyme disease using an individualized, holistic approach. You will also read numerous case histories of people who finally found answers and solutions after years of consulting conventional physicians and getting neither. In the process, you will discover the many factors that can contribute to the development of these disorders—factors frequently ignored or overlooked by mainstream medicine.

Best of all, this book can start you on your path to full recovery. I'm here to tell you that you don't have to endure your illness, no matter what you've heard before. This book will show you how you can join the other success stories and leave your chronic fatigue, fibromyalgia, environmental illness, and/or Lyme disease behind.

God bless,
*Burton Goldberg*

# User's Guide

One of the features of this book is that it is interactive, thanks to the following eight icons:

This means you can turn to the listed pages elsewhere in this book for more information on the topic.

This tells you where to contact a physician, group, or publication, or how to obtain substances mentioned in the text. This is an editorial service to our readers. Most importantly, the use of this icon empowers you right now, by giving you a source to acquire something vital to your health, quickly and easily. Whenever possible, we give you complete contact information for all substances mentioned in the text. All items are based on recommendations from the clinical practice of physicians in this book. The publisher has no financial interest in any clinic, physician, or product discussed in this book.

Many times the text mentions a medical term that requires explanation. We don't want to interrupt the text, so instead we put the explanation in the margins under this icon. This gives you the option of proceeding with the text or taking a moment to learn more about an important term. You will find some of the key definitions repeated at different places in the book so you don't have to search for the definition.

This sign tells you there may be some risks, uncertainties, side effects, or special contraindications regarding a procedure or substance.
*Pay close attention to these icons.*

 This icon asks you to give a particular point special attention in your thinking. It is important to the overall discussion at hand.

 This icon highlights a particularly noteworthy point and bids you to remember it.

 In many cases, alternative medicine is far less expensive than conventional treatments. This icon means that the widespread acceptance of the therapy or substance under discussion could save considerable health-care money.

 More research on this topic would be valuable and should be encouraged to further substantiate or clinically prove a promising possibility of benefit to many.

# one

# Related Epidemics

*Chronic Fatigue Syndrome, Fibromyalgia,*
*Environmental Illness, and Lyme Disease*

When the first cases of chronic fatigue syndrome (CFS) were identified in the 1980s among patients in a small Nevada town, the strange disease—marked principally by deep fatigue and muscle aches—was dubbed "Yuppie flu." It seemed to be concentrated among young, affluent white professionals. Due to this and to the seemingly subjective nature of the symptoms, CFS was the butt of jokes and its sufferers were often not taken seriously by many physicians. A decade later, CFS had become an epidemic across all ethnic and demographic barriers. It is now recognized as a severe, debilitating illness, although the dismissive attitude persists among some doctors.

Despite the eventual recognition of the disorder, conventional medicine still does not know what causes chronic fatigue syndrome—blaming it variously on the Epstein-Barr virus, candidiasis (fungal overgrowth), and the herpes virus—and has no answers for treating it. Meanwhile, the number of cases continues to rise. In fact, government health agencies have spent far too much time and attention on devising supposedly accurate descriptive terms and diagnostic categories for chronic fatigue rather than on figuring out successful ways to eliminate the problem.

The U.S. Centers for Disease Control and Prevention (CDC), based in Atlanta, Georgia, offers a typically conservative estimate of four to ten cases per 100,000 adults (which translates to 10,440 to 26,100 Americans),[1] but other sources place the numbers much higher. According to Murray R. Susser, M.D., a physician practicing in Santa Monica, California, chronic fatigue syndrome (also known as chronic fatigue and

## The Multiple Factors That Contribute to Chronic Fatigue Syndrome

- Multiple infections
  (viruses, candidiasis, parasites)                    See chapter 3

- Immune dysfunction                                    See chapter 4

- Thyroid problems                                      See chapter 6

- Toxicity (from environment, food,                     See chapters 5 and 7
  dental amalgams, and drugs)

- Enzyme deficiency                                     See chapter 8

- Underlying allergies                                  See chapter 9

- Nutritional deficiency                                See chapter 10

- Lifestyle (stress, psychological/                     See chapter 11
  emotional factors)

- Lyme disease                                          See chapter 15

immune dysfunction syndrome, CFIDS) afflicts an estimated three million Americans and possibly 90 million people worldwide.

Jesse A. Stoff, M.D., coauthor of *Chronic Fatigue Syndrome: The Hidden Epidemic*, believes it is even more widespread; he estimates that the number of people with CFS in North America alone exceeds by four million the number of people with AIDS.[2] The CDC reports that 80% of diagnosed cases are women, the majority of whom are white and between the ages of 25 and 45. However, these figures reflect underreporting among nonwhite populations.[3] In addition to the United States, CFS has been reported widely in Canada, New Zealand, Australia, Europe, South Africa, Russia, Japan, and Iceland.[4]

A new study probing the extent of CFS occurrence in the nonwhite population suggests that possibly 10% of that population is "highly fatigued." A survey by the San Francisco Department of Health of 16,000 residents of San Francisco revealed that 2% had suffered from unexplained fatigue for at least six months and 10% of these met the criteria for chronic fatigue syndrome as defined by the CDC.

When the numbers were extrapolated to all of San Francisco, it suggested that 14,600 residents were "highly fatigued, extremely tired, or exhausted," according to the study directors. This number was considered to be 20 times higher than previous official estimates and was consistent with similar surveys in Chicago, Illinois, and Seattle, Washington, as well as England and Australia.

The San Francisco survey also found that for every 100 whites with CFS symptoms, there were 144 African Americans and 157 Latinos, but only 64 Asians reporting the same. The symptoms were most prevalent among women, aged 30 to 39. No single type of job was associated with the incidence of chronic fatigue, nor did it seem to cluster in households, which would have suggested a contagious aspect. Contrary to earlier assumptions, the syndrome seemed to affect more people (by a factor of about 30%) with incomes under $40,000 than those with incomes exceeding this amount.[5]

## Required Symptoms for a Diagnosis of Chronic Fatigue

In March 1988, the CDC released criteria for a diagnosis of CFS; it revised these in 1994 to encompass the broader symptom spectrum of those afflicted. In order to be diagnosed with CFS, a person has to be suffering from these symptoms:

1) New, unexplained, persistent, or relapsing chronic fatigue that is not a consequence of exertion, not resolved by bed rest, and severe enough to significantly reduce previous daily activity; and

2) four or more of the following symptoms for at least six months:
   - Unexplained or new headaches
   - Short-term memory or concentration impairment
   - Muscle pain
   - Pain in multiple joints unaccompanied by redness or swelling
   - Unrefreshing sleep
   - Postexertion malaise that lasts for longer than 24 hours
   - Sore throat
   - Tender lymph nodes in the neck or armpits

In fact, fatigue in general, whether it is chronic or episodic, is increasingly a problem in the United States. It is estimated that 24% of the general adult population of the United States has experienced fatigue lasting two weeks or longer; of these people, 59% to 64% reported no known medical cause. One study showed that 24% of primary care patients had experienced prolonged fatigue of at least one month's duration; some reported their fatigue lasted more than six months.[6]

## Closely Related Severe Chronic Fatigue States

Two close relatives of chronic fatigue syndrome—fibromyalgia and environmental illness—are also becoming more prevalent. Fibromyalgia (from *fibro*, or connective tissue, and *myalgia*, or muscle pain) is a painful muscle disorder in which the thin film or tissue (myofascia) holding muscle together becomes tightened or thickened, causing pain. Also called fibrositis, fibromyalgia shares many of the same symptoms as CFS, including debilitating fatigue, muscle and joint pain, sleeping disorders, depression, anxiety, mental confusion, and digestive problems. Jacob Teitelbaum, M.D., a specialist in the two syndromes, calls CFS the "drop-dead" flu and fibromyalgia the "aching-all-over" disease. Given the similarity that these descriptive names embody, Dr. Teitelbaum prefers to put CFS and fibromyalgia in a single category he calls severe chronic fatigue states.[7]

An estimated three to six million Americans suffer from fibromyalgia, 86% of whom are women. The level of disability caused by fibromyalgia is severe enough that 25.3% of women and 27% of men affected are unable to work, according to a recent study.[8]

### *The Official Definition of Fibromyalgia*

In 1990, the American College of Rheumatology (ACR) established the following diagnostic criteria for fibromyalgia. According to the ACR, there must be widespread pain of at least three months' duration in 11 out of 18 tender muscle sites, as follows:

- *Occiput* (on the head): bilateral (on both sides), at the suboccipital muscle insertion
- *Lower Cervical:* bilateral, at the anterior aspects of the intertransverse spaces of cervical (neck) vertebrae C5 to C7
- *Trapezius* (upper back): bilateral, at the midpoint of the upper border
- *Supraspinatus* (shoulder blades): bilateral, at origins above the scapula near the medial border
- *Second Rib:* bilateral, at the second costochondral junctions just lateral to the junctions on the upper surfaces
- *Lateral Epicondyle* (top of the thigh bone, or humerus): bilateral, 2 cm distal to the epicondyle
- *Gluteal* (buttocks): bilateral, in upper quadrants of buttocks in anterior fold of muscles
- *Knee:* bilateral, at the medial fat pad proximal to the joint line

The symptoms of environmental illness similarly overlap those of both CFS and fibromyalgia. Also known as multiple chemical sensitiv-

## Symptom Chart of the Three Related Epidemics

**Chronic Fatigue**

allergies
anxiety
brain fog and confusion
cough
decreased appetite
depression
digestive disorders
dizziness
dry eyes and mouth
general stiffness
headaches
increased thirst
irritability
joint and muscle pain
low body temperature
low-grade fever
memory loss
muscle weakness
nausea
night sweats
PMS (women)
poor concentration
prolonged fatigue after exertion
rashes
recurring infections
severe fatigue
sleep problems
sore throat
swollen lymph nodes
visual blurring

**Fibromyalgia**

allergies
anxiety
carpal tunnel syndrome
depression
dizziness
dry eyes alternating with watery eyes
dysmenorrhea (women)
exercise intolerance
fingernail ridges
general fatigue
general stiffness
headaches
heightened sensitivity to light, sound, smell, touch
"hurting all over"
irritability
irritable bowel symptoms
mood swings
numbness or tingling sensations
sensitivity to cold
sleeping disorders
tender skin
widespread muscle and joint pain

**Environmental Illness**

anxiety
asthma
coughing or wheezing
depression
digestive problems
fatigue
headaches
infections
irritability
mood swings
multiple allergies
multiple chemical sensitivities
muscle pain and/or weakness
weight loss

ity, the syndrome involves numerous and extensive allergies, often to nearly everything in one's environment and to such a degree that many sufferers must isolate themselves in their homes and avoid exposure to such commonplace items as chemically treated building materials, plastics, synthetic carpets, newsprint, perfume, soap, and car exhaust, to name a few. Since the sensitivities seem to be focused on (although not limited to) manufactured products, many people view environmental illness as a response to the increasing level of toxins in our environment.

Some practitioners believe that environmental illness is an extreme extension or outcome of prolonged chronic fatigue syndrome. Shari Lieberman, Ph.D., C.N.S., a nutritional specialist based in New York City, is among them. She has treated several hundred people with chronic fatigue syndrome to date and reports: "I see patients with envi-

According to the American College of Rheumatology, when a patient has widespread pain of at least three months' duration in 11 out of 18 tender muscle sites (as pictured above), they're diagnosed as having fibromyalgia.

ronmental sensitivities who have come to me after three to five years of chronic fatigue. If they've only had CFS for six months, they don't tend to have environmental sensitivities."

The primary sufferers of CFS, fibromyalgia, and environmental illness are women, and all three disorders share the dubious distinction of being poorly understood by the medical profession. Although fibromyalgia was first described by a physician in 1816 and classified as a distinct disorder (a painful arthritic condition) in 1904, it did not receive recognition as the debilitating condition it is until fairly recently; in 1987, the American Medical Association cited it as a disabling illness.[9]

However, a misconception in the medical community that fibromyalgia is caused by deconditioning—muscles becoming weak and limp as a result of inactivity—has added to the painful burden of those who suffer from the disorder. This blaming of the victim is singularly unhelpful to the patient's state of mind and is also medically inaccurate—most fibromyalgia sufferers were highly active people—overachievers, in fact—when the condition struck.

Environmental illness is less widely acknowledged as a physical disorder than fibromyalgia and CFS, but this is changing as its growing occurrence makes it a phenomenon that can no longer be ignored. All three conditions have frequently been misdiagnosed as depression, and patients have often been told "it's all in your head." Some doctors still refuse to even admit the existence of the three syndromes. Fortunately, their numbers are dwindling as the number of the afflicted rises.

However, with the overlap of symptoms, it can be difficult to determine which syndrome a person has and, indeed, an individual may be suffering from all three. Alternative medicine—the approach of this book—finds it more useful to identify the systemic imbalances that are producing the symptoms rather than trying to fit the individual into one of the three conventional diagnostic categories. This approach also stems from the alternative medicine model of addressing the sources of illness rather than just treating symptoms; the latter practice only produces temporary relief at best. The conventional medical solution for fibromyalgia—painkillers—is a prime example of symptom-driven treatment, with little understanding of causes and equally slim chances of therapeutic success.

Although this book focuses predominantly on chronic fatigue syndrome, the alternative medicine view is that the three disorders share

## Chemical Exposure as a Factor in CFS

According to the Centers for Disease Control (CDC), exposure to toxic chemicals rules out a diagnosis of CFS. However, a recent study of 22 people who met the CDC criteria for CFS, and 17 people who had CFS symptoms but whose history of chemical exposure precluded a CFS diagnosis, found that there was no significant difference between the two groups in terms of their blood level of chlorinated hydrocarbons, notably HCB and DDE.

Chlorinated hydrocarbons, also known as organochlorines, are chemical compounds formed by a carbon-to-chlorine bond. HCB is a widely used pesticide and DDE is a byproduct of the metabolism of DDT, another common pesticide. Both the CFS group and the group with CFS symptoms and known chemical exposure had significantly higher organochlorine levels than the control group of 34 non-CFS subjects. The researchers concluded that toxic chemical exposure may play a causal role in CFS. They also concluded that the CDC's exclusion of a toxic exposure history from the criteria for CFS is not valid.

Source: Dunstan, R. H., et al. "A Preliminary Investigation of Chlorinated Hydrocarbons and Chronic Fatigue Syndrome." *Medical Journal of Australia* 163:6 (September 18, 1995), 294–297.

> The primary sufferers of CFS, fibromyalgia, and environmental illness are women, and all three disorders share the dubious distinction of being poorly understood by the medical profession.

the same cluster of underlying causes. Therefore, learning about the causes of CFS and how to address these causes in treatment (as discussed here) is equally useful for people with fibromyalgia and environmental illness. The multiple causes of the three syndromes—and, therefore, the necessity for a combination of treatment methods—make them ideal candidates for alternative medicine's multimodal approach to healing. This means many symptoms require multiple therapies to unravel them.

## Treating the Individual

As a syndrome, CFS presents an array of symptoms that may appear unrelated. But according to alternative medicine, all are products of an underlying imbalance in the body produced by multiple simultaneous infections and accompanying physical, mental, and environmental factors.

Specifically, Dr. Susser states that CFS develops as a result of a combination of nutritional deficiency; acquired toxicity (from environment, food, dental amalgams, dental infections, and/or drugs); poor stress-coping abilities; acquired systemic infections (often due to excessive use of antibiotics causing candidiasis and parasite overgrowth); and a vicious cycle of lowered immune function, allergy, more infection, and further depleted energy reserves. These factors will be explored in depth in the chapters that follow.

It is essential to understand the factors involved in the onset of CFS in each person because CFS is never caused by one thing alone and no two people have exactly the same causal factors. This individualized diagnostic approach is particularly important in the case of CFS because, along with fibromyalgia and environmental illness, it shares symptoms with diseases such as multiple sclerosis and lupus.[10] Misdiagnosis is common and creates additional pain and frustration, which could likely have been avoided by an individualized approach to the patient.

In the following section, Dr. Stoff details the multiple causes of CFS (in the context of relating a CFS case) and demonstrates how it can be successfully reversed using a treatment plan tailored to the individual's needs. Dr. Stoff's case will frame this book's approach to reversing

## Concise Definitions of the Three Related Epidemics

**Chronic fatigue syndrome (CFS)** is an umbrella term for a multiple-symptom disorder characterized most commonly by the sudden onset of extreme, debilitating fatigue, pain in the muscles and joints, headaches, and poor concentration. The fatigue is not alleviated by rest and results in a substantial reduction in previous levels of daily activity. CFS is often cyclical, with periods of relative health followed by debilitation. Other symptoms include depression, anxiety, digestive disorders, memory loss, allergies, recurring infections, and low-grade fever. According to the CDC, CFS predominantly affects white women, 25–45 years old.

**Fibromyalgia** is a multiple-symptom syndrome primarily involving widespread muscle pain (myalgia) that can be debilitating in its severity. The pain seems to be caused by the tightening and thickening of the myofascia, the thin film of tissue that holds the muscle together. Typical tender sites include the neck, upper back, rib cage, hips, and knees. Other symptoms include general fatigue and stiffness, insomnia and sleeping disorders, anxiety, depression, mood swings, allergies, carpal tunnel syndrome,

headaches, the sense of "hurting all over," tender skin, numbness, irritable bowel symptoms, dizziness, and exercise intolerance. Post-traumatic fibromyalgia is believed to develop after a fall, whiplash, or back strain, whereas primary fibromyalgia has an uncertain origin. The majority of fibromyalgia sufferers are women between the ages of 34 and 56.

**Environmental illness** is a multiple-symptom, debilitating, chronic disorder involving prolonged, heightened, and often incapacitating allergies or sensitivities to numerous common substances found in one's environment. Symptoms may include headaches, fatigue, muscle pain and/or weakness, coughing or wheezing, asthma, weight loss, infections, and emotional fluctuations, depression, and irritability. The illness is sometimes referred to as "twentieth century disease" because patients become allergic to and functionally incompatible with many products and substances found in the modern world, such as car exhaust, synthetic carpets, plywood and other building materials, cleaning agents, office machines, and plastics, among others.

chronic fatigue syndrome. The chapters that follow will be extensions and commentaries on Dr. Stoff's insights and protocols.

# The "Whole Patient" Approach to Chronic Fatigue Syndrome

Successfully treating illnesses such as chronic fatigue, AIDS, and cancer is Dr. Stoff's specialty. He draws upon a wide range of alternative medicine therapies to accomplish this, including nutrition, homeopathy, Chinese herbs, Anthroposophic medicines, relaxation techniques, guided imagery, and massage, among others. "Health is restored to the whole patient, not just the body," Dr. Stoff says.

The goal of Dr. Stoff's treatment approach is to help each person achieve a working balance between physical healing and the emotional,

> Misdiagnosis of chronic fatigue syndrome is common and creates additional pain and frustration, which could likely have been avoided by an individualized approach to the patient.

mental, and spiritual aspects of their life. "We assist and encourage the patient to take an active role in the healing process," Dr. Stoff explains.

The first step before designing a treatment plan is extensive testing. Dr. Stoff believes in evaluations of a patient's blood, urine, and stool, consultations with staff physicians and specialists, and an assessment of a client's innate healing resources and state of mind. The new patient will spend an hour with Dr. Stoff during this process.

Next, the patient meets with an immunologist and expert in guided imagery who will often prepare instructional tapes for clients, taking them through the stages of generating mental images of healing. Then a naturopathic physician trained in acupuncture, herbs, homeopathy, and structural/energy work provides a nutritional assessment and some counseling.

Finally, the new patient talks with one of several staff psychologists, who assesses the patient's self-image and attitude about the illness. There may be psychological or unconscious factors, such as secondary gain or codependency, that make it advantageous for the patient to remain sick. "Most importantly, what we want to know is this: what are this person's perceived roadblocks to healing?" Dr. Stoff says. "Through close collaboration among our staff members, we provide an individualized and comprehensive treatment program based on an in-depth understanding of each of our patients."

Quite often, Dr. Stoff's team gets a patient who has received the "proverbial million-dollar workup" from conventional medicine, but still has no clear diagnosis. The tests Dr. Stoff runs are targeted at discovering the level of function of the various systems in a patient's body. For example, the results of a test for levels of T and B immune cells, called lymphocytes (SEE QUICK DEFINITION), tell Dr. Stoff whether the person's immune system is fighting a chronic viral infection and, if so, which type. The more details Dr. Stoff has about a patient's immune system and the status of its different cells, the better he is able to design an effective treatment plan.

Dr. Stoff checks the patient's organic acid levels (found in the urine) as a gauge of how well his or her system can detoxify itself. "Our extensive laboratory tests show us where the patient's problems lie. That way I can tell, for example, if the person has an underlying autoimmune problem." (An autoimmune disorder is one in which the immune system attacks the body's own tissues; examples include multiple sclerosis, rheumatoid arthritis, lupus, diabetes mellitus, and chronic thyroiditis. Some physicians, including Dr. Stoff, put CFS in this category as well.)

Not infrequently, Dr. Stoff discovers that a patient actually has cancer, misdiagnosed as chronic fatigue syndrome. Often, conventional doctors fail to do a complete series of tests and come up with a chronic fatigue syndrome diagnosis because it seems to fit the variety of symptoms, according to Dr. Stoff. But this can be misleading and sometimes simply wrong, not to mention fatal. "As much as possible, we try to approach the patient without any blinders on. I don't just rubber-stamp another doctor's diagnosis," he says.

Nor is the final prescription out of a therapeutic cookbook: "We may see a hundred women with CFS, but the treatment protocol will be different for each. We don't have any canned protocols that we take off the shelf just because a person has a presumed diagnosis." The clinic's staff meets to discuss their findings and together come up with an overall treatment plan. "We don't miss a trick," says Dr. Stoff. "That's how we consistently get good results." Customarily, a patient's complete evaluation and initial treatment prescription can last for two days. If the patient has cancer or a serious autoimmune problem, it may require he or she receive a month of daily intravenous treatments.

 For more information about **urine tests** and **stool analyses**, see chapter 2, Testing. For more about **psychological factors in CFS**, see chapter 11, Healing Psychological and Emotional Factors.

 A **lymphocyte** is a form of white blood cell, representing 25% of the total count, whose numbers increase during infection. Lymphocytes, produced in the bone marrow, come in two forms: B cells, which produce antibodies to neutralize foreign matter in the blood, and T cells, which mature in the thymus gland (behind the breastbone) and perform many functions in the body's immune response.

## Paul's Case: Down and Out with Chronic Fatigue

Paul came to Dr. Stoff's clinic suffering from chronic fatigue syndrome. The 39-year-old former missionary was so exhausted that some days he even lacked the energy to get out of bed. Paul had a constant sore throat, swollen glands, recurrent low-grade fever, muscle and joint aches, headaches, chronic indigestion, sleeping disorders, depression, and problems with memory, concentration, and focus. He was tired all the time, took frequent naps, and often could not keep his eyes open in the mornings.

Dr. Stoff learned that during Paul's time as a missionary he had often skipped meals even though he was performing strenuous physical work. His body had become undernourished and continual stress regarding money problems further depleted his system. Although Paul's work had been in the back country of South America, Dr. Stoff's blood, urine, and stool tests did not reveal the presence of any exotic tropical or parasitic infections. But Paul did have high levels of Epstein-Barr virus (SEE QUICK DEFINITION), which is commonly associated with chronic fatigue syndrome. In addition, his inadequate diet, high physical demands, and stress had left his system seriously deficient in many amino acids and essential fatty acids.

Even more serious, Paul's basic biological rhythms and hormonal cycles were out of balance. For example, his levels of adrenocorticotropic hormone (ACTH, secreted by the pituitary gland and vital for adrenal gland health) were undetectable; his dehydroepiandrosterone (DHEA—SEE QUICK DEFINITION) level was almost negligible; his cortisol (SEE QUICK DEFINITION) levels were too high; and he had multiple enzyme (SEE QUICK DEFINITION) failures based in his pancreas, which made his system unable to absorb nutrients from foods or supplements. "Paul's immune system wasn't working properly because his body could no longer regulate these natural, deep-set cycles," explains Dr. Stoff.

Paul's treatment program had many facets. First, Dr. Stoff administered a series of Anthroposophic (SEE QUICK

DEFINITION) remedies (*Echinacea Argentum*, to stimulate the immune system; *Apis Belladonna*, to work against inflammations; and *Cardus Marianus*, to detoxify the liver) through a single injection every day for ten days. Next, he put Paul on a multivitamin and an acidophilus supplement. To help regulate his biological cycles and promote sleep, he recommended melatonin (a brain hormone from the pineal gland) at the initial dose of 9 mg at bedtime, then gradually lowering it to 3 mg daily. Dr. Stoff also started Paul on a commercial amino acid formula called Amino-virox (two capsules, three times daily, taken 30 minutes before meals) and a multinutrient supplement called Immune Boosters (three capsules daily, with meals).

One treatment goal was to balance the relationship between two vital brain chemicals, the neurotransmitters (SEE QUICK DEFINITION) sero-

 **Cortisol** is a hormone secreted by the adrenal glands which are located atop the kidneys. Cortisol secretion (as well as the adrenal gland's other hormones, DHEA, adrenaline, and aldosterone) occurs in daily cycles, peaking in the morning and having the lowest values at night. Cortisol promotes protein building, regulates insulin and glycogen synthesis, and helps produce prostaglandins. Under conditions of stress, high amounts of cortisol are released; chronic excess secretion is associated with obesity and suppressed thyroid function. Imbalances in cortisol secretion are linked with low energy, muscle dysfunction, impaired bone repair, thyroid dysfunction, immune system depression, sleep disorders, poor skin regeneration, and decreased growth hormone uptake.

**Enzymes** are specialized living proteins fundamental to all living processes in the body, necessary for every chemical reaction and the normal activity of our organs, tissues, fluids, and cells. There are hundreds of thousands of different enzymes. Among their many other functions, certain enzymes enable the body to digest and assimilate food. There are special enzymes for digesting proteins, carbohydrates, fats, and plant fibers; specifically, protease digests proteins, amylase digests carbohy-

drates, lipase digests fats, cellulase digests fiber, and disaccharidase digests sugars.

**Anthroposophic medicine** is an extension of conventional Western medicine developed by Austrian scientist Rudolf Steiner, in conjunction with European physicians, in the 1920s. It is based on a spiritual model of the human being and its medicines are extensions of homeopathic remedies. In the United States there are about 60 practitioners—all M.D.s— plus hundreds of nurses and adjunctive therapists, but in German-speaking countries there are thousands of practitioners. In addition, there are several major hospitals in Germany and Switzerland devoted exclusively to this medical approach.

A **neurotransmitter** is a brain chemical with the specific function of enabling communications between brain cells. Chief among the 100 identified to date are acetylcholine, gamma-aminobutyric acid (GABA), serotonin, dopamine, and norepinephrine. Acetylcholine is required for short-term memory and all muscle contractions. GABA works to stop excess nerve signals and thus keeps brain firings from getting out of control. Serotonin does the same and helps produce sleep, regulate pain, and influence mood, although too much serotonin can produce depression. Norepinephrine is an excitatory neurotransmitter.

Jesse Stoff, O. M.D.

Based on Dr. Stoff's experience, the return to health involves three stages: First, you must deal with whatever viruses or other pathogens are involved. Second, you have to repair the cellular and systemic damage. Third, the patient must "learn the lessons of the disease" so that the same lifestyle and emotional patterns are not repeated in the future.

tonin and dopamine, which, in turn, would reset Paul's biocycles. To counter Paul's depression, promote sleep, and increase his levels of serotonin, Dr. Stoff prescribed 5-hydroxy-tryptophan, a form of the amino acid L-tryptophan (100 mg at bedtime). To restore his depleted levels of dopamine, Dr. Stoff prescribed a form of the amino acid L-tyrosine, and activated vitamin B6 (peridoxyl-s-phosphate). To address Paul's enzyme deficiencies and to increase his nutrient absorption, Dr. Stoff prescribed an enzyme formula called Absorbaid.

After three days on this program, Paul began to feel much better and his energy levels were markedly improved, indicating that his body was resetting its biological clock. A month later, Dr. Stoff added a natural form of DHEA (100 mg, taken at dinner) to Paul's regimen. In all, it took about 18 months before Paul was fully recovered. Normally, chronic fatigue syndrome patients recover faster, "but Paul was so nutritionally depleted that it took much longer," says Dr. Stoff.

Dr. Stoff has successfully treated more than 1,500 cases of chronic fatigue syndrome. Based on his experience, the return to health involves three stages. First, you must deal with whatever viruses or other pathogens are involved. Second, you have to repair the cellular and systemic damage. Third, the patient must "learn the lessons of the disease" so that the same lifestyle and emotional patterns are not repeated in the future. Paul had to learn how to pace himself, maintain his priorities, and "gain insight into the deeper sig-

**EDITOR'S NOTE** **Jesse Stoff, M.D.,** is medical director of Immune Therapies, International. From 1985 to 1991 Dr. Stoff was editor of the *Journal of Anthroposophic Medicine,* and from 1986 to 1991 he was vice president of the Physicians' Association for Anthroposophic Medicine. Dr. Stoff is co-author of *Chronic Fatigue Syndrome: The Hidden Epidemic* (Harper-Collins, 1992). To contact Jesse Stoff, M.D.: Immune Therapies International, Southwest Professional Plaza, 2122 North Craycroft Road, Tuscon, AZ 85712; tel: (866) 937-3450. Website: www.drstoff.com.

nificance" of his illness. To better enable him to do this, Dr. Stoff's staff taught Paul guided visualization techniques and gave him stress-reduction counseling.

The goal, says Dr. Stoff, "is to get the person feeling a hundred and ten percent improved without taking any supplements, but this third stage, when they're fully functional, feeling great, and without symptoms, takes the longest to achieve. Until then, things slowly but progressively improve." In general, most of Dr. Stoff's chronic fatigue patients "do well fairly quickly if they follow our directions." As for Paul, once he was cured he left for Russia to do missionary work.

## Mapping the Multiple Causes of CFS

Paul's case illustrates the complexity of chronic fatigue syndrome and the need to address that complexity if treatment is going to be successful. As with many other illnesses, the conventional medical establishment searches for a single cause of CFS. It should be obvious that this limited focus does not apply to the picture of Paul and the majority of CFS patients, for whom illness was the result of the convergence of numerous factors.

Alternative physicians regard the idea of seeking a single cause of CFS as misguided. "There has been a search for bacterial, viral, or fungal activity," says Dr. Leon Chaitow, N.D., D.O., of London, England. "Since many of these—Epstein-Barr virus, herpes simplex, candidiasis—are commonly found to be present, either active or dormant, in people with CFS, whatever was found was considered to be 'the cause' of the entire syndrome." Paul's case

> For **Immune Boosters** (with different formulations of vitamins, minerals, and botanicals: breakfast, lunch, dinner; available without prescription) and **Absorbaid**, contact: Origen, LLC, 982 Stuyvesant Avenue, Union, NJ 07083; tel: (800) 765-7842. For **Amino-Virox**, contact: Tyson and Associates, 12832 South Chadron Avenue, Hawthorne, CA 90250; tel: (800) 318-9766. For **Anthroposophic medicines** (available to physicians; some may be obtained without a prescription), contact: Weleda, Inc., 175 North Route 9W, Congers, NY 10920; tel: (800) 241-1030.

and the others discussed in this book make it clear that a complex illness such as chronic fatigue results from the convergence of many layers of imbalance and dysfunction. To expect to find a single cause is medically foolish.

Like Dr. Stoff, Dr. Chaitow believes strongly that CFS is and must be treated as a multisymptomatic condition, a condition he describes as "similar to an onion in which each peeled layer reveals another layer, or symptomatic factor, underneath. Focus on immune function would be more beneficial than focus on the virus, which is simply taking advantage of the situation," he observes.

## Undoing Chronic Fatigue in Stages: The Scope of This Book

**Testing:** Before a physician can design an effective treatment plan, it is necessary to determine precisely what is happening in the patient's body. In order to repair the damaged body systems, you must first eliminate the viruses, infections, and any other factors that are weakening these systems.

Chapter 2 covers the range of testing that is useful to pinpoint the imbalances, deficiencies, infectious agents, and specific immune system weaknesses that can contribute to CFS. This includes testing for viral and bacterial infections, candidiasis, parasites, immune system function, hormonal levels, heavy metal toxicity, enzyme deficiencies, allergies, and nutritional deficiencies. Most of the testing involves simple blood, urine, and stool analyses, but your conventional doctor may not be aware of the specific parameters to investigate.

**Bacterial and Fungal Infections, Viruses, Candidiasis, and Parasites:** Research and clinical evidence has shown that parasites, candidiasis, viruses, and bacterial and fungal infections are often present in patients with chronic fatigue syndrome and related conditions. After testing to determine exactly which of these invaders are present, treatment begins with eliminating them, as a first step toward restoring the body's natural healing abilities. Chapter 3 explains how these infections can contribute to CFS and discusses an array of techniques used by leading alternative medicine practitioners to successfully rid their patients of the infectious burden on their immune systems.

**Restoring Immune Function:** A depleted immune system is a central feature of CFS. The immune system is the body's basic defensive system with which it resists infection and disease formation—it strives to keep the body immune from illness. In someone with CFS, the immune system has been operating at a constant, heightened level of activity for a prolonged period. Ironically, this seemingly heightened level of activity is marked by diminished competency; the system seems to work harder, but it is actually incapacitated. Chapter 4 describes options for fortifying your depleted immunity.

**Detoxifying the Body:** The accumulation of toxins in the body is often another feature of CFS and creates a further burden on the immune system. Whether from stress, poor diet, or chemicals in food and the environment, these toxins need to be removed from the body if the immune system is to be restored to health. Chapter 5 presents methods for removing toxins from the body, especially from the intestines.

**An Underactive Thyroid Gland:** Although an underactive thyroid was not one of the elements contributing to Paul's chronic fatigue, Dr. Stoff and other physicians have encountered this condition, known as hypothyroidism, in numerous patients diagnosed with CFS. While hypothyroidism is technically considered a separate illness and not a cause of CFS, many CFS patients have not been properly tested for thyroid problems, and distinct categorization of the two illnesses is not necessarily of benefit to the patient. Hypothyroidism may be one of the many factors contributing to a person's CFS.

In chapter 6, you will learn how the thyroid gland and the hormones it produces are integral to the maintenance of your energy levels and to the health of all of your body systems. Stephen Langer, M.D., and Raphael Kellman, M.D., two alternative medicine practitioners who specialize in treating the thyroid, detail cases from their patient files illustrating their successful reversal of hypothyroidism and the associated chronic fatigue.

**Mercury in the Mouth Can Lead to CFS:** Another hidden factor that often contributes to CFS is mercury toxicity from dental fillings. Again, though Paul's illness did not involve this particular element, it is often a component in CFS. The mercury that most people in the United States have in their teeth is actually classified by the Environmental Protection Agency as a hazardous waste. In chapter 7, biological dentists and other alternative physicians explain the effects of mercury on the body and relate case histories of chronic fatigue patients whose illnesses were turned around after mercury-amalgam filling removal.

**Enzyme Deficiency:** As Dr. Stoff discovered in the tests he ran on Paul, enzyme deficiencies were interfering with Paul's absorption of nutrients from food and supplements. Enzymes are needed to digest food; when they are deficient, numerous problems develop in the gastrointestinal system and eventually in the immune system. Without the necessary fuel, his already weakened body was further depleted. In chapter 8, enzyme experts Maile Pouls, Ph.D., and Lita Lee, Ph.D., describe the far-reaching effects of enzyme deficiencies and their vital role in intestinal health, and how a precise program of enzyme and other nutrient supplementation can help reverse serious health problems such as chronic fatigue syndrome.

## Other Factors That Can Generate Fatigue

Fatigue can result from a variety of conditions other than chronic fatigue syndrome, according to Leon Chaitow, N.D., D.O. These include:

- **Adrenal insufficiency** caused by excessive stress and/or the overuse of stimulants (tea, coffee, chocolate, cola, alcohol, tobacco, drugs)
- **Anemia** (low levels of iron or vitamin B12 in the blood result in anemia; a blood test can verify this diagnosis)
- **Candidiasis** (often misdiagnosed as CFS in women)
- **Cardiovascular causes** (if breathlessness and/or chest pain on exertion accompanies fatigue, the heart may be involved)
- **Chronic ill-health** (many chronic diseases have fatigue as a symptom)
- **Depression**
- **Diabetes**
- **Headaches**
- **Hypoglycemia** (low blood sugar)
- **Obesity**
- **Premenstrual syndrome (PMS)** (the connection will be obvious if fatigue occurs at the same time in the monthly cycle)
- **Sleep disturbance or inadequate sleep**
- **Stress**

A number of the causes listed above are also symptoms of chronic fatigue syndrome. This highlights the circularity of symptoms and illness. Depression is both a symptom and a cause of fatigue, as are headaches, candidiasis, PMS, poor stress-coping skills, and sleep disorders. The presence of these factors can produce a downward spiral of illness and it becomes difficult to tell which came first, the fatigue or the other exhibited symptoms.

*Underlying Allergies:* One of the symptoms shared by CFS, fibromyalgia, and environmental illness is allergies; in the case of the latter, the allergies are so severe as to be debilitating. In chapter 9, Milton Hammerly, M.D., describes how hidden allergies and related intestinal imbalance can perpetuate CFS. Devi Nambudripad, D.C., L.Ac., R.N., Ph.D., presents cases in which chronic fatigue was reversed by getting rid of allergies using her Nambudripad Allergy Elimination Technique (NAET). Finally, Susan Lange, O.M.D., L.Ac., recounts the story of her own recovery from environmental illness—the ultimate allergy—and explains the "sick building syndrome."

*Nutritional Deficiencies Weaken the Immune System:* Like most CFS patients, Paul had numerous nutritional deficiencies. In his case, they were the result of an inadequate diet, enzyme deficiencies, the heavy physical demands of his work, and stress. Once the underlying factors that are producing the deficiencies are identified and treated, it is necessary, according to Dr. Stoff and other alternative physicians, to replenish the body's supply of vitamins, minerals, amino acids, and other essential nutrients. This will help bolster the immune system and give the body the strength to begin healing itself. Chapter 10 details the nutrients that are commonly deficient in chronic fatigue conditions and those useful in fortifying the immune system.

# From the Vapors to Soldier's Heart to Tahoe Flu: A Brief History of Chronic Fatigue

The first cases of chronic fatigue syndrome may have occurred in the nineteenth century in the form of "the vapors," followed in the early twentieth century by a malady of World War I veterans called "soldier's heart." It wasn't until the mid-1980s, however, that the disorder received widespread attention as the result of a virtual epidemic in the small Lake Tahoe resort town of Incline Village, Nevada.

Beginning early in 1984, Daniel Peterson, M.D., and Paul Cheney, M.D., were baffled by the several patients a day who came to their office suffering from persistent extreme fatigue and whole-body muscle aches. Later it was learned that doctors across the country were treating patients for similar symptoms, but nowhere was the disease as prevalent in a population as in Incline Village.

By June of 1985, the number of afflicted patients consulting Drs. Peterson and Cheney was 90; by August the number had risen to 150. The CDC ignored the situation until the doctors sent them 12 samples of the Tahoe patients' blood, all of which tested abnormally high for the Epstein-Barr virus (EBV) antibodies, as had samples from other sources. These results prompted the CDC to launch an investigation, which did not lead to the discovery of why the disorder was so concentrated in Incline Village, but did eventually result in its classification as a recognized illness. In addition, the CDC investigators came to the conclusion that Epstein-Barr was not necessarily the source. The patients involved also had high antibody levels for cytomegalovirus and herpes simplex. Later, other viruses were pinpointed in connection to the disease as well. Meanwhile, the numbers of those affected in Incline Village had risen to nearly 200 out of the town's population of 20,000.

Variously labeled Tahoe flu, chronic Epstein-Barr, or chronic mononucleosis, in 1987, the elusive illness was given the official name of chronic fatigue syndrome (CFS) by the CDC; in 1988, the CDC released guidelines for its diagnosis (see "Required Symptoms for a Diagnosis of Chronic Fatigue," p. 3). A glib reporter dubbed CFS the "Yuppie flu" as a result of the published demographics—at that time, those seeking medical help for CFS were predominantly white and upper middle-class. While CFS still tends to be an adult disease and affects more women than men, the epidemic has since become more democratic, leaving no one exempt.

As a footnote, Drs. Cheney and Peterson were repaid for bringing the epidemic to official and public attention by being labeled as quacks in their own community. Many people preferred to believe this was an imaginary illness and blamed the doctors for perpetuating patients' fantasies and hypochondria—and, in the process, scaring away the tourist trade that was the town's economic backbone. Dr. Cheney moved his practice to North Carolina, where patients from all over the country came to consult with him.

Source: Straus, S., M.D. Chronic Fatigue Syndrome NIH Publication 90-3059 (Washington: U.S. Department of Health and Human Services, Public Health Service, 1990), 5. Johnson, Hillary. Osler's Web: Inside the Labyrinth of the Chronic Fatigue Syndrome Epidemic (New York: Penguin Books, 1996). Southern Medical Journal 88:10 (October 1995), 994–995. Cowley, Geoffrey, et al. "Chronic Fatigue Syndrome: A Modern Medical Mystery." Newsweek (November 12, 1990). National Institutes of Health Website: www.niaid .nih.gov/factsheets/cfs .htm.

# Drugs Whose Side Effects Resemble Symptoms of Chronic Fatigue

According to the *Physicians' Desk Reference*, the following drugs can produce side effects similar or identical to symptoms associated with chronic fatigue syndrome. If you are taking any of these drugs, they may be compounding or even producing your symptoms. (Percentages refer to individuals affected.)

Accutane Capsules
  (approximately 1 in 20)

Actimmune (14%)

Alferon N Injection (6% to 14%)

Anafranil Capsules (35% to 39%)

Aredia for Injection (up to 12%)

Atrofen Tablets (2% to 4%)

Blocadren Tablets (3.4% to 5%)

BuSpar (4%)

Cardura Tablets (12%)

Cartrol Tablets (7.1%)

Catapres to TTS (4% to 6%)

Centrax Capsules (11.6%)

CHEMET (succimer) Capsules
  (5.2% to 15.7%)

Combipres Tablets (about 4%)

Cordarone Tablets (4% to 9%)

Dantrium Capsules (among the most
  frequent)

Depo-Provera Contraceptive Injection
  (more than 5%)

Desyrel and Desyrel Dividose
  (5.7% to 11.3%)

DynaCirc Capsules (0.4% to 3.9%)

Engerix to B Unit to Dose Vials (14%)

Epogen for Injection (9% to 25%)

Ergamisol Tablets (6%)

Ethmozine Tablets (3.1% to 5.9%)

Fludara for Injection (10% to 38%)

Foscavir Injection (More than 5%)

Hismanal Tablets (4.2%)

Hivid Tablets (less than 1% to 34%)

Hylorel Tablets (25.7% to 63.6%)

Hytrin Tablets (11.3%)

Intron A (18% to 84%)

Kerlone Tablets (2.9% to 9.7%)

Lariam Tablets (among the most
  frequent)

Leucovorin Calcium for Injection
  (2% to 13%)

Levatol (4.4%)

Lopid Tablets (3.8%)

Lopressor Ampuls, Tablets (10%),

HCT Tablets (10 in 100 patients)

Lozol Tablets (greater than or
  equal to 5%)

Ludiomil Tablets (4%)

Marplan Tablets (among the most
  frequent)

Mesnex Injection (33%)

Mexitil Capsules (1.9% to 3.8%)

Mykrox Tablets (4.4%)

NebuPent for Inhalation Solution
(53% to 72%)

Neupogen for Injection (11%)

Nipent for Injection (29%)

Nolvadex Tablets (3.8%)

Normodyne Injection, Tablets
(2% to 10%)

Norpace Capsules, CR Capsules
(3% to 9%)

Norvasc Tablets (4.5%)

Parlodel Capsules, SnapTabs
(1% to 7%)

Polygam, Immune Globulin
Intravenous (Human) (3% to 6%)

Prinivil Tablets (3.3%)

Prinzide Tablets (3.7%)

Procardia XL Extended Release
Tablets (5.9%)

Procrit for Injection (9% to 13%)

Proleukin for Injection (53%)

Prozac Pulvules and Liquid, Oral
Solution (4.2%)

Reglan Injectable, Syrup, Tablets
(10%)

Roferon-A Injection (89% to 95%)

Rowasa Rectal Suppositories, Rectal
Suspension Enema (3.4%)

Rythmol Tablets (1.8% to 6%)

Sectral Capsules (11%)

Seldane Tablets (2.9% to 4.5%)

Supprelin Injection (1% to 10%)

Tambocor Tablets (7.7%)

Tegison Capsules (50% to 75%)

Tenex Tablets (3% to 12%)

Tenoretic Tablets (0.6% to 26%)

Tenormin Tablets and I.V. Injection
(0.6% to 26%)

Toprol XL Tablets (about 10 of 100
patients)

Trandate Injection (1% to 10%),
Tablets (2% to 11%)

Valrelease Capsules (among the
most common)

Vaseretic Tablets (3.9%)

Visken Tablets (8%)

Wellbutrin Tablets (5%)

Xanax Tablets (48.6%)

Zebeta Tablets (6.6% to 8.2%)

Zestoretic (3.7%)

Zestril Tablets (3.3%)

Zoloft Tablets (10.6%)

***Healing the Psychological Side of CFS:*** Dr. Stoff mentioned that people with CFS need to "learn the lessons of the disease" in order not to repeat the emotional, psychological, and lifestyle patterns that contributed to their illness. He provided Paul with the tools of guided-visualization and stress-reduction counseling to gain these insights. In chapter 11, clinical cases from alternative medicine physicians illustrate how lifestyle choices, psychological factors, and suppressed emotions can contribute to CFS. You will learn how homeopathy, traditional Chinese medicine, flower remedies, and color therapy can assist in resolving the psychological and emotional aspects of illness. You will also learn more about the relationship between CFS and depression, the main psychological/emotional symptom of the syndrome.

***Herbal Medicine Can Help Treat Causes and Symptoms:*** There are a variety of herbs that can be of assistance in the treatment of CFS by both addressing underlying causes and providing symptomatic relief. An example of the former are herbs that support and strengthen the immune system or adrenal glands. In the latter category, herbs can offer relief from the array of CFS symptoms ranging from fatigue to muscle aches. They have the advantage over conventional medications of doing so without side effects. Chapter 12 offers a compendium of herbs, with research presenting evidence of their efficacy in particular applications.

***Other Holistic Therapies Can Also Be Helpful:*** Because of the complexity of symptoms that often accompany CFS and its related conditions, many practitioners of alternative medicine employ additional therapies as part of a comprehensive treatment plan. In chapters 13 and 14, you will learn more about these therapies.

***Ruling Out Lyme Disease:*** As previously mentioned, Lyme disease has become pandemic across the United States. Despite this, it often goes undetected, masked by a wide range of symptoms that can easily be misdiagnosed as other diseases, including CFS, fibromyalgia, and environmental illness. In chapter 15, you will learn how alternative physicians screen for Lyme disease, and how they are treating it.

By the time you have finished these chapters, you will have a comprehensive view of CFS and many practical recommendations for putting an end to your chronic fatigue, including a list of helpful physicians and organizations that can further help you.

# two

# Testing

*The Key to Understanding
the Causes of Chronic Fatigue*

As chronic fatigue syndrome expert Jesse Stoff, M.D., explained in chapter 1, using a variety of medical tests to find out the interlinking causes of a patient's CFS is the essential first step to formulating an effective treatment plan. But, because no single standard medical test exists to detect chronic fatigue syndrome in all its complexity, an accurate diagnosis depends on a history of illness that fits the pattern of CFS, along with ruling out all other conditions with similar symptoms. These include multiple sclerosis, systemic lupus erythematosus, cancer, unresolved hepatitis B or C, sleep apnea, narcolepsy, alcohol or substance abuse, side effects of medication, severe obesity, and such psychiatric illnesses as major depressive disorder, schizophrenia, bipolar disorder, dementia, and eating disorders (anorexia and bulimia).[1]

Getting a clear symptom picture is often difficult, due to the tendency of CFS symptoms to fluctuate in degree and severity, not only over a period of weeks or months, but even from day to day. A cyclical pattern of illness and reasonable health is the result. Frequently, after a severe bout of CFS, a patient resumes normal activity and exercise, only to relapse into extreme fatigue after a period of time. But if a number of CFS symptoms persist for six months, and other causes have been eliminated, it is considered likely that the person has CFS.[2]

A careful medical history, a physical examination, and the selected laboratory tests highlighted in this chapter can pinpoint specific infections often associated with CFS and provide the physician with an inventory of the pattern of symptoms. This may be the surest way to diagnose the illness, says Leon Chaitow, N.D., D.O., of London, England.

> A careful medical history, a physical examination, and laboratory tests can pinpoint specific infections often associated with CFS and provide an inventory of the pattern of symptoms, which may be the surest way to diagnose the illness.

In addition to the well-known symptoms of CFS, Murray R. Susser, M.D., of Santa Monica, California, notes that in CFS patients—unlike in healthy people—brain circulation gets worse after exercise. Therefore, as part of getting a complete symptomatic picture, he tests patients after exercise for decreased blood circulation in the brain. He also tests the cortisol level in the blood, which also decreases in CFS patients after exercise. Low levels of this hormone (vital for dealing with stress) suggest the likelihood of CFS.[3]

## Testing for the Underlying Causes

As discussed in Chapter 1, alternative medicine physicians are less focused on getting a definitive diagnosis of CFS (aside from eliminating other disorders) than they are in gathering as much information as possible on the underlying causes that are producing the patient's symptoms. Without this information, any treatment program is guesswork. For this reason, depending on the individual's symptoms, it may be wise to test for the following: candidiasis, parasites, bacterial and viral infections, immune system abnormalities, hormonal imbalances and deficiencies, heavy metal toxicity, enzyme deficiencies, allergies, nutritional deficiencies, and Lyme disease.

### Electrodermal Screening: Versatile Energy Testing

Electrodermal screening (EDS) is a quick method for identifying most of these conditions, especially ones involving toxic or allergic substances. A blunt, noninvasive electric probe is placed at specific points on the patient's hands, face, or feet, corresponding to acupuncture points at the beginning or end of energy meridians. Minute electrical discharges from these points serve as information signals about the condition of the body's organs and systems, useful for the physician in evaluation and in developing a treatment plan.

The normal waiting period for laboratory analysis is avoided through the immediate feedback provided by this computerized testing of the body's organs and systems via acupuncture points. As a cross-reference, specific blood, urine, and stool analyses can be ordered to serve as confirmation of electrodermal results. By quickly pinpointing problems, EDS can prevent unnecessary, guesswork testing. For example, if EDS indicates that a person has a specific type of parasite, running a stool analysis for that parasite eliminates the often long process of trial-and-error testing to see whether parasites, in general, are a problem. EDS can also be helpful in determining the body's tolerance to medications or remedies that may be prescribed.

EDS serves as a "data acquisition process" in which the trained practitioner conducts an "interview" with the patient's organs and tissues, gathering information about the basic functional status of those systems and their energy pathways, according to James Hoyt Clark of Orem, Utah, an EDS inventor and educator. As such, EDS is an investigational—not a diagnostic—procedure, because it requires the physician's knowledge of acupuncture, physiology, and therapeutic substances to interpret the energy imbalances, establish their precise focus, and select the most appropriate therapeutic response.

EDS can indicate the degree of stress that is affecting an organ and can monitor the progress of therapy, avoiding trial and error and general guesswork. Depending on how EDS devices are calibrated, initial readings above 60 can indicate an inflammation somewhere in the body, while readings below 45 can often indicate physiological changes brought

## Tests Covered in This Chapter

- Electrodermal Screening
- Anti-Candida Antibodies Panel
- Stool Analysis
- Urine Analysis
- CBC Blood Test Report
- Immune System Testing
  - T and B Cell Panel
  - Natural Killer Cell Function
  - Nitrogen Balance
  - Biological Terrain Assessment
- Hormone Testing
  - Saliva Assay Report
  - TRH Test (thyroid)
  - Adrenal Stress Index
  - DHEA Challenge Test
- Heavy Metal Toxicity Screening
  - ToxMet Screen
- Testing for Enzyme Deficiencies
  - Loomis Urinalysis
- Allergy Testing
  - NAET
  - Skin Testing
  - IgG ELISA Test
- Testing for Nutritional Deficiencies
  - Individualized Optimal Nutrition
  - Functional Intracellular Analysis
  - Pantox Antioxidant Profile
  - Oxidative Protection Screen

> Alternative medicine physicians are less focused on getting a definitive diagnosis of CFS than they are in gathering as much information as possible on the underlying causes that are producing the patient's symptoms.

about by a degenerative process. The physician's task is to find a single substance or combination of substances that will balance the point, which means bringing its EDS reading back close to 50. For example, the pancreas readings for a person with diabetes will become balanced when the correct and appropriate dose of insulin is placed within the EDS circuit.

The more sophisticated EDS devices, such as the Orion system developed by James Hoyt Clark, contain an inventory of energy signals corresponding to several thousand different substances. (The Orion system is programmed with information for about 56,000 substances.) These include most of the homeopathic remedies; grass, weed, and tree pollens; foods; toxic chemicals; dental materials; molds; bacteria; healthy and diseased organ states; and conventional drugs.

 For more information about the **Orion System and EDS seminars**, contact: Star Tech Health Services, LLC., 1219 South 1840 West, Orem, Utah 84058; tel: (888) 229-1114. Website: www.startechhealth.com.

 For more about **allergies**, see chapter 9, Addressing the Allergy Connection.

"The EDS device is not diagnostic; it doesn't pick the remedy," explains Bruce Shelton, M.D., M.D.(H), Di.Hom., founder and director of the Allergy Center in Phoenix, Arizona. Dr. Shelton routinely uses EDS as a front-line testing procedure to identify multiple toxins and allergens in his patients. "I use the device as a yes/no meter for what I'm thinking about the patient." EDS only indicates, based on the operator's skillful input, whether a given substance will balance a condition. "When a substance balances the symptoms highlighted by EDS, it means you need it as a remedy," says Dr. Shelton.

## Testing for Candidiasis, Parasites, and Bacterial and Viral Infections

While the presence of multiple infections often associated with CFS may not provide definitive proof that a person has the illness, knowing what the body is contending with is the first step in treatment design. "The

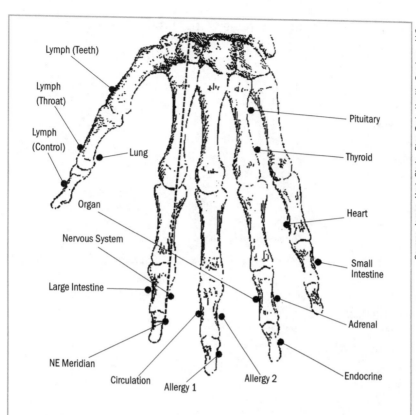

Lymph (Teeth)

Lymph (Throat)

Lymph (Control)

Lung

Organ

Nervous System

Large Intestine

NE Meridian

Circulation

Allergy 1

Allergy 2

Pituitary

Thyroid

Heart

Small Intestine

Adrenal

Endocrine

Source: James Hoyt Clark, Star Tech Health Services, LLC., 1219 South 1840 West, Orem, Utah 84058; tel: (888) 229-1114.

Electrodermal screening probes specific points on the hands (indicated by black dots) to gather information about the health function or possible toxicity of organs and body systems. These points are part of the acupuncture meridians.

most common infections we find are yeast [*Candida albicans*] and parasites," reports Dr. Susser. "We also find hidden bacterial infections such as Lyme disease [*Borrelia burgdorferi*] and abscesses in the teeth, and sometimes chronic prostatitis, chronic sinusitis, and chronic gastritis." Elevated antibody levels (activated immune proteins) to certain viruses are frequently found in the blood of CFS patients. These include Epstein-Barr, cytomegalovirus, human herpes virus 6 (HHV6), herpes simplex, rubella, and enteroviruses such as Coxsackie.

## The Anti-Candida Antibodies Panel

As mentioned above, electrodermal screening can identify the presence of most of these infectious agents. Follow-up blood tests or other labo-

## A Sampling of Substances Whose Effect on the Body Can Be Pinpointed with Electrodermal Screening

alcohol products

amino acids

animal danders

Ayurvedic herbs

blossoming flowers

cacti and succulents

chemicals

Chinese/Japanese herbs

cleaners

colors and dyes

dental products

digestive enzymes

endocrines

environmental agents

essential oils

flower essences

food

gems/minerals

geopathic agents

grasses, weeds

habit-forming drugs

homeopathics—combinations

homeopathics — drainage

homeopathics—polychrest

homeopathics—singles

hormones

insects

metals

miasms

minerals

molds/fungi

nosodes (homeopathic remedies made from a disease product)

parasites

pesticides

phenolic resins

sarcodes (sections of healthy tissue used in homeopathic remedies)

shrubs

snakes

spiders

tree pollens

veterinary viruses

vitamins

ratory workups can quantify the presence of these agents. Candidiasis, an overgrowth of the yeastlike fungus *Candida albicans* (a normal flora of the skin, mouth, intestinal tract, and vagina), can be determined by stool or blood analyses. One blood test, called the Anti-Candida Antibodies Panel, measures the levels of the IgG and IgM antibodies (SEE QUICK DEFINITION) against *Candida*; the IgG levels indicate both past and ongoing infection, while the IgM may be a truer reflection of present infection.

### Parasites

Another factor that may be weakening the CFS patient's immune system from the inside is parasites. The human body may harbor unwelcome residents that are harmful to health—literally eating us from the inside, using our nutrients and often plugging up our lymphatic vessels. The possible presence of parasites in the body, mostly in the intestines, is a little-appreciated but major health problem, according to nutrition educator Ann Louise Gittleman.[4] People assume they are vulnerable to parasites only if they travel in tropical areas, but this is a dangerous mis-

| Antibodies | Normal | Abnormal | Reference Range |
|---|---|---|---|
| IgG | 500.0 | | (REF. RANGE 500-8000) |
| IgM | 50.0 | | (REF. RANGE 50-3000) |
| IgA | 50.0 | | (REF. RANGE 50-8000) |
| Candida Antigen | 2.0 | | (REF. RANGE 0-10) |
| Immune Complex | 1200.0 | | (REF. RANGE 0 - 7000) |

The Anti-Candida Antibodies Panel measures the levels of key immune defense proteins, or antibodies (the immunoglobulins IgG and IgM), against the yeast *Candida albicans*.

conception, says Gittleman, since parasites can easily be contracted regardless of the geographic region in which a person lives.

Undiagnosed parasitic infections (from microscopic protozoa to various species of worms) may account for a great deal of the otherwise unexplained diseases currently besetting America, and some health experts estimate that parasitic infection affects as much as 25% to 50% of our nation's population. Parasites tend to reside in the intestines, but they can also migrate to the blood, lymph, heart, liver, gallbladder, pancreas, spleen, eyes, and brain. They can produce numerous symptoms, including constipation, diarrhea, gas, bloating, irritable bowel syndrome, joint and muscle aches, allergies, anemia, skin problems, sleep disturbances, chronic fatigue, and gradual immune dysfunction.

According to Gittleman's research, parasite damage can be extensive. Parasites can destroy cells faster than they can

**QUICK DEFINITION**

An **antibody** is a protein molecule containing about 20,000 atoms, made from amino acids by B lymphocyte cells in the lymph tissue and set in motion by the immune system against a specific foreign protein, or antigen. An antibody, also referred to as an immunoglobulin, may be found in the blood, lymph, colostrum, saliva, and the gastrointestinal and urinary tracts, usually within three days after the first encounter with an antigen. The antibody binds tightly with the antigen as a preliminary step to removing it from the system or destroying it.

An **antigen** is any biological substance (a toxin, virus, fungus, bacterium, amoeba, or other protein) that the body identifies as foreign and dangerous to itself. As such, an antigen induces a state of cellular sensitivity or immune reaction that seeks to neutralize, remove, or destroy the antigen by dispatching antibodies against it.

For the **Anti-Candida Antibodies Panel**, contact: Great Smokies Diagnostic Laboratory, 63 Zillicoa Street, Asheville, NC 28801; tel: (800) 522-4762. Website: www.gsdl.com.

## A Dental Marker of Chronic Fatigue?

One of the primary setbacks to treating chronic fatigue syndrome has been the lack of a specific medical "marker" that would indicate a clinical way to diagnose the syndrome. Burke A. Cunha, M.D., chief of the Infectious Disease Division of Winthrop-University Hospital in Mineola, New York, has discovered arch-shaped, bright red membrane tissue in the back of CFS patients' mouths. Located on both sides of the mouth next to the back molars, these "crimson crescents," as Dr. Cunha calls them, intensify in color as the patient's condition worsens, and fade as the patient improves.

Dr. Cunha states that the crescents appear in 80% of CFS patients but show up in less than 5% of non-CFS patients with sore throats, and not at all in patients with mononucleosis or strep throat. He states, "If your patient has crimson crescents, you now can say his condition is probably chronic fatigue syndrome."* Although Dr. Cunha's findings have not been confirmed by other health practitioners, the existence of such a marker for CFS bears further investigation.

---

*Straus, S., M.D. *Chronic Fatigue Syndrome* NIH Publication 90-3059 (Washington: U.S. Department of Health and Human Services, Public Health Service, 1990), 5.

be regenerated; they can release toxins that damage tissues, resulting in pain and inflammation; and, over time, they can depress, even exhaust, the immune system. Of the dozens of specific parasites of concern to human health, the major groupings include microscopic protozoa, roundworms, pinworms, hookworms (Nematoda), tapeworms (Cestoda), and flukes (Trematoda).

Parasitic infection, however, is as difficult to diagnose as chronic fatigue syndrome itself. One of the main problems related to the study of parasitic infections and their link to systemic illness is the fact that "most parasitology laboratories fail to find the majority of intestinal parasites in stool specimens submitted to them," according to the *Journal of Advancement in Medicine*.[5] David Casemore, M.D., of the Public Health Laboratories in Bodewuddan, Rhyh, England, adds that parasitic infection "is almost certainly under-detected, possibly by a factor of ten or more."[6] Steven Bailey, N.D., of Portland, Oregon, reports that one patient with AIDS required examination of 12 stool samples before giardiasis (infection with the protozoan *Giardia lambia*) was diagnosed.[7] Unfortunately, this is not an unusual occurrence.

According to Martin Lee, Ph.D., director of Great Smokies Diagnostic Laboratory in Asheville, North Carolina, many doctors, hospitals, and laboratories fail to diagnose parasitic infection because they rarely allow the time for careful analysis or multiple procedures using stool specimens collected over several days. Dr. Lee suggests that if you suspect you may have an intestinal parasite, or just want to be tested as a preventative measure, make sure your physician, hospital, or lab follows the guidelines set by the U.S. Centers for Disease Control and Prevention (CDC) and the *Manual of Clinical Microbiology*.

The Comprehensive Digestive Stool Analysis described below provides useful indications of general parasitic activity. Immunofluorescent staining can also be used to detect parasites. This technique uses antibodies tagged with fluorescent dyes, which make them highly visible under the microscope. As they attack specific parasites, the antibodies will show up only where there is a parasitic presence.

## What a Stool Analysis Can Indicate

In addition to parasites, there are many other intestinal factors that may be playing a role in your illness. A healthy digestive system is central to the maintenance of overall health. Problems that begin in the intestines have far-reaching effects on the body and can contribute to the development of a variety of serious illnesses. Digestive problems—such as diarrhea, constipation, irritable bowel syndrome, bloating, gas, or indigestion—are usually part of the symptom picture in CFS, fibromyalgia, and environmental illness.

Understanding how well, or poorly, food is digested, and measuring other parameters of intestinal health in a patient with one of these disorders can provide therapeutic insights and point the way to healing. Stool analysis is an effective method for determining digestive disorders. The following is a glossary of terms used in this type of analysis along with an explanation of what each of the values can tell you:

 For information about the **Comprehensive Digestive Stool Analysis**, contact: Great Smokies Diagnostic Laboratory, 63 Zillicoa Street, Asheville, NC 28801; tel: (800) 522-4762. Website: www.gsdl.com.

*Dysbiosis Index:* Intestinal dysbiosis refers to an imbalance of intestinal flora. Specifically, these flora include friendly, beneficial bacteria called probiotics (for example, *Lactobacillus acidophilus* and *Bifidobacterium bifidum*) and unfriendly or harmful bacteria (for example, *Pseudomonas aeruginosa*). In dysbiosis, the unfriendly bacteria predominate; they begin fermentation, producing toxic by-products that interfere with normal elimination cycle. The dysbiosis index reflects the balance of friendly and pathogenic bacteria, and those markers—such as pH and short-chain fatty acids (SCFAs)—related to the flora.

### Colonic Environment

**Lactobacillus and Bifidobacteria:** These bacteria are involved in vitamin synthesis and the detoxification of procarcinogens (substances that

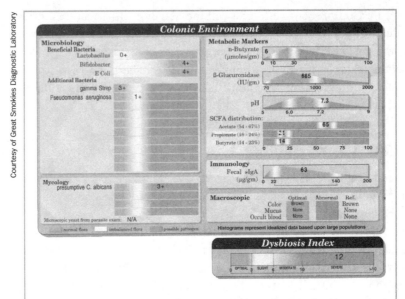

The stool analysis provides important information about the health status of the intestines and their function, especially regarding the population of numerous bacteria, both helpful and pathogenic. This relationship, when it is imbalanced, is called dysbiosis; in the analysis shown, the level of dysbiosis is slight.

become carcinogenic or cancer-causing); they also support the immune system. Deficiencies of *Lactobacillus* have been linked with a higher risk for various chronic diseases.

**Gamma Streptococcus:** This is a bacteria normal to the intestines; its presence in the analysis is not an indication of digestive imbalance.

**Candida albicans:** The intestinal tract normally contains small amounts of this yeast. In some cases, however, wide use of antibiotics or birth-control pills and a high-carbohydrate diet may cause an overgrowth of the *Candida* yeast, causing a condition called candidiasis. Overgrowth of *Candida albicans* and other intestinal yeasts has been linked to food allergies, migraines, vaginitis, irritable bowel syndrome, indigestion, and asthma.

**Pseudomonas aeruginosa:** Associated with wound infections, infected burn lesions, and urinary tract infections, this bacterium causes infections in the context of a weakened immune system and produces a characteristic blue pus. These problems do not normally occur in the colon; however, *P. aeruginosa* in the colon may or may not be symptomatic. If symptomatic, it may contribute to diarrhea and inflammation.

*Macroscopic (appearance):* Yellow to green stools may indicate diarrhea and a bowel sterilized by antibiotics; black or red may reflect bleeding in the gastrointestinal tract; tan or grey can indicate a blockage of the common bile duct; presence of mucus or pus can point to irritable bowel syndrome, polyps, diverticulitis, or intestinal wall inflammation; and occult blood may result from eating too much red meat, or may indicate either hemorrhoids or colon cancer.

*pH:* This is a reflection of the acid/alkaline balance in the colon. The preferred range is 6.0 (mildly acidic) to 7.2 (mildly alkaline). Fecal pH reflects the status of colonic digestive processes, SCFAs (see below), beneficial bacteria, and bacterial metabolism. An elevated fecal pH is associated with a higher risk of colitis and colon cancer.

*N-butyrate:* This SCFA is a form of butyric acid, a primary energy source for the colon cells; it must be present in adequate amounts for healthy metabolism (energy, nutrient, and water release from foods) in the colon. Butyric acid is needed to digest SCFAs. Low levels of N-butyrate are associated with a higher risk of colon cancer.

*Total SCFA:* Short-chain fatty acids—such as acetate, propionate, N-butyrate, and valerate—are produced when the colon ferments soluble fibers. SCFAs are important because they provide 70% of the energy needed by the cells lining the colon.

*SCFA distribution:* Elevated levels of SCFAs can indicate poor nutrient absorption in the colon or bacterial overgrowth; decreased levels suggest a lack of dietary fiber, unbalanced metabolic processes, or dysbiosis. The key factor here is the ratio among the four SCFAs, which usually remains relatively constant in healthy individuals but can shift noticeably when metabolism becomes disordered.

*Beta-glucuronidase:* This is an enzyme produced by various bacteria in the colon. Elevated levels may result from bacterial overgrowth, an abnormal intestinal pH, too much dietary fat (especially from meat), or low levels of beneficial bacteria. Elevated levels can increase bioactivation of carcinogens in the bowel, thus increasing the risk of colon cancer.

*Fecal sIgA:* Fecal secretory IgA is a specialized immunoglobulin, one of a class of five specially designed antibody proteins produced in the spleen, bone marrow, or lymph tissue. They are involved in the immune system's defense response to foreign substances. Fecal sIgA

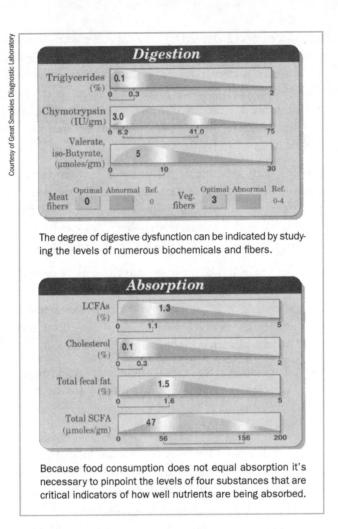

The degree of digestive dysfunction can be indicated by studying the levels of numerous biochemicals and fibers.

Because food consumption does not equal absorption it's necessary to pinpoint the levels of four substances that are critical indicators of how well nutrients are being absorbed.

serves as the first line of defense against invading pathogens, toxins, and food allergens in the intestines. Low levels mean an increased susceptibility to infection and food allergies.

## Measures of Digestive Dysfunction

*Triglycerides:* Most dietary fats are triglycerides—a term that denotes their chemical structure. During digestion, lipase, a pancreatic enzyme, breaks triglycerides down into glycerol and free fatty acids. Elevated fecal triglyceride levels indicate incomplete fat metabolism and possible problems in the pancreas.

***Chymotrypsin:*** Relative levels of this digestive enzyme, produced in the intestines, can indicate the patient's enzyme status and activity. Decreased levels mean the pancreas is not releasing enough enzymes and/or that the stomach is low on digestive acids, which are needed to activate chymotrypsin. Elevated levels suggest a rapid transit time (the speed at which fecal matter moves through the intestines).

***Valerate and iso-butyrate:*** Valerate and iso-butyrate are SCFAs produced when intestinal bacteria ferment protein. Elevated levels indicate that the protein was not digested properly in the stomach and intestines.

***Meat and vegetable fibers:*** These are crude microscopic markers for digestive function. Elevated levels may indicate inadequate chewing, stomach acid, or digestive enzymes.

### Measures of Absorption

***LCFAs:*** Long-chain fatty acids are normally absorbed directly by intestinal mucosa. Elevated levels reflect malabsorption of fats, a result of maldigestion or inflammation of the lining of the small intestine.

***Cholesterol:*** Cholesterol in the feces comes from either dietary fats or the breakdown of the cells lining the intestines. Generally, fecal cholesterol levels remain stable, despite dietary intake; elevated fecal levels suggest malabsorption or irritation of the mucosal lining.

***Total fecal fat:*** This represents the sum of all fats or lipids, except for SCFAs, and can indicate either maldigestion or malabsorption.

# What a Urine Analysis Reveals

A urine analysis provides another window into what precisely is happening in a CFS patient's body. Again, chronic digestive problems are often associated with CFS and a 24-hour urine analysis can pinpoint what is going wrong in digestion. Then the appropriate therapies can be implemented to help break the cycle of CFS in which imbalances in one system of the body feed imbalances in another.

 For information about receiving a **urine analysis**, contact: Dr. Lita Lee, P.O. Box 516, Lowell, OR 97452; tel: (541) 937-1123. Website: www.litalee.com.

For the test, a patient's total urine output is collected over a 24-hour period, then analyzed in a laboratory for the status of key biochemical

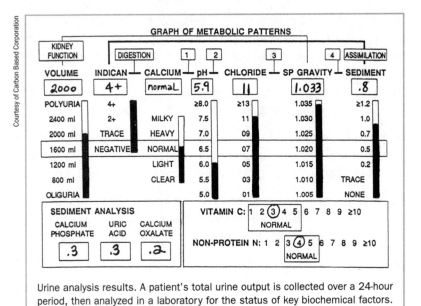

**GRAPH OF METABOLIC PATTERNS**

| KIDNEY FUNCTION | DIGESTION | | 1 | 2 | | 3 | | 4 | ASSIMILATION |

| VOLUME | INDICAN | CALCIUM | pH | CHLORIDE | SP GRAVITY | SEDIMENT |
|---|---|---|---|---|---|---|
| **2000** | **4+** | **normaL** | **5.9** | **11** | **1.033** | **.8** |

| VOLUME | INDICAN | CALCIUM | pH | CHLORIDE | SP GRAVITY | SEDIMENT |
|---|---|---|---|---|---|---|
| POLYURIA | 4+ | | ≥8.0 | ≥13 | 1.035 | ≥1.2 |
| 2400 ml | 2+ | MILKY | 7.5 | 11 | 1.030 | 1.0 |
| 2000 ml | TRACE | HEAVY | 7.0 | 09 | 1.025 | 0.7 |
| 1600 ml | NEGATIVE | NORMAL | 6.5 | 07 | 1.020 | 0.5 |
| 1200 ml | | LIGHT | 6.0 | 05 | 1.015 | 0.2 |
| 800 ml | | CLEAR | 5.5 | 03 | 1.010 | TRACE |
| OLIGURIA | | | 5.0 | 01 | 1.005 | NONE |

**SEDIMENT ANALYSIS**

| CALCIUM PHOSPHATE | URIC ACID | CALCIUM OXALATE |
|---|---|---|
| **.3** | **.3** | **.2** |

**VITAMIN C:** 1 2 ③ 4 5 6 7 8 9 ≥10
NORMAL

**NON-PROTEIN N:** 1 2 3 ④ 5 6 7 8 9 ≥10
NORMAL

Urine analysis results. A patient's total urine output is collected over a 24-hour period, then analyzed in a laboratory for the status of key biochemical factors.

factors. These can include kidney function; levels of bowel toxicity; pH; vitamin C, calcium, and other essential nutrients; and how the body is handling proteins, fats, and carbohydrates. The following specific values are measured in urine analysis:

*Volume:* The total urine output—which may be normal, excessive (polyuria), or minimal (oliguria) in relationship to the specific gravity (see below)—indicates how well the kidneys are functioning.

*Indican:* This indicates the degree of toxicity, putrefaction, gas, and fermentation in the intestines. Indican comes from putrefying proteins in the large intestine that are kicked back into the blood and excreted through the kidneys. Indican is extremely toxic and causes many symptoms; the higher the level, the greater the intestinal toxemia or inflammation in the digestive tract. Readings as close to zero as possible are desirable.

*pH:* Based on hydrogen ion concentration, this value indicates the degree of urine acidity versus alkalinity on a scale of zero to 14, with urine pH usually ranging from 4.5 to 8.0 and 7.0 being neutral.

*Chlorides:* These are salt residues in the urine; the measured values give information on salt intake and assimilation.

**Specific gravity:** This value measures the weight of total dissolved substances (solutes) in the urine against an equal amount of water to determine the general water content (hydration) of the body. A normal reading of 1.020 means the urine is 20% heavier than water. Values typically range from 1.005 to 1.030; a high reading indicates solute concentration and kidney stress.

**Total sediment analysis:** This indicates the amount of dissolved organic and mineral substances remaining in the urine after digestion; an optimal total reading for the three sediment categories is 0.5.

**Calcium phosphate:** This reading indicates the status of carbohydrate digestion; a level of 0.5 signifies normal carbohydrate digestion.

**Uric acid:** Levels of uric acid signify the status of protein digestion; optimal digestion yields a reading of 0.

**Calcium oxalate:** This value indicates the status of fat digestion; a reading of 0 signifies optimal fat digestion.

**Vitamin C:** Levels of vitamin C indicate body reserves of this key nutrient; a reading of 1 is high, 2 to 5 normal, and 6 to 10 deficient.

## The Complete Blood Count as a Guide to Therapy

In addition to comprehensive stool and urine analyses, blood tests can reveal important information about a person's biochemical status and, as with the other tests, serve as an invaluable guide to developing the most effective, individually tailored treatment program. However, the standard blood tests of conventional medical practice do not necessarily provide a complete picture.

With this in mind, in 1985 Mark A. Schauss developed a new method for making optimum, practical use of information revealed by the standard blood test. His Carbon Based Corporation (CBC) offers a Cell-Mate™ Blood Test Report that gives both doctors and patients an inexpensive, user-friendly five-part formulation of the information, opening "a therapeutic window" to the patient's unique biochemistry, says Schauss. The test also empowers users to take more control of their health care by allowing them to make more informed decisions.

The CBC CellMate™ Blood Test's Basic Status Report alphabetically lists the detected amounts of about 44 substances—such as cholesterol, lymphocytes, sodium, and bilirubin—normally found in the

> The CBC Blood Test Report can "depict a patient's potential disease patterns, that is, whether abnormalities in their blood indicate a predisposition toward a certain disease."

blood. It also ranks these items according to their relative deviation from the mean value. Schauss calls this ranking "Percentage Status"; it indicates, by percentage, how much higher or lower the client's readings are than the statistical norm. For example, Schauss explains, normal sodium levels range from 135 to 145, so a one-point deviation is substantial, as there are only ten points for normalcy. In contrast, normal triglycerides range from zero to 250, so a one-point change there is not significant. The goal, says Schauss, is to provide a statistical context and normative comparison for the test results as measured against agreed-upon standards of what is normal.

The Blood Test's Panel Report groups the results according to 14 biochemical considerations, such as electrolytes, kidney function, acid or alkaline pH, nitrogen, and protein. "You can review each of the panels at a glance for unbalanced patterns in your patient's blood chemistry," says Schauss. The Disease Indicators Report compares the total blood status to indicators of any of 140 diseases. Known disease patterns, as revealed in a blood analysis, are correlated with the individual's results. For example, the test might indicate a 62.5% match for myasthenia gravis, a 40% match for folic acid deficiency, and a 33.3% match for angina pectoris.

According to Carbon Based Corporation, the CBC Blood Test Report can "depict a patient's potential disease patterns, that is, whether abnormalities in their blood indicate a predisposition toward a certain disease. On the lookout for that disease, a physician can investigate further, perhaps stopping the disease before it strikes. By predicting these patterns, the test offers a new outlook toward preventive medicine."

 For more information about the **CBC** CellMate™ **Blood Test Report**, contact: Carbon Based Corporation, 920 Incline Way, Suite 2C, Incline Village, NV 89451; tel: (702) 832-8485; fax: (702) 832-8488. Website: www.carbonbased.com.

The Drug Interactions Report identifies potential aggravating effects if the patient were to use any of hundreds of conventional drugs. For example, if one's total bilirubin is out

of balance, the use of aspirin, penicillin, niacin, or streptomycin is contraindicated because these would further the imbalance. Finally, the Biochemical Pharmacology Report suggests which supplements are indicated
for the given abnormal blood chemistry; the exact dosages are left to a
physician to determine. Carbon Based Corporation delivers the five-part
report to clients within 48 hours.

## Testing the Immune System

Measuring the activity of the immune system is a vital component in
determining the level and kind of disease involved and thus the type of
support needed to restore immune strength. Certain levels of T and B
immune cells (lymphocytes) can indicate a chronic virus and identify the
strain. According to Charles W. Lapp, M.D., of Raleigh, North Carolina, immune testing of CFS patients often reveals, in addition to
increased T-cell activity, abnormal levels and impaired function of natural killer cells (foreign-protein destroyers) and the presence of autoantibodies (antibodies that attack the body's own cells) such as the anti-
thryroid autoantibody.

Highly elevated levels of lymphokines or cytokines (interleukin 1, 2,
and 3) may also be in evidence. Lymphokines are released by lymphocytes, and cytokines by lymphocytes and other cells, in response to specific antigens (foreign disease-producing substances). Lymphokines
assist cellular immunity by stimulating macrophages—the immune system's vacuum cleaners. Cytokines combat local and systemic inflammation. Dr. Lapp reports that extremely high levels of interleukin 1 and 2
are usually seen only in CFS, AIDS, and blood-related malignancies.[8]

Jesse Stoff, M.D., of Tucson, Arizona, relies on standard blood tests
to establish the state of a patient's biochemistry and immune function
and provide the information needed to design an individualized treatment program targeting the specific deficiencies or areas of weakness.
The tests he runs most frequently are a T and B Cell Panel, natural killer
(NK) cell function, and nitrogen balance.

*The T and B Cell Panel:* This test, Dr. Stoff says, provides information on
about 25 immune system components and the structural status of an
individual's immune system. Some viruses and other infections are also
detected by this test. The T and B Cell Panel and the blood test for
NK cell function are relatively inexpensive standard laboratory tests

> It's important to note that if the natural killer cells lack the biochemical support [from nutrients] that they need to work appropriately, stimulating them will get you nowhere.
>
> —*Jesse Stoff, M.D.*

that any physician can order. Through these tests, the clinician can locate the breach in the person's immune system defense and whether the deficiency is in T, B, or NK cells. Then you can determine which immunomodulators (substances that can regulate, or modulate, the activities of the immune system) will work best to close the breach.

Testing nitrogen balance reveals the ratios between amino acids (protein building blocks). "Having amino acids in the correct ratios is akin to giving the NK cells the biochemical 'teeth' they need to perform their work," Dr. Stoff explains. "It's important to note that if the natural killer cells lack the biochemical support [from nutrients] that they need to work appropriately, stimulating them will get you nowhere."

 For more on **immunomodulators for strengthening the immune system**, see chapter 4, Restoring Immune Vitality.

The principles of immunomodulation can also be useful for individuals who may not be sick but want to keep their immune system in top working order. All you need is one simple blood test to measure natural killer cell function; an NK cell function test typically costs about $200. If your NK values are normal, then you have no need to worry, but if they are subnormal, you will have valuable diagnostic information that a physician can use to help restore your immune system to an optimal level.

If your results are below normal, further testing is advisable—a T and B Cell Panel will tell you whether there is a viral trigger—to determine where the problems originate. Then, immunomodulating supplementation can help reverse the underlying weakness before it becomes a full-blown illness. This kind of early monitoring can potentially prevent many cases of chronic fatigue syndrome and related chronic diseases because it tests for precisely the factors involved in CFS: multiple infections, impaired NK function, and a variety of other immune deficiencies.

# The Major Players in Your Immune System

The immune system guards the body against foreign, disease-producing substances. Its "workers" are various white blood cells.

A **lymphocyte** is a specialized form of white blood cell, representing 25% to 40% of the total blood count, whose numbers increase during viral infection and when a person is fighting cancer. Lymphocytes are produced in the bone marrow; the two most abundant forms are B cells and T cells.

**B cells** mature in the bone marrow and produce antibodies to neutralize foreign cells (this is known as humoral immunity). B cells account for 10% to 15% of all lymphocytes.

**T cells** mature in the thymus gland and react to and destroy specific invading antigens (this is known as cell-mediated immunity); 75% to 80% of lymphocytes are T cells. T cells are predisposed to respond to specific foreign substances (antigens) or infections.

**Helper T cells** (also known as T4 or CD4 cells) secrete immune proteins (particularly the interleukins and interferon) to stimulate B cells and macrophages, and activate Killer T cells; they account for 60% to 75% of T cells.

**Killer T** cells (T8 or CD8 cells) bind to the specific invader and secrete enzymes to destroy it; they account for 25% to 30% of T cells.

**Suppressor T cells** prevent excessive immune reactions by suppressing antibody activity.

**Natural Killer (NK)** cells are a type of non-specific, free-ranging lymphocyte that is neither a B nor T cell. Unlike other lymphocytes, NK cells are not activated by a specific antigen—they can recognize and quickly destroy any antigen on first contact. They have potent cell-killing activity, being "armed" with an estimated 100 different biochemical poisons for destroying foreign cells. As with antibodies, their role is surveillance: they rid the body of aberrant or foreign cells before they can grow and produce cancer or infection. NK cells account for 5% to 10% of all lymphocytes. An estimated 65% of normal healthy individuals have NK cell function between 30 and 160, 20% between 20 and 29, 10% between 161 and 250, and 5% less than 20.

**Macrophages** are a form of white blood cell (originally produced in the bone marrow and called monocytes) that can literally swallow germs and foreign proteins, then release an enzyme that chemically either damages or kills the substance. The name means "big" (macro) "swallower" or "eater" (phage). Macrophages are the vacuum cleaners and filter feeders of the immune system, ingesting everything that is not normal healthy tissue, even old body cells.

An **antibody** is a protein molecule containing about 20,000 atoms, made from amino acids by B lymphocyte cells in the lymph tissue and set in motion by the immune system against a specific foreign protein or antigen.

## *Biological Terrain Assessment: Analysis at the Cellular Level*

The Biological Terrain Assessment (BTA) analysis is a ten-minute test conducted by a computerized device called the BTA S-2000. The device uses a pen-shaped microelectrode to determine pH, resistivity, and redox values in blood, saliva, and urine. ("Redox" is an abbreviation of oxidation-reduction potential; this refers to the degree of "oxidative stress" on the body, or how much free-radical burden [oxidation of tissues] the body is exposed to.) Samples of blood (0.5 ml), saliva (0.5 ml), and first-morning urine are obtained following a 12- to 14-hour fast. If a person eats an acid-producing, alkaline-producing, salty, or antioxidant food (SEE QUICK DEFINITION) just before BTA, the testing will reflect more about the ingested food than about the body's baseline condition.

The underlying philosophy that explains the value of the BTA originated with French biologist Louis Claude Vincent, Ph.D., who discovered that the key to healing was not the use of powerful drugs but, rather, knowing the patient's biochemistry and the optimal conditions. He called these the "terrain" of body function.

The term "biological terrain" is used to describe the conditions, general health, and activity level of cells. This includes the status of microorganisms at the cellular level: some are beneficial to life and health, others are not. Each type of bacteria, fungus, or virus thrives in a precise biochemical medium. Viruses require a fairly alkaline environment to function, whereas fungi favor a more acidic environment; bacteria can thrive under various conditions, but their growth is best stimulated by a high-sugar environment. An excess of toxins in one's diet and environment tends to increase the production of acid within cells, forcing the body to compensate by producing a strong alkaline chemical reaction in the blood, which, in turn, tends to favor the growth of fungi.

Dr. Vincent concluded that the components of the blood, urine, and saliva afford insight into the way the body functions. By monitoring bio-

**QUICK DEFINITION**

An **antioxidant** (meaning "against oxidation") is a natural biochemical substance that protects living cells against damage from harmful free radicals. Antioxidants work against the process of oxidation—the robbing of electrons from substances. If unblocked or left uncontrolled, oxidation can lead to cellular aging, degeneration, arthritis, heart disease, cancer, and other illnesses. Antioxidants in the body react readily with oxygen breakdown products and free radicals, neutralizing them before they can damage the body. Antioxidant nutrients include vitamins A, C, and E, beta carotene, selenium, coenzyme Q10, pycnogenol (grape seed extract), L-glutathione, superoxide dismutase, and bioflavonoids. Plant antioxidants include *Ginkgo biloba* and garlic. When antioxidants are taken in combination, the effect is stronger than when they are used individually.

## An Immunological Test to Indicate Chronic Fatigue

Jay Levy, M.D., of the Division of Hematology and Oncology at the University of California, San Francisco, has developed an immunological test that distinguishes patients with CFS from healthy people and from those with other disorders having similar symptoms, such as systemic lupus erythematosus, documented depression, acute viral-like illness, and prolonged fatigue without other CFS criteria.[a]

Dr. Levy emphasizes that the test is not yet diagnostic, but it is used as a kind of prescreening to identify possible CFS candidates for further study. Dr. Levy and his colleagues have found that the immune systems of people with CFS, unlike those of healthy people, are in a constant overactive state and never return to a normal operating level. This overactivity is what is behind the deep fatigue; paradoxically, this heightened activity overlays a condition of dysfunction and immune incompetency.

In this test, CFS patients with the most severe symptoms (based on a study sample of 147 patients) tend to have increased activation markers on CD8 cells, with reduced numbers of CD8 suppressor cells. This reveals the immune imbalance: one aspect is inappropriately activated, the other exists in insufficient numbers. The test involves monitoring CD8 cells (the proteins on killer T cells that are attacked by viruses). "Most noteworthy is the statistical evidence that an individual with two or more of the CD8 cell subset alterations has a high probability (90%) of having active CFS," says Dr. Levy.[b]

---

[a]Landay, Alan L., Carol Jessop, Evelyne T. Lennette, and Jay A. Levy, "Chronic Fatigue Syndrome: Clinical Condition Associated With Immune Activation." *The Lancet* 338:8769 (September 21, 1991), 707–712.

[b]"Diagnostic Blood Test for CFIDS?" *CFIDS Treatment News* 2:1 (Spring 1991), 3. Landay, Alan L., Carol Jessop, Evelyne T. Lennette, and Jay A. Levy. "Chronic Fatigue Syndrome: Clinical Condition Associated with Immune Activation." *The Lancet* 338:8769 (September 21, 1991), 707–712. Levy, Jay, M.D. Personal correspondence. Division of Hematology and Oncology, Department of Medicine, University of California at San Francisco (October 1997).

chemical changes in these fluids and by making appropriate changes in diet, lifestyle, and medical treatment, health can be reestablished and disease processes retarded or possibly reversed. In the pioneering tradition of Dr. Vincent, naturopathic physician and chiropractor Robert Greenberg, D.C., N.M.D., of the Whole Health Centre in Chesterfield, Missouri, developed BTA to better enable him to determine the optimal conditions for a specific patient's internal environment.

According to Dr. Greenberg, the healthy body must satisfy three criteria to function at the highest level: (1) optimal pH (acid-base balance); (2) optimal redox (oxidation-reduction potential); and (3) resistivity (the opposite of electrical conductivity). Through BTA, these factors are measured in blood, urine, and saliva to yield a total of nine measures.

"The pH reading tells us whether enzymatic activity in the body is occurring properly and if digestion and absorption of vitamins and other nutrients is adequate," says Dr. Greenberg. "It can also alert us to the potential presence of environmental or industrial contaminants, substances that prove very damaging to the body's delicate chemistry." In general, the urine is a better indicator of pH changes than the blood, because the blood's pH level is very tightly controlled; however, both measures together, along with salivary pH, give a more complete picture of the body's chemical balance.

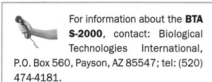
For information about the **BTA S-2000**, contact: Biological Technologies International, P.O. Box 560, Payson, AZ 85547; tel: (520) 474-4181.

For more on **cellular terrain**, see chapter 4, Restoring Immune Vitality.

Values of the second factor, oxidation-reduction potential (abbreviated as redox), can compromise health. "Because of the effects of stress, poor air, poor food quality, and lack of aerobic exercise typical of most Americans, these values are generally much lower than they should be to sustain a healthy body," says Dr. Greenberg. "If the values remain low for extended periods of time, the person will be more susceptible to cancer and other illnesses."

The third factor, resistivity, is a measure of a tissue's resistance to the flow of electrical current—as opposed to conductivity, which indicates the ability to transmit or conduct electrical current through a cell, nerve, or muscle. With low resistivity (high conductivity), there is typically a congestion or buildup of mineral salts. High resistivity (low conductivity) indicates a lack of minerals, which raises the need to further evaluate the individual for specific deficiencies of these vital elements.

"Urine is a good indicator of the body's secretory ability and toxic load on cells," says Dr. Greenberg. "Blood is a good indicator of toxicity and oxygen balance, while saliva offers insight into a person's digestive capacities." Taken together and analyzed by means of the BTA S-1000, these measures provide a benchmark for determining whether or not someone is getting healthier. "The goal is to move the body toward the optimal benchmark, which is the same regardless of age, weight, and sex," Dr. Greenberg explains. "We find that people who attain these benchmarks seem capable of maintaining sound health indefinitely."

The therapeutic approach indicated by BTA findings will vary greatly from one patient to the next. "BTA may uncover inadequate enzymatic secretions in one person and chronic and degenerative stress in another," Dr. Greenberg explains. "As a result, they are placed on different nutritional and lifestyle modification programs and require unique nutritional support or therapies. When the patient's body chemistry is balanced and maintained with a healthy diet, proper vitamin and mineral supplementation, and adequate amounts of exercise and rest, the body can remain healthy and nourish a vibrant immune system to protect and sustain it."

Many patients who undergo BTA came into their doctor's offices with reports of "normal" laboratory values, based on a blood test and other standard tests. Yet these same individuals display illness both objectively and subjectively, even though their standard blood results do not show it. "Often potent influences exist within the patient's system, which can include pollutants, environmental poisons, parasites, viruses, fungi, invasive microbes, lack of adequate vitamins and minerals, lack of oxygen, and excessive carbon dioxide," says Dr. Greenberg. Most standard laboratory tests are incapable of detecting these elements; as a result, many patients remain sick, while their doctors contend that nothing more can be done.

For example, Dr. Greenberg evaluated Susan, 36, who had frequent outbreaks of debilitating herpes sores in her mouth. During an episode, they would become so numerous that Susan

## A Primer on Cellular Terrain

The term **pH**, which means "potential hydrogen," represents a scale for the relative acidity or alkalinity of a solution. Acidity is measured as a pH of 0.1 to 6.9 and alkalinity as a pH of 7.1 to 14; a pH of 7.0 is considered neutral. The numbers refer to how many hydrogen atoms are present compared to an ideal or standard solution. Normally, blood is slightly alkaline, at 7.35 to 7.45; urine pH can range from 4.8 to 7.5, although normal is closer to 7.0.

**Acid-base metabolism** refers to the metabolic processes that maintain the balance of acids and bases (alkalines) in body fluids. Acids release hydrogen ions, while bases accept them. The total number of these hydrogen ions present determines the pH of a fluid. Too many hydrogen ions (a pH below 7.0) produce an acidic state called acidosis; too few hydrogen ions (a pH above 7.0) cause an alkaline excess called alkalosis; both can lead to illness.

**Oxidation-reduction** is the basic chemical mechanism in the cell by which energy is produced from foods. Electrons (negatively charged particles in an atom) are removed from one atom, resulting in "oxidation" of this first atom, and then are added or transferred to another atom, resulting in "reduction" of this second atom. This continual process of energy metabolism is actually a flow of electrons, or a minute electrical current, within the cell.

had trouble eating and drinking. She had consulted many physicians and tried all the drugs they prescribed, but nothing helped her. "We did a Biological Terrain Assessment and discovered a cellular picture that looked very much like a heavy metal profile," says Dr. Greenberg. On this basis, he ordered a hair analysis and 24-hour urine test, both of which

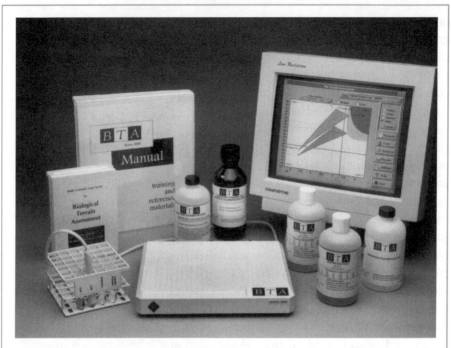

The Biological Terrain Assessment unit analyzes blood, urine, and saliva samples and displays information about an individual's cellular health on its monitor.

revealed that Susan had high concentrations of mercury, probably leached into her tissues from her dental amalgams. She had all her mercury amalgams replaced and in the last 18 months has not had a single herpes sore, says Dr. Greenberg.

## Testing Hormone Levels

Hormone (SEE QUICK DEFINITION) imbalances are common in CFS; the adrenal hormones DHEA (SEE QUICK DEFINITION) and cortisol, and the hormone ACTH (adrenocorticotropic hormone, secreted by the pituitary gland and essential for adrenal health) are frequently implicated in the disorder. Since the adrenal glands play a central role in maintaining the body's energy levels, when these glands are functioning poorly, the result is fatigue. Low amounts of melatonin—the pineal-gland hormone that regulates the body's sleep cycle—may also be contributing to the overall symptom picture of CFS.

An underactive thyroid, a condition called hypothyroidism, is another important component to consider when investigating the causes of your chronic fatigue. As you will learn in chapter 6, thyroid problems often go undiagnosed; for someone with CFS, eliminating or confirming the thyroid as a factor should be included in any initial diagnosis.

Initial testing and subsequent monitoring of hormone levels in the blood provide specific guidelines for supplementation in order to restore hormonal balance in the body—one component in overcoming chronic fatigue. In addition to standard blood testing, the Aeron LifeCycles Saliva Assay Report, TRH test for thyroid function, Adrenal Stress Index, and DHEA Challenge Test can provide further useful information.

## Saliva Assay Report

"The concept of hormone replacement therapy is the first long-term concept related to antiaging medicine," states John Kells, president of Aeron LifeCycles in San Leandro, California, a laboratory that offers a saliva-based test for measuring levels of eight different hormones. Most of the key hormones in our bodies—estrogen, testosterone, DHEA—decline as we age, leaving us more susceptible to reduced physiological functioning and possibly disease. The goal of hormone replacement is to prevent illness and enhance the quality of life, says Kells, but he notes that "there is a fair bit about this that is not yet known."

There is no evidence, he says, "that people will necessarily live longer if they replace hormones in decline, but experts in this field are hopeful that [those who are treated] will live disease-free longer and will not succumb to the early onset of disease that many now believe is associated

**QUICK DEFINITION**

**Hormones** are the chemical messengers of the endocrine system; through an intricate communication system, they impose order among the body's estimated 50 trillion cells. Examples include the "male" sex hormone (testosterone), the "female" sex hormones (estrogen and progesterone), melatonin (pineal), growth hormone (pituitary), and DHEA (adrenal).

**DHEA** (dehydroepiandrosterone) is naturally produced by the human adrenal glands and gonads, with optimal levels occurring around age 20 for women and age 25 for men. After those ages, DHEA levels gradually decline so that a person 80 years old produces only a fraction of the DHEA they did when they were 20. As an antioxidant, a hormone regulator, and the building block from which estrogen and testosterone are produced, DHEA is vital to health. Low DHEA levels have been associated with cancer, diabetes, multiple sclerosis, hypertension, obesity, AIDS, heart disease, Alzheimer's, and immune dysfunction illnesses. Test subjects using supplemental DHEA reported improved sleeping patterns, better memory, an improved ability to cope with stress, decreased joint pain, increases in lean muscle, and decreases in body fat. No serious side effects have been reported to date, although acne, oily skin, facial hair growth on women, deepening of the voice, irritability, insomnia, and fatigue have been reported with high DHEA doses.

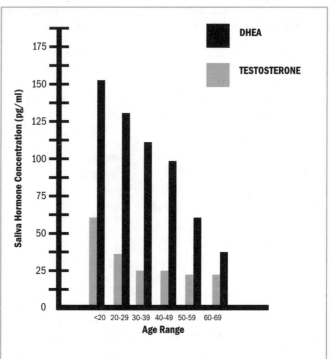

The Aeron LifeCycles Saliva Assay Report provides graphs of individual hormone levels. This chart shows the age-dependent range of testosterone and DHEA in females. The graph clearly shows how DHEA and testosterone levels decline with age.

with decline in body function and hormone levels." If you maintain these levels, you will probably slow down the aging process, says Kells. There are age-associated optimal levels of progesterone, estradiol, estriol, estrogen, and cortisol; Aeron LifeCycles uses these as a reference point in their saliva assay, Kells explains. These target values can then be used as a dosage guideline for supplementation. "The goal is to try to bring the hormone levels back up to a level that existed in our physiological youth."

The Aeron LifeCycles Saliva Assay Report, which can be ordered by both laypeople and physicians, provides graphs of individual hormone levels. Changing levels can be plotted over time on the same graph if supplementation or subsequent testing is done. Although hormones are present in saliva only in fractional amounts compared to the amounts in blood, "clinically relevant and highly accurate levels of hormones can be determined in saliva," says Kells. "Saliva testing provides a means to establish whether or not your hormone levels are within the expected normal range for your age."

The saliva assay has several advantages over traditional blood testing for hormones. It is painless and noninvasive, and tests can be performed simply, at any time or place. As DHEA, cortisol, estrogen, progesterone, and testosterone levels are highest in the morning, it is far more convenient to test them at home and immediately ship the saliva sample to Aeron's laboratory than to drive to a physician's office to have them tested—possibly at a later time, when levels have naturally fallen off.

Because the saliva test is less expensive than blood tests, you can do frequent testing to monitor changes (brought on by interventions such as diet, exercise, herbs, stress reduction, or acupuncture) and to adjust dosages of over-the-counter hormones such as DHEA or mela-

 For more information about the **Aeron LifeCycles Saliva Assay Report**, contact: Aeron LifeCycles Clinical Laboratory, 1933 Davis Street, Suite 310, San Leandro, CA 94577; tel: (800) 631-7900. Website: www.aeron.com.

tonin, Kells says. In general, Kells explains that it is best to establish a baseline level of saliva hormones first; then, after intervention (which can include hormone supplementation), test a second time to measure the changes.

## TRH: The Gold Standard of Thyroid Tests

A major contributing factor to the development of chronic fatigue is often an underactive thyroid gland, an endocrine gland located in the neck. Here the CFS patient is confronted with two obstacles: first, many doctors pay little or no attention to the thyroid; second, standard tests for thyroid function are often misleading. Many patients who should be tested are not, due to traditional medicine's low awareness of the importance of thyroid function; if they're fortunate enough to have a thyroid test, they may get "normal" results, because most standard tests are not sensitive enough to identify hypothyroidism. The result is often an erroneous diagnosis.

The TRH (thyrotrophin-releasing hormone) test is a far more sensitive laboratory measure than routine thyroid blood tests and can show conclusively that a patient is suffering from an underactive thyroid, explains Raphael Kellman, M.D., director of the Kellman Center for Progressive Medicine in New York City. Dr. Kellman specializes in thy-

> Many patients who should be tested are not, due to traditional medicine's low awareness of the importance of thyroid function; if they're fortunate enough to have a thyroid test, they may get "normal" results because most standard tests are not sensitive enough to identify hypothyroidism.

roid-related cases and uses the test regularly in his clinical practice. "Our center has seen hundreds of patients whose routine thyroid tests revealed nothing, but who then failed the TRH stimulation test, allowing us to make the appropriate diagnosis. In patients I've seen with three or more typical symptoms of hypothyroidism, 35% to 40% have tested 'normal' in standard tests, while TRH tests show they have an underactive thyroid."

The TRH is an inexpensive test, costing about $100, says Dr. Kellman. First, through a simple blood test, the physician measures the patient's level of TSH (thyroid-stimulating hormone); second, the patient receives an injection of TRH (a completely harmless synthetic hormone modeled after the TRH secreted by the hypothalamus gland in the brain); finally, 25 minutes later blood is drawn again to remeasure the TSH. The TRH injection stimulates the pituitary gland, which produces thyroid-stimulating hormone; if the thyroid is underfunctioning, the pituitary gland will secrete excess TSH upon stimulation. If the second TSH blood test measures are high (above 10), it indicates that the patient's thyroid is underactive. A TSH reading of 15 is suspicious, while 20 strongly points to hypothyroidism, according to Dr. Kellman.

 For a **Complete Thyroid Panel** (includes rT3, T3, T3/rT3 ratio, T4, and TSH), contact: Meridian Valley Clinical Laboratory, 515 West Harrison Street, Suite 9, Kent, WA 98032; tel: (253) 859-8700. Website: www.meridianvalleylab.com. The Thyroid Panel must be ordered by a physician.

"Routine testing assumes that if TSH is high, then thyroid hormone must be low, but in these tests a high TSH is only detectable in cases of extreme abnormalities," Dr. Kellman explains. "The TRH test reveals a deeper physiological level by looking at the function of the thyroid and by measuring abnormal function levels, as compared to standard blood tests and the TSH test, which measures only pathology." The TRH test was once widely used by American physicians, but was replaced by the

> The standard blood tests measuring thyroid levels are ineffectual.
>
> —*Raphael Kellman, M.D.*

quicker, easier TSH. "In the age of assembly-line medicine, doctors jettisoned the TRH because it is cumbersome and time-consuming, and opted for the easy route," comments Dr. Kellman. "But this is a grave mistake of modern medicine, causing needless suffering for many people. The standard blood tests measuring thyroid levels are ineffectual."

Understanding the utility of the TRH test has implications for several of today's leading health problems, Dr. Kellman points out. For example, he estimates that 50% of people reporting chronic fatigue actually have an undiagnosed underactive thyroid. Depression, a common symptom of CFS, is also linked with abnormal TRH results and an underactive thyroid, he says. For those who have received a diagnosis of hypothyroidism, the TRH can be used to monitor medication dosage. "If you are currently on thyroid medication yet still complain of fatigue, the TRH test can tell us if you are being medicated properly," Dr. Kellman explains. "Many lives have been changed—and healed—from this one test."

The thyroid gland

Copyright © 1989-97 by TechPool Studios, Inc. USA

 For more about **the thyroid gland, its hormones, and its role in chronic fatigue**, see chapter 6, Reversing Hidden Thyroid Problems.

### Adrenal Stress Index (Saliva Test)

Symptoms commonly associated with chronic fatigue syndrome—such as lack of energy, headaches, sleep disturbances, low body temperature, and muscle and joint pain—can all be caused by an imbalance in the adrenal glands. Located above each kidney, the adrenal glands secrete key stress hormones such as cortisol, DHEA, and adrenaline. Levels of these hormones are often abnormal in people with CFS, which could also be defined as a continual stress response. The Adrenal Stress Index (ASI), a simple, noninvasive test, can pinpoint whether an imbalance in

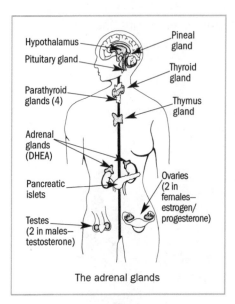

Hypothalamus

Pituitary gland

Parathyroid glands (4)

Adrenal glands (DHEA)

Pancreatic islets

Testes (2 in males— testosterone)

Pineal gland

Thyroid gland

Thymus gland

Ovaries (2 in females— estrogen/ progesterone)

The adrenal glands

For information on the **Adrenal Stress Index saliva test** and the **DHEA Challenge Test**, contact: Diagnos-Tech, Inc., 6620 South 192nd Place, J-104, Kent, WA 98032; tel: (800) 878-3787. Website: www.diagnostechs .com.

the adrenal glands might be contributing to CFS.

The adrenal glands do not secrete their hormones at a constant level throughout the day; instead, hormones are released in a cycle, with the highest volume in the morning and the lowest at night. This 24-hour cycle, known as the circadian rhythm, can influence a variety of body functions, from immune response to quality of sleep. If the adrenal glands secrete hormones improperly (due to an abnormal adrenal rhythm), fatigue and muscle pain may result.

The ASI saliva test evaluates how well one's adrenal glands are functioning by tracking the 24-hour cycle. Four saliva samples, taken at intervals throughout the day, are used to reconstruct the adrenal rhythm in the laboratory and determine whether the three main stress hormones are being secreted in proper proportion to each other, and at the right times. Based on the results, a physician can prescribe the appropriate treatment to restore the balance of hormones and correct the circadian rhythm.

### DHEA Challenge Test (Saliva Test)

DHEA hormone levels are often low in people with CFS, and taking a DHEA supplement to raise the levels is relatively easy. However, while many people taking DHEA report significant improvement in sleeping patterns, energy level, and ability to cope with stress, some people actually experience the opposite effect. Depending upon a person's genetic make-up, a certain amount of DHEA from a supplement may be converted by the body into the hormones testosterone and estradiol (a type of estrogen). If you are genetically predisposed to convert DHEA, you may experience unwanted side effects with supplementation as a result of the increased amounts of testosterone and estradiol. These side effects can include fatigue, insomnia, irritability, acne, oily skin, deepening of the voice, and an increase in body hair.

Through a simple saliva sample, the DHEA Challenge Test determines whether, in your particular case, DHEA supplements would improve or worsen your health. The test works by measuring levels of the two hormones (testosterone and estradiol) in the saliva both before and after a five- to seven-day treatment with the DHEA hormone (15 mg for women, 25 mg for men). If your testosterone and estradiol levels are too high following this "challenge" to the system, continuing to take DHEA supplements is probably not advisable.

# Testing for Heavy Metal Toxicity

Increasingly, practitioners of alternative medicine find that chronic low-level exposure to a variety of toxic heavy metals poses serious health dangers if the toxins are allowed to stay in the body. These toxins are commonly found in our food, water, and air, as well as in cooking utensils, cosmetics, auto exhaust, tobacco smoke, many of the building materials and fabrics in our work and living environments, and dental materials in our teeth (mercury amalgam fillings).

Typical symptoms of heavy metal toxicity include nervous system disorders, depression, fatigue, skin rashes, high blood pressure, hyperactivity, nausea, irritability, and headaches, as well as more serious conditions including autism, intelligence deficits, and cancer. Testing for heavy metal toxicity can identify which metals are present in the body and in what amounts. On the basis of this information, a physician is able to develop an individualized detoxification and nutritional prescription program both to eliminate the toxic metals from the system and to restore depleted essential nutrients.

### ToxMet Screen

The ToxMet Screen, from MetaMetrix Medical Laboratory, provides an inexpensive but detailed analysis of the levels of specific heavy metals in a patient's system, based on a urine sample. ToxMet tests for levels of four highly toxic heavy metals (arsenic, cadmium, lead, and mercury); it also reports on levels for ten potentially toxic elements, such as aluminum, bismuth, boron, nickel, and strontium. Finally, information is gathered on a patient's status regarding 14 essential metals and minerals, such as copper, calcium, chromium, molybdenum, selenium, and vanadium. When test results exceed limits believed to be safe, the report indicates a "high" concentration. For example, one patient was high in arsenic (65 units compared to a high limit of 40) and cadmium (3.7 compared to the limit of 2). ToxMet also indicated that this patient had high levels of calcium, magnesium, manganese, and zinc.

## Testing for Enzyme Deficiencies

Many CFS patients have depleted enzyme levels, which means they are unable to properly absorb the nutrients from food and supplements, thus contributing to prolonging their overall symptoms. Enzymes (SEE QUICK DEFINITION), essential in the breakdown of nutrients and the clearing of toxins in the blood, come from two sources: they are manufactured in the pancreas and we get them from our food. If our food doesn't contain the necessary enzymes—which is often the case in the standard American diet of highly processed foods—then the pancreas must work overtime to produce more enzymes. This taxes the pancreas and also depletes the number of enzymes available to circulate in the blood and clear toxins. When this state of affairs is prolonged, digestive and absorption problems develop and toxins accumulate beyond the body's ability to eliminate them. Therefore, before implementing dietary changes and a regimen of nutritional supplements as part of a total treatment program, it is advisable to determine if enzyme deficiencies are present. Without investigating this possibility, the most careful diet and highest-quality supplements will have little or no effect.

**Enzymes** are specialized living proteins fundamental to all living processes in the body, necessary for every chemical reaction and the normal activity of our organs, tissues, fluids, and cells. There are hundreds of thousands of different enzymes. Among their many other functions, certain enzymes enable the body to digest and assimilate food. There are special enzymes for digesting proteins, carbohydrates, fats, and plant fibers; specifically, protease digests proteins, amylase digests carbohydrates, lipase digests fats, cellulase digests fiber, and disaccharidase digests sugars.

A 24-hour urine analysis is all that is required to determine one's enzyme status. Specific parameters of the test reveal the status of digestive function in three food groups: protein, carbohydrates, and fats. Abnormal values in uric acid indicate a deficiency of protease, the enzyme that digests protein. If calcium phosphate values are abnormal, it means there is a deficiency of amylase, the enzyme that digests carbohydrates. Lastly, the calcium oxalate component is linked to lipase, the enzyme that digests fats. (See "What a Urine Analysis Reveals," pp. 35–37.)

## Loomis Urinalysis

In her work as an enzyme therapist, Lita Lee, Ph.D., of Lowell, Oregon, relies on the urinalysis developed by Charles Loomis, D.C., founder and president of 21st Century Nutrition in Madison, Wisconsin. She emphasizes that a 24-hour urine sample is the only way to pinpoint enzyme deficiencies. In addition to enzyme deficiencies, the Loomis test isolates digestive disorders and nutrient deficiencies. For the test, Dr. Lee asks clients to avoid taking vitamins, minerals, enzymes, herbs, or other supplements for at least a day before the test and during the 24-hour testing period. No dietary changes are necessary, she

 For information on **Loomis urinalysis**, contact: 21st Century Nutrition, 6421 Enterprise Lane, Madison, WI 53719; tel: (608) 273-8115. Website: www.loomisenzymes.com.

says. The client collects urine in a sterile container, noting the total urine volume eliminated (in cups, or other units of measure) each time, along with any symptoms experienced while urinating. The sample is then analyzed by a technician who specializes in Loomis urinalysis.

# Allergy Testing

Allergies are a characteristic component of CFS, fibromyalgia, and environmental illness. Identifying and taking steps to eliminate these allergies or avoiding exposure to the offending substances is a vital part of reducing the burden on the immune system. In the case of environmental illness, the extent of the allergies presents a daunting prospect, but the level of disability created by the constant allergic reaction makes the process of identification all the more necessary. There are numerous tests to identify allergens, or allergy-causing substances, but two of the most effective are the Nambudripad Allergy Elimination Technique (NAET) and electrodermal screening. Other, more conventional tests include skin testing and the IgG ELISA (enzyme-linked immunoabsorbent assay) test.

## Nambudripad Allergy Elimination Technique (NAET)

Developed by Devi Nambudripad, D.C., L.Ac., R.N., Ph.D., this method of both detecting and permanently eliminating allergies and sensitivities combines applied kinesiology's (SEE QUICK DEFINITION) muscle response testing with acupuncture and chiropractic. To identify an allergen, the patient holds a vial containing the suspected allergy-causing substance in one hand while the practitioner tests the muscle strength of the patient's arm or leg. A weak muscle response indicates an allergy or sensitivity to that substance. Treatment involves the patient again holding the substance while the NAET practitioner uses acupuncture or acupressure to reprogram the way the body responds to the substance, thereby removing the allergic charge.

"Because your energy pathways are unblocked while you are holding the substance during the acupuncture treatment, your body stops reacting to it," Dr. Nambudripad explains. "This, in turn, leads your brain to stop viewing the substance as harmful." Once the treatment is complete, patients are then instructed to avoid exposure to the substance for 25 to 30 hours, after which time it should no longer cause an allergic reaction.

**Applied kinesiology**, developed by George Goodheart, D.C., of Grosse Pointe Woods, Michigan, is the study of the relationship between muscle dysfunction (weak muscles) and related organ or gland dysfunction. Applied kinesiology employs a simple strength-resistance test on a specific indicator muscle that is related to the organ or part of the body that is being tested. If the muscle tests strong, maintaining its resistance, this indicates health; if it tests weak, this can mean infection or dysfunction. For example, the deltoid muscle in the shoulder is related to the lungs and therefore is a good indicator of any problems there.

For more on **NAET**, see chapter 9, Addressing the Allergy Connection.

### Electrodermal Screening (EDS)

Electrodermal screening is widely used in Europe, and to an increasing extent in the United States, to test for both food and environmental allergies, and to determine what remedy to use to properly neutralize the allergic reaction. "A small [painless] current of electricity is introduced at specific acupuncture points on the patient," explains Fuller Royal, M.D., of Las Vegas, Nevada. "Various allergens are then introduced into the circuitry, enabling the physician to determine any change in the way the patient reacts to the current." Dr. Royal states that EDS allows him to accurately test for a full spectrum of allergens, and that the entire battery of tests can be done in an hour. According to Dr. Royal, a reading of 50 on a scale of 100 is normal and "a reading of over 50 means allergens are present," he says. "As they are found, various treatment doses are also added into the circuit and the correct treatment will bring the reading back down to 50."

## Skin Testing

"Skin testing is one of the most consistent methods of testing people for pollen, mold, dust, chemical, and other environmental allergies," says Richard Wilkinson, M.D., who practices environmental medicine in Yakima, Washington. He recommends Serial Endpoint Titration (SET) testing, which is far more accurate than the more commonly used scratch test. The scratch test consists of lightly scratching the skin and placing a dilution of a suspected allergen in that spot. If it raises a wheal (an irritated bump) within 15 minutes, allergy is confirmed. Compared to NAET or EDS, however, using the SET method to identify one's full range of allergies is potentially a long and uncomfortable process.

During a SET test, a diluted form of a potential allergen is injected just below the skin. The body immediately reacts to the introduction of this foreign substance by forming a wheal about four millimeters in diameter. In the next ten minutes, the wheal will grow according to the severity of the immune reaction. Ten minutes after the injection, the wheal is measured again. A wheal of seven millimeters or larger indicates that the patient has an allergy, while a smaller wheal indicates that no allergy is present.

If the patient tests positive for allergy, the process can then be repeated with increasingly diluted forms of the allergen. These new tests show how severely the body reacts to varying amounts of the substance. SET is one of the few tests that can evaluate your degree of sensitivity to a known allergen; NAET is another.

## The IgG ELISA Test

Most allergy tests only measure the presence of IgE (immunoglobulin E [SEE QUICK DEFINITION]) antibodies, while most food allergies are dealt with in the body by the IgG (immunoglobulin G) antibodies. The IgG ELISA (enzyme-linked immunoabsorbent assay) test offers new hope for food allergy sufferers. It is currently the only commercially available test of its kind for delayed food allergies.

An **immunoglobulin** is one of a class of five specially designed antibody proteins produced in the spleen, bone marrow, or lymph tissue and involved in the immune system's defense response to foreign substances. The main types of immunoglobulins, grouped according to their concentration in the blood, are IgG (80%), IgA (10% to 15%), IgM (5% to 10%), IgD (less than 0.1%), IgE (less than 0.01%). Technically, all antibodies are immunoglobulins.

"We know that one of the fundamental causes behind food allergies is the penetration of undigested or partially digested food from the digestive tract into the bloodstream," explains James Braly, M.D., founder and past medical director of Immuno Laboratories in Fort Lauderdale, Florida. "With the IgG ELISA test, we

 For more information about the **IgG ELISA test**, contact Immuno Laboratories, 1620 West Oakland Park Boulevard, Fort Lauderdale, FL 33311; tel: (800) 231-9197. Website: www.immunolabs.com.

can measure the actual presence of specific foods and their specific IgG antibodies in the blood to precisely determine which foods a person is allergic to." Convenient and automated, the IgG ELISA test involves computer analysis of a blood sample for the presence of IgG antibodies against over 100 foods. The test can be done through the mail, as long as samples reach testing labs within 72 hours after the blood is drawn.

## Tests to Identify Nutritional Deficiencies

Nutritional deficiencies are usually a feature of chronic fatigue syndrome, fibromyalgia, and environmental illness. Such deficiencies can be due to impaired digestion (as a result of the multiple infections involved), poor diet, stress, environmental toxins, or a combination of any or all of these factors. Specific nutritional deficiencies can contribute to certain CFS symptoms. For example, a lack of amino acids (SEE QUICK DEFINITION), which are the protein building blocks of neurotransmitters (SEE QUICK DEFINITION), can lead to depleted levels of these essential chemical messengers in the brain. Such a deficiency has been linked to depression, anxiety, and other mood disorders.

As with other aspects of treatment, in order to design an effective program of nutritional supplementation, it is necessary to identify all deficiencies. Thorough testing can avoid prescribing the wrong supplement and save time and expense in the long term. Among the laboratory tests for nutrient status, the four discussed below are relatively inexpensive and provide detailed, practical information.

### Individualized Optimal Nutrition (ION)

Using a blood and a urine sample, the ION (Individualized Optimal Nutrition) Panel from MetaMetrix measures 150 biochemical components. The test is highly useful for physicians who need detailed biochemical assessment of patients who have chronic fatigue or other immune disorders, multiple chemical sensitivities, cancer, heart disease, learning difficulties, or obesity. Specifically, ION checks for nutritional status in categories including vitamins, minerals, amino acids, fatty and organic acids, lipid peroxides, general blood chemistries (cholesterol, thyroid hormone, glucose), and antioxidants. In each category, a patient's levels are compared with predetermined limits.

Based on the individual's test results, ION can provide supplement recommendations. For the antioxidant panel, for example, ION provides a precisely tailored blend of 16 substances, from coenzyme Q10 and copper citrate to beta carotene and vitamin C. ION also summarizes the test results and places them into nine categories according to disease risk, such as cardiovascular, liver function, intestinal balance, energy, digestive disorders, and thyroid status. In each case, an individual's biochemical status is contrasted against a healthy norm. The total ION test of seven panels typically costs between $600 and $1,000. Individual panels may also be ordered.

 **Amino acids** are the basic building blocks of the over 40,000 different proteins in the body, including enzymes, hormones, and the key chemical messenger molecules called neurotransmitters. Eight amino acids cannot be made by the body and must be obtained through the diet; others are produced in the body, but not always in sufficient amounts. The body's main "amino acid pool" consists of alanine, arginine, aspargine, aspartic acid, carnitine, citrulline, cysteine, cystine, gamma-aminobutyric acid (GABA), glutamic acid, glutamine, glycine, histidine, isoleucine, leucine, lysine, methionine, ornithine, phenylalanine, proline, serine, taurine, threonine, tryptophan, tyrosine, and valine.

A **neurotransmitter** is a brain chemical with the specific function of enabling communications to happen between brain cells. Chief among the 100 neurotransmitters identified to date are acetylcholine, dopamine, GABA, norepinephrine, and serotonin.

## FIA (Functional Intracellular Analysis)

These tests—the Comprehensive Profile 3000, B-Complex Profile 1100, Primary Profile 1500, Cardiovascular Profile 1600, and Antioxidants Profile 1400—measure the function of key vitamins, minerals, antioxidants, amino acids, fatty acids, and metabolites (choline, inositol) at the cellular level. They also assess the status of carbohydrate metabolism in terms of insulin function and fructose intolerance. The FIA measures how these micronutrients are actually functioning within the activities of living white blood cells, rather than simply measuring the micronutrient levels in the blood (which may or may not provide useful information about cell metabolism). More specifically, FIA assesses the amount of cell growth for metabolically active lymphocytes (a type of white blood cell) as a way of identifying micronutrient deficiencies that are known to interfere with growth or immune function in the cells. These tests typically cost $300 or less.

### Pantox Antioxidant Profile

Using a small blood sample, this diagnostic screen measures the status of more than 20 nutritional factors as a way of determining the body's antioxidant defense system. It then compares the results against a database of 7,000 normal, healthy profiles. Specifically, the screen reports on lipoproteins (cholesterol, triglycerides), fat-soluble antioxidants (vitamins A and E, carotenoids, coenzyme Q10), water-soluble antioxidants (vitamin C, uric acid, bilirubin), and iron balance. The test helps determine whether you are getting the right antioxidants in the correct amounts. The Pantox Profile is displayed in bar graphs with accompanying explanatory medical text, telling you whether your levels of a specific nutrient are low and pose a health risk. The test cost to patients is about $300 and is often covered by health insurance, including Medicare.

It is important to realize that just because you consume a nutrient does not mean your body has assimilated it or that it is present and active in your bloodstream. The stress produced by the heightened activity of free radicals can seriously deplete your reserves of antioxidants, despite a healthy diet and nutritional supplementation delivered imprecisely, explains Pantox Laboratories director Charles A. Thomas, Jr., Ph.D. The practical goal, he says, is for "an individual to take steps to change one's levels so as to join others who are experiencing a lower rate of degenerative diseases."

For more information about **ION**, contact: MetaMetrix Medical Laboratory, 4855 Peachtree Industrial Boulevard, Suite 201, Norcross, GA 30092; tel: (800) 221-4640. Website: www.metametrix.com. For **Functional Intracellular Analysis**, contact: SpectraCell Laboratories, Inc., 7051 Portwest Drive, Suite 100, Houston, TX 77024; tel: (800) 227-5227. Website: www.spectracell.com. **The Pantox Antioxidant Profile** must be ordered by a licensed health-care practitioner. Contact: Pantox Laboratories, 4622 Santa Fe Street, San Diego, CA 92109; tel: (888) 726-8698. Website: www.pantox.com. **Oxidative Protection Screen** must also be ordered by a licensed health-care practitioner. Contact: Antibody Assay Laboratories, 1715 East Wilshire #715, Santa Ana, CA 92705; tel: (800) 522-2611. Website: www.aalrl.com.

### Oxidative Protection Screen

The Oxidative Protection Screen from Antibody Assay Laboratories, of Santa Ana, California, can provide your physician with an actual biochemical analysis of how well your body is handling free radicals. This information is valuable for a physician in assessing a patient's overall health, the degree of antioxidant protection the patient has, and the possible need for further nutrient supplementation. When lipids (fatty acids and other oily organic compounds) are damaged by free radicals, they form lipid peroxides that circulate in the blood. Using a drawn blood sample from a patient, the lab test determines the amount of lipid peroxides in the plasma; these numbers vary with age and gender.

For a 20-year-old woman, for example, the normal range is 1.28 to 1.69 micromole/liter, but for a 60-year-old female, it is 2.15 to 2.82 micromole/liter. An elevated amount, beyond this range, indicates a high production of free radicals; the lower the amount of lipid peroxides, the stronger the antioxidant protection. The Total Oxidative Protection Index (TOPI) will indicate the system's overall ability to withstand the attack of free radicals and thus the patient's individual degree of oxidative protection. The normal range here is 45% to 63%; ranges above 63% indicate a high degree of antioxidant protection and health.

# three

# Eliminating Viruses, Infections, Candidiasis, and Parasites

Parasites, candidiasis, viruses, and other infections are often present in patients with chronic fatigue syndrome. Whether these infections in combination are the cause of CFS or opportunistic invaders of a weakened immune system has not been conclusively demonstrated, but in either case, compromised immunity is a central feature of the syndrome, and the infections involved perpetuate and deepen immune dysfunction by further taxing an already overloaded system. As a result, an immune-strengthening protocol is integral to the CFS treatment programs of many alternative medicine physicians.

Some researchers and doctors still hold stubbornly to the view that a single virus is behind CFS. The conventional medical profession has tended to focus on the herpes family of viruses, which includes Epstein-Barr and oral and genital herpes. The Epstein-Barr virus (EBV; SEE QUICK DEFINITION) has received the most attention because its symptoms are duplicated in CFS sufferers, who usually also test high for levels of EBV antibodies—immune proteins mobilized to defend the body against EBV molecules. In the early days of the CFS epidemic (the 1980s), conventional doctors assumed—and some insisted—that EBV was the cause of chronic fatigue syndrome. When patients with CFS started turning up without elevated levels of EBV, conventional physicians eventually changed their thinking on causality.

Even the National Institutes of Health (NIH) admits that there is no clear-cut evidence that the Epstein-Barr virus, or any other virus, is the

> One of the hallmarks of alternative medicine thinking and practice is that there is rarely, if ever, a single cause of any illness; diseases develop out of multiple converging imbalances and deficiencies.

primary cause of CFS. The NIH reports that recent studies found that acyclovir, a drug that blocks multiplication of the Epstein-Barr virus, is ineffective in CFS patients.[1] So to focus on only EBV is a mistaken approach. One of the hallmarks of alternative medicine thinking and practice is that there is rarely, if ever, a single cause of any illness; diseases develop out of multiple converging imbalances and deficiencies.

## Infectious Agents: The Chicken or the Egg?

The wide-ranging, complex symptomology of CFS patients indicates that the disorder is caused by more than EBV alone. Murray R. Susser, M.D., of Santa Monica, California, concedes that EBV may indeed be a major factor in CFS cases, but poses the possibility that EBV (dormant or suppressed) might be reactivated due to other weaknesses in immune function.[2]

"CFS can start with ordinary viral infections, such as those that cause respiratory infections, like the common cold and flus," he explains. "There are 2,300 viruses that can cause a cold or flu and if one of those hits you and your body isn't able to get rid of it, then you have a chronic infection. In CFS, we often get hidden viral, parasite, and yeast infections that are results of a weakened immune system. One infection puts demand on the immune system, which can't kick it, and another infection may join in, leading from one to another in a domino effect. With this constant infection, CFS behaves like the flu that never got better."

 **Epstein-Barr virus (EBV)** is a herpes-like virus thought to be the cause of infectious mononucleosis and Burkitt's lymphoma. It is contracted through the cells in the lining of the mouth and throat, and can therefore be spread by sharing of utensils, kissing, and unsanitary habits. EBV symptoms, frequently duplicated in other conditions, include debilitating fatigue, fever, swollen glands, arthritic symptoms, multiple allergies, and difficulties in concentrating. People with chronic fatigue syndrome often have a high level of EBV antibodies in their blood, but EBV is no longer regarded (as it was in the 1980s) as the sole, or even necessarily a contributing, cause for chronic fatigue.

> In CFS, we often get hidden parasite, yeast, and viral infections that are results of a weakened immune system. One infection puts demand on the immune system, which can't kick it, and another infection may join in, leading from one to another in a domino effect.
>
> —*Murray Susser, M.D.*

Some of the infections in this domino effect may be retroviruses, a group that includes the leukemia and AIDS viruses, and that recent research has linked to CFS, reports Dr. Susser.[3] Sinusitis (inflammation of the sinuses, which may be caused by a virus, bacteria, or allergies) is also common in cases of CFS.

Other factors may leave the body vulnerable to infections, parasites (SEE QUICK DEFINITION), or an overgrowth of the *Candida albicans* fungus. For example, poor digestion is a contributing cause of parasitic infection. "Someone who has a low acid level [a measure of the pH, or general chemical balance] in his stomach won't digest food properly, so whatever parasites come through in the food won't get sterilized out," says Maoshing Ni, D.O.M., Ph.D., L.Ac., president of Yo San University in Marina del Rey, California. "That's what hydrochloric acid [digestive acid in the stomach] does—it sterilizes the food and kills off all the germs. When it's not effective at doing that, the parasites get passed along into the intestines." A complicating factor of parasitic infection is that most people who have parasites don't know it.

 **Parasites** are any organisms that live off another organism (called a host), and draw nourishment from it. Common forms of parasites are the protozoa (single-cell organisms), arthropods (insects), and worms that infect the body and cause major damage to tissues and organs. Protozoan parasites include *Giardia lamblia*, which causes giardiasis; *Entamoeba histolytica*, which produces dysentery; and *Cryptosporidium*, a cause of diarrhea, particularly in people with immunologic diseases such as AIDS. The most common arthropod parasites are lice, mites, ticks, and fleas. Worm parasites include pinworms, roundworms, tapeworms, whipworms, *Trichinella spiralis* (worms usually acquired by eating tainted pork), hookworms, guinea worms, and filaria (threadlike worms that inhabit the blood and tissues).

Parasitic infection can, in turn, lead to candidiasis. This overgrowth of *Candida albicans* in the intestinal tract is often found as a complication of giardiasis (infection with the protozoan *Giardia lamblia*, a highly contagious and virulent unicellular organism found mostly in the contaminated waters of lakes, streams, and oceans).

## The Insider's View of Stomach pH

The term pH, which means "potential hydrogen," represents a scale for the relative acidity or alkalinity of a solution. Acidity is measured as a pH of 0.1 to 6.9, and alkalinity as a pH of 7.1 to 14; a pH of 7.0 is considered neutral. The numbers refer to how many hydrogen atoms are present compared to an ideal or standard solution. Normally, blood is slightly alkaline, at 7.35 to 7.45; urine pH can range from 4.8 to 7.5, although normal is closer to 7.0.

An effective way to determine the pH in the stomach is the Heidelberg pH capsule system. According to its manufacturer, this "tubeless gastric analysis" is a way of showing abnormal conditions of acidity or alkalinity in the stomach or small intestines.

A miniature electronic transmitter is put inside a small capsule made of polyacrylate (which is inert and indigestible). The patient swallows this; once in the stomach, the capsule transmits, by radio signals, continuous and/or changing values for the pH of that area. The capsule is active for about 22 hours after ingestion. These recordings of the pH fluctuations are displayed in graph form, called a gastrogram. The stomach's pH can be challenged by introducing an alkalinizing drink such as sodium bicarbonate; the gastrointestinal system's response to this challenge offers valuable information about its health.

The technique was developed in the 1950s by German researcher Hans G. Nöller, M.D., professor of pediatrics at the University of Heidelberg. Dr. Nöller sought an alternative to the invasive, uncomfortable stomach tube procedure commonly used by gastroenterologists to assess stomach and small-intestine function. Since its invention, over 200 scientific studies have reported on the Heidelberg pH capsule's application for a variety of gastrointestinal conditions.

 For information about the **Hedelberg pH capsule system**, contact: Heidelberg International, Inc., 933 Beasley Street, Blairsville, GA 30512; (706) 745-9698.

Like CFS itself, candidiasis is reaching epidemic proportions in the United States.

Considered an opportunistic infection (one that develops when the body is compromised by other infections), candidiasis has serious consequences because it increases gut permeability to undigested foods and bowel toxins. These can then enter the bloodstream, where they induce an immune response and promote intolerance of or sensitivities to common foods. The reverse can also occur—continual allergic reactions in the body and the circulation of allergens create an ideal environment for candidiasis.

Both candidiasis and parasites are often the result of an excessive use of antibiotics, which kill much of the body's important intestinal flora, thereby inviting opportunistic infections. Leon Chaitow, N.D., D.O., of London, England, describes the likely candidate for *Candida* overgrowth as someone whose medical history includes any of the following: steroid hormone medication (such as cortisone or corticosteroids), which are often prescribed for skin conditions such as rashes, eczema, or psoriasis; prolonged or repeated use of antibiotics, which are frequently given for urinary and ear infections, sinusitis, bronchitis, and other infections; ulcer medications (such as Tagamet and Zantac); and oral contraceptives.

While candidiasis is more commonly linked to CFS, parasites are frequently overlooked as a contributing factor; even when testing is ordered, it often fails to detect them (see chapter 2, Testing). As evidence of parasite involvement in CFS, Leo Galland, M.D., of New York City, reports that 82% of those who suffered from chronic fatigue syndrome were cured of their symptoms when treated for parasitic infection. In one study, over one-third of the CFS patients tested were found to be infected with *Giardia lamblia*.[4]

 For more about **candidiasis** and **allergies**, see chapter 9, Addressing the Allergy Connection.

The clinical profile of parasitic infection resembles that of CFS: chronic fatigue, joint and muscle pain, immune dysfunction, allergies, skin conditions such as rashes and hives, nervousness, and digestive problems. Dr. Galland's research indicates that major health problems can be caused by even a mild parasitic infection. Consequently, his view is that any person with unexplained fatigue, multiple allergies (especially to food), and chronic gastrointestinal complaints—such as bloating, diarrhea, abdominal pain, flatulence, or chronic constipation—should be screened for intestinal parasites.

Prolonged viral or bacterial infection, candidiasis, and parasites tax the immune system and contribute to malabsorption of nutrients, which results in nutritional deficiencies. Obviously, eliminating this drain on the body is a treatment priority. To accomplish this, many alternative medicine doctors employ a two-pronged approach: targeting the infectious agents and bolstering the immune system so that it can fulfill its purpose of fighting off such agents.

**Murray Susser, M.D.**: 2730 Wilshire Boulevard, Suite #1110, Santa Monica, CA 90403; tel: (310) 453-4424. **Leo Galland, M.D.**: 133 East 73rd Street, New York, NY 10021; tel: (212) 861-9000. **William Campbell Douglass, M.D.**: 7100 Peachtree-Dunwoody Road, Suite #100, Atlanta, GA 30328; tel: (770) 668-0432.

Detoxification therapy to rid the body of an accumulation of toxins from a variety of sources may be a component of both. Chapter 5 discusses detoxification methods along

## Is Chronic Fatigue the New Face of Polio?

Just as tuberculosis, once believed to have been eradicated by modern medicine, has now returned in more virulent, drug-resistant strains, so may polio be with us again in a disguised form. We may be mistakenly calling it chronic fatigue syndrome (U.S.) or myalgic encephalomyelitis (England). According to William Campbell Douglass, M.D., editor of the medical newsletter *Second Opinion*, polio is more common than ever and may actually be caused by the polio vaccination. This intriguing and potentially electrifying theory is based on information Dr. Douglass gleaned from several clinical studies.

Dr. Douglass argues that the Salk and Sabin vaccines, widely administered to children in the 1950s for poliomyelitis, did not eliminate polio at all, but forced it to change its form. While the vaccines suppressed the polio virus, the virus was replaced by genetically similar ones, such as Coxsackie virus, which is often found in elevated levels in CFS patients. The Coxsackie family of viruses, first isolated in 1948, consists of 29 different strains and is linked to numerous illnesses. When physicians first began identifying these viruses in the blood of CFS patients, they failed to discern their connection with polio.

The sustained use of polio vaccines for over 40 years has resulted in "at least 72 viral strains that can cause polio-like diseases," says Dr. Douglass. Before the polio vaccines, there were only three polio viruses. He notes that he was not the first to point to evidence of "the changing of polio rather than the elimination of it." As early as 1934, cases of "atypical" polio were reported in Los Angeles, and "abortive poliomyelitis" was reported in Switzerland in 1939.

Dr. Douglass suggests that the trend towards the emergence of a new polio—its predominant symptom changing from infantile paralysis to adult muscle weakness—has rapidly increased since the polio vaccines were introduced. "We now know that chronic fatigue syndrome is not a new disease, but simply an 'aborted form' of the more serious paralytic polio," he states. If Dr. Douglass's speculations prove correct, the credibility of conventional medicine's mass vaccination program will be seriously undermined. It is hardly a public-health benefit if a vaccine simply modifies an existing disease, forcing it to take another form in the next generation of patients. The indiscriminate use of vaccines may prove to be as counterproductive as has the overprescription of antibiotics.

with alternative medicine techniques for rebuilding the immune system in general. In this chapter, we focus on treating the specific viral infections, candidiasis, and parasites using the two-pronged approach.

## Treating Viral and Bacterial Infections

Viruses do not respond to antibiotics, so these drugs are only prescribed for bacterial infections or to prevent a bacterial infection from developing in the immune-weakened environment created by a virus. Although alternative medicine physicians sometimes employ antibiotic treatment, they generally try to avoid doing so because of the further problems antibiotics create in the body, such as destroying the beneficial intestinal flora along with the infection-causing bacteria, thus creating a prime environment for candidiasis and parasites.

In addition to strengthening the immune system to bolster the body's own defense mechanisms against disease-producing microorganisms, alternative medicine employs antimicrobial herbs to reduce the viral and bacterial load on the body. These include echinacea, goldenseal, citrus seed extract, aloe vera, and tea tree oil, among others. Pau d'arco bark, obtained from a tropical tree native to Brazil, has particularly strong antiviral qualities. (See herbal medicine treatments for candidiasis and parasites, later in this chapter.)

According to Lita Lee, Ph.D., of Lowell, Oregon, coconut oil can also be used to treat chronic fatigue patients. "Medical research on the use of coconut oil for chronic fatigue patients shows it to have an antiviral effect," she reports. In addition, it is antiallergenic and antiseptic, promotes thyroid function, regulates blood sugar, and protects mitochondria (the cells' "energy factories") against stress injuries. "Coconut oil has gotten a bad rap," Dr. Lee adds. "It is actually one of the most healthy saturated fats."

Another strong antiviral botanical is an extract of shiitake mushroom called LEM (for *Lentinus edodes mycelium*, the immature form of the fungus). Research at Yamaguchi University in Tokyo, Japan, demonstrated LEM's ability to inhibit viruses and stimulate the immune system.[5] It may stop the spread of a virus by blocking the virus's receptor sites. LEM appears to boost the immune system by stimulating macrophages and lymphocytes, both of which play an important role in protecting against toxins, viruses, and other invading microorganisms.

See chapter 4, Restoring Immune Vitality, and chapter 12, Correcting Chronic Fatigue with Herbs.

Thus far, the research on LEM's antiviral qualities has taken place in a test tube, but *HealthWatch*, the newsletter of the CFIDS (chronic fatigue and immune dysfunction syndrome) Buyers Club, reports that LEM is the "all-time best-selling nutritional supplement used by CFIDS sufferers."[6]

### An Antiviral Nutritional Program

Shari Lieberman, Ph.D., C.N.S., a well-known scientist and certified nutrition specialist, developed a multivitamin/mineral formula called Optimum Protection, which she uses (at a dosage of four tablets daily) as the basis of an antiviral, antibacterial nutritional supplement program for CFS patients. Here are the components of her program, with typical dosages (the components and dosages will vary, depending upon the individual):

**Kyolic Premium EPA:** This product is a combination of garlic and fish oil (EPA or eicosapentaenoic acid, an omega-3 essential fatty acid). "I combine these because garlic is a broad-spectrum antibiotic and fish oil is excellent for inflammation and any sort of autoimmune phenomenon," Dr. Lieberman says. "I classify CFS as an autoimmune disease." She recommends four capsules a day.

**Quercetin:** Dr. Lieberman reports that this bioflavonoid (vitamin C helper) is "an antihistamine like vitamin C, and it's great for patients who have allergies, rhinitis, sinusitis, even environmental allergies. It's also effectively antiviral. I use it with any viral syndrome, including CFS and HIV." Quercetin also has anti-inflammatory properties. Dr. Lieberman normally recommends 1,000 to 1,500 mg per day.

**N-acetyl-cysteine (NAC):** NAC is an amino acid precursor for the production of glutathione, which reduces free radical damage to DNA and prevents the depletion of other antioxidants. N-acetyl cysteine is also an antiviral and is effective in breaking up mucus as well. "I'll use NAC if the person has some upper-respiratory symptoms or if they have environmental allergies," Dr. Lieberman says. A typical dosage is 500 mg twice a day.

**Glycyrrhizinate:** An active component of licorice, glycyrrhizin is "probably the most studied antiviral compound on the planet," according to Dr. Lieberman. However, she often has difficulty obtaining it. The typical dosage for the capsules made by Jarrow Formulas is two or

## A Flu Virus May Contribute to Fibromyalgia

In a study of the possible connection between flu viruses and fibromyalgia (chronic muscle pain), nine out of ten fibromyalgia patients tested positive for antibodies to influenza type A and three out of ten in an age- and sex-matched second group of people with fibromyalgia tested positive for influenza B.* Influenza A is a viral infection that mainly affects the respiratory and autonomic nervous systems.

The sympathetic branch of the autonomic nervous system is associated with arousal and stress, increasing heart rate, blood pressure, and muscle tension. If this branch is affected by a flu virus, muscle tension would be affected. The researchers conclude that influenza A may be implicated in the development of fibromyalgia, the primary symptom of which is widespread muscle pain.

*Tyler, Allen N., M.D., N.D., D.C. "Influenza A Virus: A Possible Precipitating Factor in Fibromyalgia?" *Alternative Medicine Review* 2:2 (1997).

three daily. Glycgel (made by Thorne Research) is in gel form; the typical dosage is ½ teaspoon twice a day.

*Echinacea:* As mentioned above, echinacea is known for its antimicrobial qualities. Dr. Lieberman favors Echinaguard, a tincture form of echinacea. She normally recommends 30 to 50 drops once a day, in an ongoing cycle of four days on, four days off.

*Coenzyme Q10:* Coenzyme Q10 is a substance not made by the human body, but found naturally in sardines, salmon, mackerel, and beef heart. "Coenzyme Q10 is 100% for energy. It increases the oxygen consumption of your cells and is crucial for making ATP [adenosine triphosphate]," states Dr. Lieberman. A typical dosage is 100 mg once or twice daily.

*Maitake D-Fraction:* The above supplements are the basics of Dr. Lieberman's program. If the patient is experiencing predominantly viral symptoms, she then adds maitake D-fraction to the regimen. This is an extract of the antiviral maitake mushroom, one of the medicinal mushrooms (shiitake and reishi are others) known to have powerful immune-enhancing effects. This tincture can be mixed with the Echinaguard at the same typical dosage, 30 to 50 drops once a day, four days on, four days off.

*Acidophilus:* Acidophilus is one of the beneficial bacteria that inhabit the human gastrointestinal tract and are essential for proper nutrient assimilation. The human body contains several trillion beneficial bacteria comprising over 400 species, all necessary for health. Among the more well-known are *Lactobacillus acidophilus* and *Bifidobacterium bifidum*. Overly acidic bodily conditions, chronic constipation or diarrhea, dietary imbalances, consumption of highly processed foods, and excessive use of antibiotics and hormonal drugs can interfere with probiotic function and even reduce the number of these microbes, setting up conditions for illness.

If a person has gastrointestinal problems, which is true of 50% of Dr. Lieberman's CFS patients, then she includes the powdered, refrigerated variety of acidophilus to help restore intestinal balance, at a dosage of ½ teaspoon once or twice a day, mixed with water or juice or sprinkled on food.

*Aloe Vera:* This herb is also useful for gastrointestinal complaints. "Aloe vera is soothing, can ease inflammation, and has natural plant enzymes that help with digestion," says Dr. Lieberman. She recommends ¼ cup, twice daily. For the patient whose system is severely weakened by CFS and who has irritable bowel symptoms, Dr. Lieberman starts the program at low dosages and gradually builds to the full amount. "A patient's stomach may be so bad that they can't tolerate the full dose of vitamins until you clear the irritable bowel," she says.

One of her main approaches for healing digestive problems is to take patients off dairy and gluten (a vegetable protein found in wheat, rye, oats, and barley). "I have found gluten to be extremely deleterious to immune function, certainly in patients with

 **Shari Lieberman, Ph.D., C.N.S.,** is available by appointment only. To schedule an appointment, call 212-929-3152. **Optimum Protection, Kyolic Premium EPA,** and the other products mentioned above are available from health-food stores.

CFS and other autoimmune disorders," says Dr. Lieberman. In addition, "viruses love fat and sugar," she observes, so cutting them out of the diet is also part of the antiviral program.

### Treating CFS and Fibromyalgia with Transfer Factors

As the preceding pages have already made clear, one of the most important keys to preventing and treating chronic fatigue syndrome, fibromyalgia, and other similar disorders is bolstering immune function, so that the immune system is able to readily respond to immunosuppressive agents—such as viruses, bacteria, and infectious pathogens—without exhausting itself. In recent years, an increasing number of alternative medicine practitioners are accomplishing this goal through the use of transfer factors (TFs), so called because they are capable of literally "transferring immunity."

Transfer factors were discovered in the late 1940s by H. Sherwood Lawrence, M.D., while he was researching tuberculosis. In the course of his research, Dr. Lawrence discovered that one person's immunity could be transferred to another patient using low molecular weight extracts derived from the healthy person's white blood cells. He named these extracts "transfer factors."[7]

Subsequent research by Dr. Lawrence and other scientists revealed that transfer factors are essential aspects of the immune systems of even the most primitive species, and that they are universally effective, even when derived from one species and administered to another.[8] Dr. Lawrence and other early researchers also knew that an immune response had been transferred because of the way TFs work. Derived from a host—either a human or an animal testing positive for a specific antigen (SEE QUICK DEFINI-

TION)—transfer factors are administered to recipients who test negative for the same antigen. In early experiments, Dr. Lawrence and others observed that when persons received antigen-specific transfer factors, they became skin-positive for that antigen, whereas before the transfer they had been skin-negative. The positive response, evidenced by skin irritation, proved that the immune response had occurred, and that the recipient's immune system had gained knowledge of the specific antigen.

 An **antigen** is a term applied to any substance that induces immune response or sensitivity after coming into contact with body cells. Antigens are molecules that are part of invading disease agents, like viruses and bacteria, which physicians often refer to as "foreign substances."

There are two basic concepts to understand about transfer factors: (1) immune response *can* be transferred, and (2) a transfer factor recipient receives an immune benefit *without receiving any antibodies*, since transfer factors contain no antibodies, only extremely small, low-molecular-weight proteins. This raises the question: What kind of immunological information is transferred from the host to the recipient when transfer factors are used?

Practitioners who use transfer factors answer that question by describing the immune system that receives transfer factors as "having gone to school." Transfer factors help to "educate," or modulate, the recipient's immune system, teaching it to recognize specific antigens and communicating the knowledge that they are present, thus stimulating the proper immune response. In this regard, transfer factors act as catalysts for the immune system, causing the appropriate immune response to occur without being consumed in the process—unlike antibodies, which are used up when they attach themselves to invading foreign substances.

Transfer factors were originally administered by injection, but later studies proved they were just as effective when taken orally.[9] Transfer factors do not, themselves, cure specific diseases involving the antigens they contain, but TFs made with specific antigens do appear to be more efficient at educating the immune system than other nonspecific substances known to boost immunity.

TFs are produced from either filtered leukocytes and lymphocytes from the blood, or from colostrum, the first breast-milk secretion that female mammals supply to their offspring. "Colostrum is the original transfer factor," states Jo Anne Whitaker, M.D., F.A.A.P., director of the Bowen Research and Training Institute in Palm Harbor, Florida, who uses TFs in her practice. She notes that a human baby's first exposure to transferred immune response comes from colostrum it receives from

## How Transfer Factors Are Prepared

Transfer factors (TFs) act as immunomodulators, and recent research suggest that TFs may work directly at the level of DNA polymerization processes, creating larger molecules from smaller ones. The TFs themselves are tiny protein molecules known as oligoribonucleotide peptides, that are one-seventh to one-fiftieth the size of antibodies.

TFs are derived either from colostrum or from filtered leukocytes and lymphocytes from the blood. Chisolm Biological Laboratory (CBL), a leader in the manufacture of TFs, uses purified dialyzable leukocyte extracts (DLE-TFs) derived from the white blood cells of chickens. "Dialyzable" means that the white blood cell protein materials have passed through dialysis filtration and are extremely small, which ensures that there is no risk of infection in human recipients with animal host antigens.

Each batch of CBL TF is prepared through a series of processes. First, the host blood cells are removed, then white blood cells (WBCs) are separated out by a mechanical centrifugation technique. Next, the WBCs are broken apart by freeze-thawing and sound waves (sonication), after which the broken-up cells are sent through dialysis filtration to yield a low molecular weight extract that is then further fractionated and purified.

A sample of the TF extract is first tested for sterility and absence of toxins, then for potency. This TF sample is then introduced into yet another large production group, and the process is repeated. The extract material, produced by passing TF extract through several purification stages, ensures the greatest safety and efficacy of the final product. To date, no adverse side effects have been reported from the use of TF, even when TFs are administered in extremely high dosages or consecutively over several years.

being breast-fed just after birth. Colostrum provides newborns with TFs, as well as antibodies from the mother, enabling them to better resist infection and disease.

According to Minter Dopson, president of Chisolm Biological Laboratory (CBL) in South Carolina, and a pioneer in the TF field for more than two decades, the usefulness of transfer factors in treating advanced health conditions such as CFS and fibromyalgia is only part of the TF story. Everyone, he points out, whether ill or not, can benefit from knowing about TFs because of the way they help bolster and maintain immunity. In order to fully protect us, the immune system must have the capability, or "cell memory," of recognizing millions of foreign substances (antigens). But, as Dopson notes, many if not all, people lack comprehensive cell memory due to environmental and internal stresses, advanced age, inherited genetic defects, or other immune cell defects. Because this is so, Dopson believes it is important to explore the benefits of taking TFs to prevent cells from "forgetting" their response before disease strikes. While a course of daily TF treatment (of varying length) helps people with serious, chronic health conditions, Dopson points out that another approach to TF treatment is to take TFs for one week out of every three-month period before cell memory is lost. This approach is called *pulsed mode*.

In 1998, CBL developed a multi-antigen-specific TF for a study of its effectiveness in treating both CFS and fibromyalgia. One person in the study was Peggy R, who had been suffering from CFS for nine years and finally ended up being bedridden for three years. Peggy used the CBL TF product for one year, and she attributes her recovery to her use of it. Prior to participating in the study, Peggy had tried many other therapies over the years, with no lasting results. As she explains, "Chronic fatigue syndrome doesn't have a one-pronged solution, but CBL's TF takes the load off."

Peggy recently completed a computer class and has been able to return to the workforce part-time. During the year that she received CBL's TF treatment, she experienced quantitative and qualitative improvement in at least three areas. Before becoming part of the study, she slept 10 to 12 hours per day; afterward, she required only 8 to 9 hours of sleep. In addition, her memory and cognition skills both improved, whereas before she was experiencing memory problems and an inability to think clearly. Finally, her energy levels were also noticeably improved, enabling her to walk for 30 to 45 minutes without a decrease in energy, whereas previously she was fatigued after only 15 minutes of walking.

 **Chisolm Biological Laboratory**, 542 Legion Road, Warrensville, SC 29851; tel: (803) 663-9777. Order line: (800) 664-1333. Website: www.chisolmbio.com.

## A Homeopathic Antiviral Program for Chronic Fatigue Syndrome

New evidence suggests that chronic fatigue can be reversed using a homeopathic (SEE QUICK DEFINITION) approach to viral therapy. According to a study of 219 case histories, nearly all patients reported significant improvement after receiving homeopathic treatments that targeted three of the main viruses—Epstein-Barr, Coxsackie virus, and cytomegalovirus—most commonly associated with chronic fatigue syndrome.

The study involved an unusually diverse group of participants. Among the 219 cases, ages ranged from 2 to 78 years, and length of symptoms extended anywhere from 1 month to 30 years. Significantly, more than half had unsuccessfully attempted treatment by another method before admission to the study. Despite this apparent diversity among participants, however, blood tests revealed that all were infected with one of these three viruses, and that many carried some combination of the three.

Researchers patterned their treatment plan on a fourfold approach previously used to successfully cure hepatitis. Participants received twice-weekly injections of four different medicinal preparations: first, a highly diluted form (nosode—SEE QUICK DEFINITION) of the virus or viruses detected by the initial blood test, to stimulate the body's immune response against the infecting agent; second, a homeopathic preparation made from extracts of live organ tissues, to improve tissue regeneration and organ function (organ therapy); third, substances given to boost the immune system in general; and fourth, complex homeopathic remedies tailored both to the disease and to the patient, according to individual presentation of symptoms.

The homeopathic remedies included any combination of the following: Heel Coenzyme compositum and Wala Betula Arnica, Heel Echinacea compositum and Wala Meteoric Iron-Phosphorus-Quartz, Heel Engystol and Wala Pancreas Meteor, Galium-Heel and oral Wala Aurum Prunus, Heel Lymphomyosot and oral Wala Skorodit, and Heel Ubichinon compositum.

After an average of five to six weeks of treatment, nearly all participants noted a significant improvement in their physical function and overall health. Because most of the patients could not afford the expense of another blood test, researchers had to rely on subjective self-reporting instead of clinical data; even so, their results are impressive. Complete recovery occurred in 82% of the cases, while the remaining 18% resolved their symptoms after a second or third series of treatments. As one long-time sufferer of CFS described his recovery, "I have been dead for ten years and now I am alive again."

The study demonstrates that complex homeopathic remedies, when used in conjunction with nosodes, organ therapy, and immune system enhancement, can provide a treatment capable of reversing chronic fatigue syndrome. "This treatment is not open-ended," the study's

 **QUICK DEFINITION**

**Homeopathy** was developed in the early 1800s by German physician Samuel Hahnemann. Today, an estimated 500 million people worldwide receive homeopathic treatment, and in Britain, homeopathy enjoys royal patronage. Homeopathy is now practiced according to two differing concepts. In classical homeopathy, only one single-component remedy is prescribed at a time, in a potency specifically adjusted to the patient; the physician waits to see the results before prescribing anything further. In complex homeopathy, a prescription involves multiple substances given at the same time, usually in low potencies.

A **homeopathic nosode** is a super-diluted remedy made as an energy imprint from a disease product—such as bacteria, tuberculosis, measles, bowel infection, influenza, and about 200 other substances. The nosode, which contains no physical trace of the disease product, stimulates the body to remove all of the residues of a particular disease that it holds, whether such residues were inherited or contracted. Only qualified homeopaths may administer a nosode.

## Human Herpes Virus-6 (HHV-6) and Its Link to CFS and Fibromyalgia

Human herpes virus-6 (HHV-6), a member of the herpes virus family, is present in nearly 100% of the adult population, but in the majority of people, symptoms either never occur or occur only during early childhood, usually before age two. The most common childhood symptom caused by HHV-6 is roseola infantum, which manifests as a rose-colored skin rash that is accompanied by fever but is not infectious. Typically, once these symptoms abate, the virus becomes dormant, but it can later be reactivated due to various immunological or environmental factors. If reactivation occurs, symptoms of HHV-6 can be much more severe, and include hepatitis, meningoencephalitis (inflammation of the brain and the membranes of the spinal cord), pneumonitis (inflammation of the lungs), and mononucleosis. Recent research indicates that HHV-6 may also be a cofactor in a variety of other disease conditions, including AIDS, cervical cancer, oral carcinoma, autism, bipolar disorder, attention deficit disorder (ADD), multiple sclerosis, fibromyalgia, and chronic fatigue syndrome.

A number of researchers—most notably W. John Martin, M.D., Ph.D., of the Center for Complex Infectious Diseases (CCID) in Rosemead, California—believe that HHV-6 plays a pivotal role in chronic fatigue syndrome, and it's Dr. Martin's view that the term CFS should be discarded altogether since, he explains, "The entity called chronic fatigue syndrome simply refers to a loose grouping of certain symptoms that are part of a much wider spectrum of the clinical manifestations of viral-induced organic brain disease [caused by HHV-6 and other viral agents]."[a] Dr. Martin calls HHV-6 and other viral agents that act similarly "stealth viruses," because, though they can cause severe ill effects at the cellular level, they typically do not cause the inflammatory response that commonly occurs when the body tries to fight off other viral agents. As a result, HHV-6, though widely prevalent, is often overlooked as a causative factor in CFS, fibromyalgia, and many other disease conditions. Thus, left untreated, HHV-6 continues to create persistent and ongoing infections that cause the immune system to remain chronically "up-regulated" or otherwise impaired, eventually to the point where it is no longer effective in maintaining health.[b]

Persons infected by a stealth virus such as HHV-6 experience systemic viral illness, according to Dr. Martin, with many of their symptoms related to dysfunction of the brain. "This merely reflects the unique susceptibility of the brain to localized viral-induced damage," Dr. Martin explains. "Significant viral damage to other organs, such as the bowel, liver, thyroid, adrenal glands, etc., can, however, add to the neurological dysfunction resulting from viral infection within the brain."[c]

For more information about the **homeopathic remedies** cited, contact: HEEL, Inc.; tel: (800) 621-7644. Website: www.heelusa.com. For **olive leaf extract** (Alive and Well for consumers; Prolive for medical professionals), contact: Allergy Research Group, tel: (800) 545-9960. Website: www.nutricology.com.

authors point out. "Rather, it will most likely result in a cure in a specified time of five to six weeks." The prospect of a CFS cure should give hope to CFS sufferers, the authors conclude, because many are understandably frustrated by endless medical treatments that result in only marginal improvement.[10]

Joseph H. Brewer, M.D., of Kansas City, Missouri, is another leading researcher investigating HHV-6. Dr. Brewer reports a strong link between the virus and CFS, fibromyalgia, and other immune disorders. Dr. Brewer has found that although latent HHV-6 infection can be easily and accurately tested using conventional diagnostic methods, "the same cannot be said for detecting active HHV-6 infection." Currently, according to Dr. Brewer, the most effective testing method for detecting active HHV-6 infection is the rapid viral culture test, available through Hemex Laboratories.[d]

To treat HHV-6 effectively, Dr. Brewer recommends a comprehensive protocol that simultaneously results in antiviral activity, immune modulation, and anticoagulation (since HHV-6 is known to cause thickening of the blood, causing strain on the heart and less effective delivery of blood-borne oxygen and nutrients to the cells). This can include antiviral drugs such as acyclovir (Zovirax), ganciclovir (Cytovene), and foscarnet (Foscavir), and blood-thinning drugs such as heparin or coumadin. But Dr. Brewer also reports successful results using transfer factors (TFs), stating that TFs have "consistently shown efficacy in the prevention and treatment of viral infections" and have "proven to be extremely safe, with virtually no significant adverse effects." In studies he has conducted on patients with chronic fatigue syndrome accompanied by chronic active HHV-6 infection, he found "significant symptom improvement, consistently negative HHV-6 blood cultures, and marked improvement in NK [natural killer cell] function" using a transfer factor derived from bovine colostrum and specific for HHV-6.[e]

Many clinicians investigating HHV-6–related disorders are also recommending the use of Wobenzym N, an oral pancreatic enzyme formula, as an effective alternative to anticoagulant drugs such as heparin and coumadin.[f]

---

[a] Martin, W. J. "Stealth Virus Infections in CFS Patients." Available from the Center for Complex Infectious Diseases (CCID), 3328 Stevens Avenue, Rosemead, CA 91770; (626) 572-7288.

[b] Ibid.

[c] Ibid.

[d] Brewer, J. "Chronic Active Human Herpes Virus-6 (HHV-6) Infection: A New Disease Paradigm." Available from Plaza Internal Medicine, 4620 JC Nichols Parkway, Suite 415, Kansas City, MO 64112; tel: (816) 531-1550.

[e] Ibid.

[f] HHV-6 and the Thin Line of Protection in Your Body." www.ImmuneSupport.com Copyright © 2000 by Pro Health, Inc.

---

 To test for **active HHV-6 infection**, contact Hemex Laboratories, 2505 West Beryl Avenue, Phoenix, AZ 85021; tel: (800) 999-2568. Website: www. hemex.com. To obtain **Wobenzym N**: Longevity Plus, 708 E. Highway 260, Bldg C-1 # F, Payson, AZ 85541; tel: (928) 472-4263. Website: www.longevityplus.net.

## Olive Leaf Extract Can Kill Viruses

Olive leaf extract may be one of the most powerful natural medicines against viral and bacterial infections. The active component of the olive leaf is oleuropein (the bitter element removed from olives when they are processed). Researchers at Upjohn, the pharmaceutical giant based in Kalamazoo, Michigan, found that the main component in oleuropein, a salt extract called calcium elenolate, is "virucidal [virus-killing] for all viruses against which it has been tested." The list of the viruses tested is impressive, including herpes, influenza A, Coxsackie, polio, encephalomyocarditis, and reovirus 3, among others. Upjohn researchers believe that calcium elenolate, interacting with the protein coat of the virus, managed to reduce the ability of these organisms to convey infections.

A study at the Volcani Institute of Agricultural Research in Rehovot, Israel, tested oleuropein's effect on a bacteria similar to *Streptococcus* and found that it effectively killed the organism. It did so by damaging the cell membrane of the bacterium, causing intracellular constituents such as phosphorus, potassium, and glutamate to leak out and impoverish the cell.[11] The olive leaf also contains natural vitamin C helpers (bioflavonoids) such as rutin, luteolin, and hesperidin, which are needed to protect against infection.

Sir Arnold Takemoto, B.S., a leading biochemist who designs nutritional programs in Scottsdale, Arizona, used olive leaf extract in his work with a rheumatologist for cases of fibromyalgia and chronic fatigue syndrome. He comments: "It's the missing link that functions as an antiviral and antiretroviral agent by slowing down the organism's reproductive cycle." Olive leaf extract, he adds, "allows the patient's immune system to go on the attack."

Donald Gay, D.C., N.D., H.M.D., based in Toronto, Canada, has also used olive leaf extract in treating chronic fatigue syndrome. "What's needed is something that rids the person of bacterial and viral infections, and now I've found the appropriate compound," states Dr. Gay. He used the extract to cure his own sinusitis, from which he had suffered for over ten years.[12]

## Treating Candidiasis

Before we discuss a range of alternative treatments for candidiasis, let's examine a case illustrating the relationship between yeast overgrowth and fibromyalgia, and consider how treating candidiasis and correcting the intestinal imbalance it creates can reverse this painful disorder.

Gary Kaplan, D.O.—a family physician, chronic pain specialist, president of the Medical Acupuncture Research Foundation in Los Angeles, California, and associate professor at Georgetown University Medical School in Washington, D.C.—explains how testing for these underlying conditions serves as a foundation for designing a therapeutic treatment program.

## Fighting the Viruses of Severe CFS with Heat Therapy

Bruce Milliman, N.D., of Seattle, Washington, reports success using hyperthermia (heat therapy) as the central element in a treatment program for severe cases of CFS. Dr. Milliman's treatment involves artificially inducing fever in order to augment the body's ability to fight viral infections. Patients must commit to a three-week course of treatment during which they stay home, get total bed rest, and undergo the fever treatment three times daily.

To induce hyperthermia, the patient soaks in a bath (as hot as is tolerable) for a full five minutes, while drinking a 12-ounce glass of tepid water mixed with 2,000 mg of vitamin C. Emerging from the bath, the patient quickly dries off and gets into a bed prepared with flannel sheets and wool blankets, placing a hot water bottle under the breast (women) or over the liver (men), and remaining under the blankets for 20 minutes. This procedure stimulates a natural fever response; the body will sweat profusely in its attempt to return to normal body temperature.

According to Dr. Milliman, fever is one of the immune system's natural adaptive mechanisms, and "turning up the thermostat" enhances immune response. He reports a 70% to 75% success rate with his patients who follow this daily protocol for the full three weeks. Dr. Milliman reports that most failures in fever therapy occur in individuals unwilling or unable to address simultaneous disorders such as yeast infections, dental amalgam reaction (to mercury), and hypothyroidism.

 This treatment must be carried out under the guidance of a qualified physician and is intended for extreme cases of CFS in which the patient is virtually incapacitated. The protocol may also be contraindicated for certain conditions, such as high blood pressure, diabetes, or endocrine problems.

## Success Story: Reversing Fibromyalgia by Treating Candidiasis and Intestinal Imbalance

Lizzy, 42, came to my office with symptoms of fibromyalgia. She complained of generalized joint pain in her hands, hips, knees, and ankles, which had begun 12 months earlier. She also had sporadic but significant fatigue and sinus problems that never completely went away after each episode. For the frequent acne she had suffered from her whole adult life, she took a conventional drug called minocycline hydrochloride (a tetracycline antibiotic) to control the outbreaks.

At one point before seeing me, Lizzy had received a diagnosis of systemic lupus erythematosus, a dangerous autoimmune disease. However, blood work performed by another physician failed to confirm this diagnosis. Lizzy followed a healthy, mostly vegetarian diet, eating only a minimum of dairy products and meat and a great deal of whole grains.

Despite her chronic pain, she exercised regularly by running and bicycling several times a week.

In the course of taking her health history, I learned that Lizzy's symptoms began shortly after a trip to Eastern Europe. In the months preceding this trip, Lizzy had been eating and sleeping poorly and was under constant stress regarding family matters. It is quite likely that in the course of her travels, Lizzy was exposed to something that set in motion an allergic reaction. In effect, you have a woman under stress who has experiences and exposures that push her over the immunological edge. The question, then, is in what area will the immune resistance break down? In Lizzy's case, it broke down in the threefold area of colonic environment, digestion, and absorption.

My job as a physician is to figure out what steps to take to unload and de-stress her system, and to bring her intestinal microflora back into balance so that her digestion and absorption processes work well and thereby restore her health. I help get things back into alignment and remove as many challenges to the body's functioning as I can so that its natural ability to heal itself is restored. Further, any significant psychological issues must be addressed as part of any comprehensive treatment program for a chronic condition.

*Analyzing Lizzy's Colonic Environment:* The relationship in time between Lizzy's travels abroad and the onset of symptoms suggested the possibility that she had picked up intestinal parasites. I requested that she send a stool sample to Great Smokies Diagnostic Laboratory for a comprehensive analysis of digestion, absorption, colonic environment, and yeast sensitivity. This test provides a great deal of information with regard to digestion of various foods, whether or not fats are being absorbed, and what digestive enzymes are present, as well as whether intestinal bacteria are in balance or whether yeasts are present in the stool. All of these factors may be contributing to a patient's symptoms.

I have found in a number of patients that parasite infestation can frequently produce an antigenic reaction that leads to generalized joint pain and sometimes asthma. The immune system judges antigens (SEE QUICK DEFINITION) to be foreign, undesirable particles and mounts an immune response to their presence. For example, I had a male patient who developed a *Giardia* infection followed by asthma symptoms, indicating an antigenic reaction; in other words, the antigenic reaction to the parasite manifested as asthma. When the *Giardia* was treated, the asthma symptoms disappeared.

An **antigen** is any biological substance (a toxin, virus, fungus, bacterium, amoeba, or other protein) that the body comes to regard as foreign and dangerous to itself. As such, an antigen induces a state of cellular sensitivity or immune reaction that seeks to neutralize, remove, or destroy the antigen by dispatching antibodies against it.

As it turned out, Lizzy did not have a parasite problem, but her intestinal flora were out of balance, as indicated by a "severe" reaction on the Dysbiosis Index (see chapter 2, "What a Stool Analysis Can Indicate," pp. 31–35). This high reading would certainly help account for her problems in digestion and absorption. Imbalances in bacterial microflora can also lead to skin problems such as rashes and acne, joint pain, and digestive problems. On a macroscopic level the test revealed that Lizzy's stools were a normal brown color with no traces of blood or mucus, but their chemical nature, or pH, was slightly too alkaline at 7.3.

Among the beneficial bacteria we expect to find in the healthy colon, Lizzy was completely deficient of *Lactobacillus* varieties although she had an optimal level of *Bifidobacteria*. Among other bacteria, Lizzy's stool showed evidence of gamma *Streptococcus* in the normal range. Of nonbeneficial microbes, her stool measured *Pseudomonas aeruginosa* beyond the acceptable limit. As a result, she was growing some strains of bacteria in her

For information about the **Comprehensive Digestive Stool Analysis,** contact: Great Smokies Diagnostic Laboratory, 63 Zillicoa Street, Asheville, NC 28801; tel: (800) 522-4762. Website: www.gsdl.com.

colon that shouldn't be there. This data, however, should be interpreted carefully—the basic tenet of all alternative medicine is that you must look at the whole picture and not single out any one piece of information. When one element shifts, everything else changes accordingly.

The most glaring fact in Lizzy's stool analysis was the high level of yeast organisms (*Candida albicans*). Her levels approached the pathogenic.

This overgrowth was behind the intestinal imbalance and many of her symptoms. To determine which prescription drugs and natural substances at what concentration would work best for her system in reducing the yeast overgrowth, I ran a second Great Smokies test called Sensitivity to Antifungal Agents. The test showed that the conventional antifungal drug Diflucan (fluconazole) was the "drug of choice."

Among the metabolic markers indicated in the stool analysis, Lizzy's levels of N-butyrate were somewhat depressed, under the preferred range of 10 to 30. This data told me that Lizzy was not metabolizing (SEE QUICK DEFINITION) her foods and extracting from them the fatty acids (such as from animal fats) her system needed. Many have observed a correlation between alkaline fecal pH and decreased levels of short-chain fatty acids (SCFAs). If you have low levels of N-butyrate, which is responsible for producing SCFAs from the metabolism of foods, then your SCFAs will be low as well. SCFAs result from the breakdown of carbohydrates and fiber; if SCFAs are in short supply, this can mean that either the proper microflora are missing from the intestines, there is too little fiber in the diet, or the stool takes too long to move through the colon.

 **Metabolism** is the biological process by which energy is extracted from the foods a person consumes, producing carbon dioxide and water as by-products for elimination. Metabolism involves hundreds of different biochemical reactions, necessitating the involvement of hundreds of different enzymes, each of which handles a specific reaction.

There are two kinds of metabolic processes constantly underway in the cells: anabolic and catabolic. In anabolic metabolism, the upbuilding phase, larger molecules are constructed by joining together smaller ones. In catabolic metabolism, the deconstructing phase, larger molecules are broken down into smaller ones. The anabolic function produces substances for cell growth and repair, while the catabolic function controls hydrolosis (digestion), disassembling food into forms the body can use for energy.

In Lizzy's case, she had a normal distribution of SCFAs, but a deficiency in total SCFAs. While the optimal range is 56 to 156, Lizzy's level was only 47. This means she was creating the right amount of SCFAs, but as a whole, she wasn't digesting or absorbing them well. Counterbalancing this, Lizzy's levels of beta-glucuronidase, an enzyme needed to digest fats and cholesterol, were solidly normal. Also, the level of her fecal sIgA was well within the normal range.

*The Status of Lizzy's Digestion and Absorption:* The quality of a patient's colonic environment is directly affected by what they eat and how well, or poorly, it is digested and absorbed. Within the category of digestion,

| Sensitivity to Antifungal Agents | | | | |
| --- | --- | --- | --- | --- |
| Minimum Inhibitory Concentration µg/ml (lowest concentration required to inhibit growth of organism) presumptive C. albicans | | | | |
| Prescriptive Agents | | Typical* | Typical* | Typical* |
| Fluconazole | <0.5 | 2 | 2 | 2 |
| Itraconazole | <0.5 | 2 | 2 | 2 |
| Ketoconazole | <0.5 | 2 | 2 | 2 |
| Nystatin | <2 | 10 | 10 | 10 |
| **Natural Substances** | | | | |
| Berberine | 160 | 160 | 160 | 160 |
| Caprylic Acid | 500 | 500 | 500 | 500 |
| Garlic | <125 | 500 | 500 | 500 |
| Sanguinaria | <8 | 160 | 160 | 160 |
| Undecylenic | 500 | 500 | 500 | 500 |
| Plant Tanins | <0.5 | 8 | 8 | 8 |
| Uva-ursi | <8 | 160 | 160 | 160 |

The Sensitivity to Antifungal Agents test indicates how the patient is likely to respond to each of a number of agents, both natural and drug-based, that are capable of producing effects against fungi.

the laboratory test provides values in three key areas: triglycerides, chymotrypsin, valerate, and isobutyrate.

Lizzy's levels were acceptable in the first and third categories, but her chymotrypsin levels were seriously low. In regard to meat and vegetable fibers, which provide another measure of digestive function, Lizzy had no traces in her stool. This was not surprising, considering her mostly vegetarian diet. In fact, if Lizzy had been eating a meat-centered diet, she would have been feeling much worse and all her stool markers would have been further imbalanced. Her system was not geared to handle meat; fortunately, she had regulated her diet on her own and kept her meat consumption to a minimum.

Within the four categories indicating absorption, Lizzy's values were mostly unacceptable. Her levels of long-chain fatty acids (LCFAs) were slightly elevated. While her fecal cholesterol levels were in the normal range, her levels of total fecal fat were at the borderline of imbalance. As just mentioned, her chymotrypsin levels (another measure of absorption) were low.

To complement the considerable data I gained from the stool analysis, I ordered a blood test for Lizzy, from which I learned that her DHEA (SEE QUICK DEFINITION) levels were low (less than 200 mg/dL). Studies have shown that restoring optimal levels of DHEA reduced joint pain

**DHEA** (dehydroepiandrosterone) is naturally produced by the human adrenal glands and gonads with optimal levels occurring around age 20 for women and age 25 for men. After those ages, DHEA levels gradually decline so that a person 80 years old produces only a fraction of the DHEA they did when they were 20. As an antioxidant, a hormone regulator, and the building block from which estrogen and testosterone are produced, DHEA is vital to health. Low DHEA levels have been associated with cancer, diabetes, multiple sclerosis, hypertension, obesity, AIDS, heart disease, Alzheimer's, and immune dysfunction illnesses. Test subjects using supplemental DHEA reported improved sleeping patterns, better memory, an improved ability to cope with stress, decreased joint pain, increases in lean muscle, and decreases in body fat. No serious side effects have been reported to date, although acne, oily skin, facial hair growth on women, deepening of the voice, irritability, insomnia, and fatigue have been reported with high DHEA doses.

**Osteopathy** is a treatment method based on the principle that the structure of the body (the musculoskeletal system) is interrelated with the function of its systems and organs, and that disruptions in one can cause problems in the other, making both subject to a wide range of disorders. After a thorough evaluation, an osteopath performs adjustments (manipulations) on the patient, which help the body to correct its structural problems. These manipulations include cranial manipulation, relax and release techniques for the muscles and soft tissues, and articulation (similar to chiropractic adjustments). Osteopathy provides relief for patients suffering from a variety of conditions including spinal and joint problems, arthritis, allergies, chronic fatigue syndrome, high blood pressure, and headaches.

in test subjects with lupus. I started Lizzy on 25 mg daily of DHEA using the Pure Encapsulations brand. I have looked at a number of DHEA products and find them to be, for the most part, unreliable in their ability to raise DHEA levels in my patients. The Pure Encapsulations formula, on the other hand, has been consistently effective.

Finally, as part of Lizzy's initial treatment plan, I suggested she start receiving osteopathic (SEE QUICK DEFINITION) manipulations and acupuncture to address the joint pain and sinusitis. After four treatments of each and daily use of DHEA, Lizzy's energy levels were better but the joint pain, especially in her hands, remained significant. It was my impression that the candidiasis in her intestines was contributing to this symptom. I started her on Diflucan, as indicated by her Sensitivity test.

I also suggested some dietary restrictions; in particular, I suggested Lizzy stay away from any foods made with wheat or yeast. Her system was unable to handle wheat; the chronic malabsorption of wheat gluten created an allergic-type reaction in her system, which then contributed to the chronic joint pain. Intolerance to wheat (called gluten enteropathy or celiac disease) is far more common than people realize. In addition, Lizzy completely eliminated meat from her diet, sensing that her system may have been reacting poorly to even the small amounts she ate. Fortunately, Lizzy had already altered her diet by the time I met her. She knew that with a digestive system out of balance, a standard meat-based American diet would make her much sicker.

After 16 days on the Diflucan, Lizzy began to show unpleasant side effects, notably an itchy rash, and I stopped the medication. Her joint pain had improved considerably, presumably as the *Candida* had been brought under control, and her energy level continued to grow. No longer taking the Diflucan, Lizzy's rash disappeared, and she began to have dramatic improvement in her joint pain, fatigue, and sinusitis. About one month later, when Lizzy ate some wheat and meat as a test to her system, the joint pain returned along with muscle pain and joint swelling. However, once she stopped eating wheat again and maintained the allergen-free diet, all of these symptoms disappeared.

Often, allergy sufferers find their symptoms are worsened by dairy products, which increase mucus production; wheat intolerance often shows up as rashes and joint pain (as we saw in Lizzy's case). Nasal congestion and symptoms of asthma often improve after wheat is eliminated from the diet. In the case of red meat, the antibiotics and steroids routinely given to animals and ingested by meat eaters can aggravate numerous symptoms. Eliminating meat from the diet often leads to a reduction of these symptoms.

 **Gary Kaplan, D.O.:** Kaplan Clinic, 5275 Lee Highway, Suite 200, Arlington, VA 22207; tel: (703) 532-4892.

In my estimation, three principal factors were responsible for throwing Lizzy's digestive system out of balance (producing the abnormal stool analysis values) and creating her symptoms: a yeast overgrowth, a wheat sensitivity, and a DHEA deficiency. By reversing these, her fibromyalgia was resolved.

## Other Alternative Medicine Treatments for Candidiasis

Successful treatment of candidiasis first requires the reduction of factors that predispose a patient to *Candida* overgrowth. Second, the patient's immune function must be strengthened. Diet, nutritional supplements, herbal medicine, Ayurvedic medicine, acupuncture, and enzyme therapy are some of the choices alternative medicine physicians employ to accomplish these ends.

Recovery from chronic candidiasis seldom takes less than three months and is usually well advanced by six months, but it can take longer to recover completely. Medical studies show that until bowel *Candida* is under control, local manifestations (such as vaginal thrush) will continue to appear. Local treatment alone (for thrush or other symptoms) is not sufficient.

## Diet

Yeast thrives on sugar, so to overcome candidiasis, sugar must be avoided in all its various forms. These include sucrose, dextrose, fructose, fruit juices, honey, maple syrup, molasses, milk products (which contain lactose), most fruit (except berries), and potatoes (their starch converts into sugar). Candidiasis patients should also stay away from all alcohol because it is composed of fermented and refined sugar. "In treating candidiasis, my basic dietary taboos are sweets, alcohol, and refined carbohydrates," reports Leyardia Black, N.D., of Lopez Island, Washington.

Meat, dairy, and poultry consumption can also foster *Candida* growth because of the large amount of antibiotics used on the animals. Traces of antibiotics given to dairy cows can later show up in milk. Organic (hormone- and antibiotic-free) meat and poultry should be consumed whenever possible. For candidiasis patients, seafood (free of mercury toxins) and vegetable protein are preferable, since they are not only antibiotic-free, but lower in fat.

Many candidiasis sufferers have allergies or sensitivities to various foods. Although *Candida albicans* yeast is not the same as yeast in foods (such as bread), a cross-reaction between food and yeast frequently occurs. As a result, foods containing or promoting yeast, such as baked goods, alcohol, and vinegar, should be avoided until possible sensitivities are clearly diagnosed.

Molds are another aspect of *Candida* sensitivity, according to Dr. Murray Susser. These include food molds (found in cheeses, grapes, mushrooms, and fermented foods) and environmental molds (found in wet climates, in damp basements, in plants, and outdoors). Mold and yeast can also exchange forms. Therefore, the ingestible molds of cheeses and fermented foods should be avoided. Avoiding food yeast and mold does not attack the *Candida* yeast itself, but is an attempt to ease stress on the immune system caused by substances that can trigger allergies.[13] Even so, avoidance of food yeast and mold should be considered on an individual basis. As Dr. Susser says, "My personal opinion is that most anti-*Candida* diets are too strict. It is unnecessary to take *Candida* patients off vinegar and mushrooms unless they are allergic to these things."

Dr. Susser advises patients to avoid yogurt because of its high sugar content, despite its high concentration of *Lactobacilli*, which suppress "bad" bacteria and keep other organisms under control. He finds that freeze-dried *acidophilus* supplements in capsule form are more effective in combating bacteria than even unsweetened raw yogurt.

## Nutritional Supplements

A general nutritional support program is frequently needed to help build up immune function and digestive efficiency, which may have become severely compromised after months or years of chronic candidiasis, according to Dr. Leon Chaitow. Specific supplementation can be helpful in reversing nutritional deficiencies and rebuilding weakened immune function.

Recommended supplements include:

- **Individual B vitamins** (increase antibody response and are used in nearly every body activity)

- **Vitamin C** (stimulates adrenaline and is essential to immune processes)

- **Vitamin E** (the lack of which depresses immune response)

- **Vitamin A** (builds resistance to infection and increases immune response)

- **Beta carotene** (a vitamin A precursor that increases T cells)

- **Antioxidants**, such as **selenium, calcium**, and **zinc** (immune system boosters useful in combating candidiasis)

- **Chromium, magnesium**, and **adrenal glandular extracts** (stimulate adrenal function)

- **Probiotic** (SEE QUICK DEFINITION) **supplements** (repopulate the intestines with "friendly" bacteria and correct the imbalance of flora created by the *Candida* overgrowth)

- **Essential fatty acids** (such as evening primrose oil) may be considered as well.[14]

As routine supplementation for treatment of candidiasis, James Braly, M.D., of Fort Lauderdale, Florida, offers the following regimen:

**QUICK DEFINITION**

**Probiotics** or friendly bacteria refers to beneficial microbes inhabiting the human gastrointestinal tract; they are essential for proper nutrient assimilation. The human body contains an estimated several trillion beneficial bacteria comprising over 400 species, all necessary for health. Among the more well-known of these are *Lactobacillus acidophilus* and *Bifidobacterium bifidum*. Overly acidic bodily conditions, chronic constipation or diarrhea, dietary imbalances, consuming highly processed foods, and the excessive use of antibiotics and hormonal drugs can interfere with probiotic function and even reduce the number of these microbes, setting up conditions for illness.

- *Vitamin C* (8 to 10 g daily)

- *Vitamin E* (one 400-IU capsule daily)

- *Evening primrose oil* (six to eight capsules daily)

- *Max EPA* (six capsules daily)

- *Pantothenic acid* (250 mg daily)

- *Taurine* (500 to 1,000 mg daily)

- *Zinc chelate* (25 to 50 mg daily)

- *Goldenseal root extract* with no less than 5% hydrastine (250 mg twice a day)

- **Lactobacillus acidophilus** (one dry teaspoon, three times daily; if allergic to milk, use nonlactose *acidophilus*)

Dr. Braly also recommends supplementation of hydrochloric acid (HCl). He notes that the aging process, alcohol abuse, food allergies, and nutrient deficiencies create a lack of HCl in the stomach, which prevents food from being digested and permits *Candida* overgrowth. Such supplementation, he says, helps restore the proper balance of intestinal flora. Dr. Braly recommends one capsule of HCl and pepsin (a digestive acid in the stomach) at the start of meals, increasing cautiously to two to four capsules with each meal if needed.

### Herbal Medicine

Herbs are often used to kill harmful yeasts and shore up immune function. They are used in teas, dried in capsules or tablets, or taken in suppository form. Herbs that contain berberain (an alkaloid found in the berbercia family) have proven particularly useful as anti-*Candida* agents. These include goldenseal, Oregon grape, and barberry.

Berberain is a natural antibiotic that acts against *Candida* overgrowth, normalizes intestinal flora, helps digestive problems, has antidiarrheal properties, and stimulates the immune system by increasing blood supply to the spleen. Soothing to inflamed mucous membranes, berberain can be taken as a tea, or in other fluid and dry forms.[15] Other antifungal and antibacterial herbs include German chamomile, aloe vera, ginger, cinnamon, rosemary, licorice, and tea tree oil.[16] Fennel, anise, ginseng, alfalfa, and red clover are also effective.

Dr. Braly's first line of attack on candidiasis is caprylic acid, a fatty acid found in coconut oil and shown to be an effective antifungal agent. Only if there is no improvement will Dr. Braly use conventional medication. Since caprylic acid is readily absorbed into the system, it should be taken in either an enteric-coated (absorbed in the small intestines rather than the stomach) or sustained-release form.

In one study, 16 patients were given 1,800 mg daily of caprylic acid (the commercial brand Capricin) for 16 days, three patients were given 2,700 mg daily, and six received 3,600 mg daily. The results were a 30% to 90% reduction in *Candida* levels among those with the 1,800 mg dosage; a 70% to 100% reduction in the three patients taking 2,700 mg; and complete elimination of *Candida* in two weeks in all of those taking 3,600 mg.[17]

Dr. Susser agrees with the use of caprylic acid, but cautions that it is far from a panacea. "It's most useful when you combine it with a good diet, allergy care, the right nutrients, acidophilus, and other treatments," he says.

As mentioned above, Dr. Braly also recommends goldenseal root extract, standardized to 5% or more of its active ingredient, hydrastine, at a dose of 250 milligrams twice daily. In a recent study, goldenseal seemed to work better in killing off *Candida* than other common anti-*Candida* therapies, adds Dr. Braly. Other fatty acids derived from olives (oleic acid) and castor beans have also been found to be useful.

Garlic, a well-known folk remedy now formulated in odorless dry powder capsules, is a particularly effective antifungal agent. It has been shown to be effective against some antibiotic-resistant organisms. In cases of vaginal candidiasis, it can used as a suppository or douche. Pau d'arco bark has long been used to treat infections and intestinal complaints and is reportedly an analgesic, antiviral, diuretic, and fungicide. However, many products claiming to contain pau d'arco have only trace amounts or use a part of the tree other than the bark.[18]

 When purchasing pau d'arco, be sure that the product contains lapachol, an organic compound found in high concentrations in pau d'arco and known for its antibiotic action.

### Ayurvedic Medicine

Ayurvedic medicine (SEE QUICK DEFINITION) considers candidiasis to be a condition caused by *ama*, the improper digestion of foods, according to Virender Sodhi, M.D. (Ayurveda), N.D., of Bellevue, Washington. Dr. Sodhi attributes this digestive malfunction, and thus candidiasis, to the widespread use of antibiotics, birth control pills, and hormones; environmental stress; and society's addiction to sugar in the diet. "Ayurvedic medicine believes that these stresses on the system cause carbohydrates to be digested improperly," he says. "Furthermore, the

**Ayurveda** is the traditional medicine of India, based on many centuries of empirical use, and founded on spiritual principles. Ayurveda describes three metabolic, constitutional, and body types (*doshas*). These are *vata* (air and ether, rooted in the intestines), *pitta* (fire and water/stomach), and *kapha* (water and earth/lungs). Ayurvedic physicians use these categories (which also have psychological aspects) as the basis for prescribing individualized formulas of herbs, diet, massage, breathing, meditation, exercise and yoga postures, and detoxification techniques.

An **immunoglobulin** is one of a class of five specially designed antibody proteins produced in the spleen, bone marrow, or lymph tissue and involved in the immune system's defense response to foreign substances. The main types of immunoglobulins, grouped according to their concentration in the blood, are: IgG (80%), IgA (10% to 15%), IgM (5% to 10%), IgD (less than 0.1%), IgE (less than 0.01%). Technically, all antibodies are immunoglobulins.

To find **practitioners of acupuncture, traditional Chinese medicine (TCM), and Ayurvedic medicine** in your area, visit the Yellow Pages Directory of Physicians at www .alternativemedicine.com.

immune system in the gut becomes worn down."

Dr. Sodhi's candidiasis protocol involves strengthening the immune system and improving digestion through stimulation of the secretory IgA, the immunoglobulin (SEE QUICK DEFINITION) or antibody found in the mucoid lining of the intestines and lungs, which may help prevent the invasion of those surfaces by disease-producing bacteria and viruses.

To address the *Candida* overgrowth and thus bolster immunity, Dr. Sodhi uses grapefruit seed oil and tannic acid, which act as antifungals and antibiotics, while *acidophilus* helps restore the balance of friendly bacteria in the intestines. Long pepper, ginger, cayenne, and the Ayurvedic herbs trikatu and neem taken a half-hour before meals increase immunoglobulin (a specific class of antibody) and digestive functions. He further recommends that his patients cleanse toxins from their systems using the *pancha karma* program, which involves herbs and dietary modification. With Dr. Sodhi's approach, candidiasis can usually be eliminated in four to six months.

### Acupuncture

William M. Cargile, B.S., D.C., F.I.A.C.A., former chairman of research for the American Association of Oriental Medicine, has successfully reversed candidiasis with acupuncture, dietary recommendations, and herbs or other supplements as needed. "Acupuncture treatment begins with the meridians [subtle energy channels] that influence genital function, spleen, and stomach," he explains. "These are *yin* [passive, receptive, cool] meridians and they correspond to areas of immune system enhancement. The goal is to normalize the metabolism of the cells in these areas." But Dr. Cargile adds that treatment is "a waste of time" if the patient does not also pay attention to nutrition, which he calls "a significant solution." (See the above section on diet.) The following case makes this point clear.

Elena, 41, was suffering from severe candidiasis when she consulted Dr. Cargile. A single mother of three children, she had chronic low-grade sore throats and was taking five antibiotic prescriptions. "This had been going on for at least three years," Dr. Cargile says. "She was constantly bloated, had colonic distension, and had such bad oral thrush it looked like she had cotton in her throat. She had clearly destroyed the balance of her intestinal flora." Dr. Cargile gave her a gargle solution of tea tree oil (an essential oil used in aromatherapy for numerous topical applications), which reduced the *Candida* pathogens in her mouth and throat. He recommended anti-*Candida* dietary changes and a douche with liquid *acidophilus*. Acupuncture treatments addressed meridians that passed through the larynx and throat. "After three treatments over a period of three weeks, she was 90% better," he states. "She had no oral *Candida* and was well on the road to recovery."

### Enzyme Therapy

Dr. Lita Lee uses plant enzyme supplements to treat yeast overgrowth. Many of her candidiasis patients come to her after unsuccessfully trying Nystatin, probiotics, homeopathics, fatty acid supplementation, and various herbs. "Certain cellulose enzymes will digest the common kinds of yeast, whereas other yeasts sometimes yield to amylase enzymes," reports Dr. Lee.

"I use a potent probiotic that contains *L. acidophilus*, *L. bifidus*, and certain cellulose enzymes, which digests yeast and reestablishes 'friendly' bowel bacteria." Dr. Lee relies upon another formula (containing protease, calcium, and magnesium) to cleanse the blood of toxic debris. This program is the most effective and fastest treatment for candidiasis Dr. Lee has discovered. "It also works well in combination with homeopathic and herbal remedies. I don't hesitate to add them to the enzyme protocol when needed," she states.

## Treating Parasitic Infections

Although antibiotics and other drugs are often used to treat parasitic infections, this approach can pose a threat to overall health by upsetting the immune system, according to Dr. Leo Galland. Those who are already immunosuppressed or chronically ill should be especially careful. Dr.

Chaitow agrees and advises pursuing a comprehensive supplement approach rather than medication. "In many cases, antiparasitic prescriptive drugs have not proved to be lastingly effective," he points out. "They may diminish symptoms for one or two months, but the symptoms later return with full force." Parasites can be fought with high-dosage probiotic substances such as *Lactobacillus acidophilus, Bifidobacterium bifidum*, and *Lactobacillus bulgaricus*. Treatment may last from eight to twelve weeks. Dr. Chaitow reports an 80% success rate in cases of seriously ill people afflicted with parasites and yeast overgrowth, using this method.

**CAUTION** "Antibiotics and other drugs are often used to treat parasitic infections, but this approach can pose a threat to one's overall health by upsetting the immune system. Those who are already immunosuppressed or chronically ill should be especially careful," says Leo Galland, M.D.

### Diet and Nutrition

If an intestinal parasitic infection is suspected, it is advisable to eliminate all uncooked foods from your diet and cook all meats until well done; soak both organic and inorganic vegetables in salted water (one tablespoon per five cups) for a minimum of 30 minutes before cooking. It is also suggested that you avoid coffee, all sugars including fruits and honey, and all milk and dairy products, with the possible exception of raw goat's milk. Raw goat's milk contains secretory IgA and IgG (immunoglobulins), which, as mentioned previously, help protect the intestinal lining from infectious agents. According to Steven Bailey, N.D., of Portland, Oregon, IgA and IgG have been found to be helpful in the treatment of parasites.

As with candidiasis, an intestinal parasitic infection may be only one element in the larger issue of suppressed immune function. A nutritional supplement program can address the restoration of both normal bowel and immune function. Nutritional supplements should include vitamin B12, vitamin A, calcium, magnesium, and the probiotics *Lactobacillus acidophilus, Bifidobacteria*, and *Lactobacillus bulgaricus*. Dr. Chaitow recommends beginning any antiparasitic protocol with high-dosage probiotics to help rebuild intestinal flora ravaged by the parasitic infestation, as well as by other opportunistic infections, such as candidiasis. Probiotics are also imperative for fighting off any further infestation.

### Herbal Medicine

The following herbal remedies are safe and effective for the treatment of parasitic infections. Any of these remedies can also be used as a pre-

## How to Avoid Parasites

There are several precautions that will help you avoid parasites:

**Food**

- Do not eat raw beef—it can be loaded with tapeworms and other parasites.
- Do not eat raw fish or sushi—you are likely to get worms if you do.
- Wash your hands after handling raw meat or fish (including shrimp)—do not put your hands near your mouth without washing them first.
- Use a separate cutting board for meat and vegetables—spores from meat can seep into the board and contaminate vegetables or anything else you put on the board.
- Wash utensils thoroughly after cutting meat.
- Wash vegetables and fruit thoroughly—particularly salad items—as they often harbor parasites. Wash in one teaspoon liquid bleach per one gallon of water. Soak for 15 to 20 minutes, then soak in fresh water for 20 minutes before refrigerating. Or, substitute a few drops of grapefruit seed extract.
- Do not drink from streams and rivers.

**Pets**

- Do not sleep near your pets—they harbor many worms and other parasites.
- Deworm your pets regularly and keep their sleeping areas clean.
- Do not let pets lick your face.
- Do not let pets eat off your dishes.

**General**

- Always wash your hands after using the toilet.
- Wash your hands after working in the garden—the soil can be contaminated with spores and parasites.

**When Traveling**

- Do not drink tap water.
- Two weeks before traveling, start taking Chinese herbs or other preventive medications and continue them while you travel.

ventive measure against parasitic infection when water or food conditions are questionable. According to Dr. Galland, it is advisable to continue any treatment regimen until at least two parasitological tests, performed one month apart on "purged stool" specimens, are negative.

*Citrus seed extract:* Citrus seed extract is highly active against viruses, protozoa, bacteria, and yeast, and has long been used in the treatment of parasitic infections. It is not absorbed into the tissue, is nontoxic and generally hypoallergenic, and can be administered for up to several months, a length of time that may be required to eliminate *Giardia* and the candidiasis that often accompanies it.

**Artemisia annua:** This is an herbal remedy of Chinese origin. Its antiprotozoal activity is especially effective against *Giardia*, but some caution is advisable.

 *Artemisia annua* should not be used during pregnancy due to the possibility that it might cause embryo toxicity.

**Before using any of the herbal remedies listed here, it is important that** you first consult with a health professional who has been properly trained in their use.

For more on **herbs**, see chapter 12, Correcting Chronic Fatigue with Herbs.

It can initially cause a worsening of symptoms, allergic reactions, and some intestinal irritation. *Artemisia annua* is often prescribed by Dr. Galland, along with citrus seed extract. It may be used with additional herbs known for their antiparasitic activity and can also be used in conjunction with conventional drug therapy.

**Artemisia absinthium:** This is one of the oldest European medicinal plants. Also known as wormwood, it was highly prized by Hippocrates and used to expel worms (an application similar to that of *Artemisia annua* in the Chinese herbal tradition). *Artemisia absinthium* taken alone can be toxic, however, and therefore should be used in combination with other herbs to nullify its toxicity.

### Traditional Chinese Medicine

In traditional Chinese medicine (TCM), Chinese herbs are the primary treatment for parasites; the type used depends on the location of the parasites in the body, according to Dr. Maoshing Ni. For intestinal parasites, the kind most often involved in chronic fatigue syndrome, purgative herbs are usually used. Pumpkin and quisqualis seeds are two common remedies. The pumpkin seeds are eaten raw; the quisqualis seeds are usually roasted. Both are taken every morning on an empty stomach, approximately 10 to 12 seeds of either type, for about two weeks. "Quisqualis and pumpkin seeds are mild and safe enough for adults and children to take daily as a preventative measure as well," says Dr. Ni.

Meliae seeds are much stronger than either pumpkin or quisqualis seeds, so they should be taken only in more severe cases. The meliae seeds paralyze the parasites for approximately eight hours, allowing the body to eliminate them through the bowels. Betel nut is another typical treatment for intestinal parasites. The nut is chewed raw like chewing tobacco.

"It can give a certain sense of euphoria, too, because it is slightly toxic," says Dr. Ni. "This is negligible, but some people might get diarrhea."

The parasite may, depending on its type, be able to get through the intestinal walls and into the bloodstream. "In situations like this you have to use some very strong antibiotic-like herbs," says Dr. Ni, "such as goldenseal and coptidis, which are antiparasitic as well."

While eliminating the parasites with herbs, Dr. Ni also strengthens

## Important Reminders During Any Parasite Treatment

Whatever treatment you employ to rid your body of parasites, the following recommendations can help ensure that the program is a success:

If you have children and/or pets, they must be treated at the same time as the adults in the household to prevent reinfection.

Drink more pure water (not from the tap) than usual to help the body flush out the dead parasites from your system: at least 64 ounces of water per day for a 150-pound adult.

Sanitize your environment. When you have almost finished treatment, wash all pajamas, bed clothes, and sheets before using them again.

Eat antiparasitic foods. According to Ann Louise Gittleman, a nutrition educator in Bozeman, Montana, these include pineapple and papaya, either as fresh juice or in supplement form, in combination with pepsin and hydrochloric acid. Avoid all meats and dairy products for at least one week. You can also use pomegranate juice (four 8-ounce glasses daily), papaya seeds, finely ground pumpkin seeds ($1/4$ to $1/2$ cup

daily), and two cloves of raw garlic daily. Do not drink the pomegranate juice for more than four to five days.

Modify your diet. For people with heavy parasitic infection, Gittleman recommends a diet composed of 25% fat, 25% protein, and 50% complex carbohydrates. You also need a regular intake of unprocessed flaxseed, safflower, sesame, or canola oils (two tablespoons daily), and vitamin A in amounts higher than RDA. Flaxseed oil is preferable because it has much higher levels of alpha-linolenic acid (an omega-3 essential fatty acid in which many people are commonly deficient) than the other oils.

Recolonize your intestines. Once you have flushed out the parasites, you need to reintroduce beneficial, friendly bacteria (probiotics) into your intestinal system, Gittleman advises. The bacterial strains most helpful here are *Lactobacillus plantarum, salvarius, acidophilus, bulgaris, bifidus,* and *Streptococcus faeceum,* which are available as nutritional supplements. *L. plantarum* is the most effective of these in combating parasite problems.

the immune system in order to get at the underlying cause of the parasitic infestation. Dr. Ni reports that nutrition and herbs such as ginseng, ligustri fruit, and schisandra berries can accomplish this. He has good success with his three-month treatment program, which addresses both parasitic infection and immune suppression.

Dr. Ni recalls treating a woman previously diagnosed with chronic fatigue syndrome, candidiasis, yeast problems, and severe stomach difficulties. "We did a stool test and found that she also had parasites. This woman was extremely underweight. When she came to see me, she weighed 86 pounds—she was five feet, four inches tall. It took about three months for us to work on nourishing her body.

"Besides using herbs to kill off the parasites, I also used them to boost her immune system, and to deal with the yeast problem and her digestive weakness. In fact, this is the reason she got the parasites in the first place. After the three-month treatment, her stool tests were normal and remained that way. All her symptoms disappeared and her weight went back up to 108 pounds."

### Ayurvedic Medicine

Ayurvedic medicine uses many natural remedies that address specific parasitic infections, according to Virender Sodhi, M.D. The most effective herbs for *Giardia*, amoebas, *Cryptosporidium*, and other protozoal intestinal parasites are bilva, neem, and berberine, which can be taken in combination, he reports. He also recommends bitter melon, as well as such nutritional support as psyllium husk, turmeric, and *L. acidophilus* for the enhancement of the intestinal microflora. It may take several months to eliminate intestinal parasites.

 Although the Ayurvedic remedies mentioned here are safe and easy to self-administer, Dr. Sodhi recommends consultation with a doctor or qualified practitioner before beginning any treatment protocol, in order to determine which of the various options will be best suited to one's individual needs and circumstances.

# four

# Restoring Immune Vitality

Along with clearing all the opportunistic infections present in chronic fatigue syndrome, it is essential to rebuild the beleaguered immune system. Having been in an overactive and dysfunctional state for a prolonged period—often for years—the immune system is in need of intensive support to return it to an optimal level of functioning and enable it to ward off current and future infection. Immunomodulation, using substances that target and adjust specific weaknesses in the immune system, and traditional Chinese medicine, a body of medical knowledge that includes acupuncture and Chinese herbal remedies, are two particularly effective alternative medicine methods for rebuilding immune strength.

Later in this chapter, you will learn about immunomodulators and other immune-building substances, as well as specific steps you can take to detoxify your body. First, let's look at how one alternative medicine physician rebuilds the immune system by focusing on detoxification of all the body's systems and by addressing both the physical and emotional aspects of the disease. A case of immune breakdown clearly illustrates the interrelationship of toxins and immunity.

## Reversing Chronic Illness with Immune Support

Often the best medicine results after the healer is healed, an event fairly common among practitioners of alternative medicine. This was the case for Constantine A. Kotsanis, M.D., medical director of the MindBody

For more information about **immune-building nutritional supplements and herbal medicine**, see chapter 8, Replenishing Enzyme Deficiencies, and chapter 10, Ending Nutritional Deficiencies with Supplements. For more on the **immune system**, see chapter 2, Testing.

Health Center International in Grapevine, Texas. Dr. Kotsanis is a board-certified specialist in nutrition, allergies, and ear, nose, and throat problems, but 17 years ago everything he knew about medicine from his conventional training failed to help him when he became unaccountably ill. Dr. Kotsanis, 38 years old at the time, was losing weight and unable to retain food in his stomach; he had diarrhea after each meal. He had consulted numerous physicians, but came back from these visits empty-handed. One physician insulted him by suggesting it was all in his head.

Dr. Kotsanis was dismayed at his declining health, his persistent allergies, and his inability to get better, even while using the best of what he knew from conventional allergy treatment. Things dragged on like this for two years, until he finally turned to his family for help. "I come from a family of health-care practitioners from Greece," says Dr. Kotsanis, who attended medical school at the University of Athens. "While most of my relatives did conventional Western medicine and a few of my uncles were surgeons, some were herbalists who treated patients with plants, vitamins, and natural remedies." Dr. Kotsanis decided to seek healing from the knowledge held in that side of his family.

**Cell therapy**, as a means of promoting physical regeneration through injecting healthy cells into the body, was developed in the 1930s by the Swiss physician Paul Niehans, M.D. Since Dr. Niehans's work, cell therapy has come to mean the injection of cellular material from endocrine glands, organs, fetuses, or embryos of various animals (and sometimes humans) to stimulate healing and to treat numerous degenerative diseases, including cancer, arthritis, atherosclerosis, chronic fatigue, eczema, mental retardation, and others. More recently, shark embryo cells, collected before they have differentiated into specific immune- or organ-building cells, have been used as the source of live cells.

After considerable reading in the field of alternative medicine, Dr. Kotsanis went to Tijuana, Mexico, to seek treatment with Wolfram M. Kühnau, M.D., a German emigré and specialist in live cell therapy (SEE QUICK DEFINITION). As a child, Dr. Kotsanis had been exposed to a dangerously high level of the pesticide DDT; as an adult, his pancreas failed to produce enough digestive enzymes. The live cell injections stimulated his sluggish organs (pancreas, liver, and stomach).

After two days on live cell therapy injections, Dr. Kotsanis experienced a turnaround in his condition. His immune system was stimulated and his

> I realized that while conventional medicine may be good for acute problems—such as life-threatening infections and trauma, as well as chronic irreversible problems requiring surgery—when it comes to chronic diseases, many conventional doctors have no idea what they are treating.
>
> — *Constantine Kotsanis, M.D.*

Constantine Kotsanis, M.D.

allergic symptoms were rapidly receding. Soon, "like magic," his symptoms were gone. Dr. Kotsanis left the Mexican clinic with a prescription for digestive enzymes and "friendly" bacteria, such as *L. acidophilus* and *L. bifidus*, to reconstitute the intestinal microflora that would facilitate better nutrient absorption.

"This experience changed my life and I started looking for more information," says Dr. Kotsanis. "I realized that while conventional medicine may be good for acute problems—such as life-threatening infections and trauma, as well as chronic irreversible problems requiring surgery—when it comes to chronic diseases, many conventional doctors have no idea what they are treating. That is why we have an obligation to look on both sides of the fence. I don't think anyone has cornered the market in medicine. All disciplines have good things to offer. The knowledgeable physician will choose the appropriate treatment that fits the person and the disease."

Dr. Kotsanis calls this multimodal approach integrative medicine and it's the order of the day at his MindBody Health Center International, where approximately 2,500 patients come for treatment each year. In addition to Dr. Kotsanis, among other practitioners at the Center are an optometrist, a clinical audiologist, an Ayurvedic counselor, and three psychotherapists and counselors. This unusual composition of medical staff reflects Dr. Kotsanis's ongoing pursuit of the best in integrative medicine.

Dr. Kotsanis adds expertise in allergy treatment, immunology, environmental medicine, orthomolecular medicine, acupuncture, homeopathy, neural kinesiology, neural therapy, and surgery. Other specialists, including osteopaths and chiropractors, consult at the Center on a rotating weekly basis, meeting with patients as needed, and imparting an "extended faculty" quality to the medical care the Center offers.

# The Major Players in Your Immune System

The immune system guards the body against foreign, disease-producing substances. Its "workers" are various white blood cells including one trillion lymphocytes and a hundred million trillion antibodies produced and secreted by the lymphocytes. Lymphocytes are found in high numbers in the lymphatic system, bone marrow, spleen, and thymus gland.

**Antibodies:** An antibody is a protein molecule containing about 20,000 atoms, made from amino acids by B lymphocyte cells in the lymph tissue and set in motion by the immune system against a specific antigen (a foreign and potentially dangerous protein). An antibody, also referred to as an immunoglobulin, may be found in the blood, lymph, colostrum, and saliva, and the gastrointestinal and urinary tracts, usually within three days after the first encounter with an antigen. The antibody binds tightly with the antigen as a preliminary for removing it from the system or destroying it.

**Lymph Nodes:** These clusters of immune tissue are part of the lymphatic system, which is the body's master drain. Acting like spongy filter bags, the lymph nodes work as filters or "inspection stations" for detecting foreign and potentially harmful substances in the lymph fluid. Cells inside the nodes examine the lymph fluid, as collected from body tissues, for foreign matter. While the body has many dozens of lymph nodes, they are mostly clustered in the neck, armpits, chest, groin, and abdomen. Lymph fluid flows through the lymphatic vessels throughout the body, helping to maintain the fluid level of cells and carrying various substances from the tissues to the blood. The human body has one to two quarts of lymph fluid, accounting for 1.5% to 3% of body weight.

**Thymus and Spleen:** The thymus, located behind the breastbone, secretes thymosin, a hormone that strengthens immune response. It also instructs certain lymphocytes to specialize their function. The spleen is like a large lymph node except that it filters blood rather than lymph fluid.

**Lymphocytes:** A lymphocyte is a form of white blood cell, representing 25% to 40% of the total count, whose numbers increase during infection. Lymphocytes, produced in the bone marrow and found in lymph nodes, come in two forms: T cells, which are matured in the thymus gland and have many functions in the body's immune response; and B cells, which produce antibodies to neutralize an antigen.

**B Cells:** B cells mature in the bone marrow and produce antibodies to neutralize foreign cells (this is known as humoral immunity). B cells account for 10% to 15% of all lymphocytes.

**T Cells:** T cells specialize their immune function to become helper (CD4), suppressor (CD8), or natural killer (CD56) cells. Helper cells facilitate the production of antibodies by the B cells. Suppressor cells suppress B-cell activity.

**Helper T Cells:** Also known as T4 or CD4 cells, helper T cells secrete hormone proteins (particularly the interleukins and interferon) to stimulate B cells and macrophages, and activate Natural Killer cells. Helper T cells account for 60% to 75% of T cells.

**Natural Killer (NK) Cells:** NK cells are a type of nonspecific, free-ranging immune cell produced in the bone marrow and matured in the thymus gland. NK cells can recognize and quickly destroy virus and cancer cells on first contact. "Armed" with an estimated 100 different biochemical poisons for killing foreign proteins, they can kill target cells without having encountered them previously. As with antibodies, their role is surveillance: to rid the body of aberrant or foreign cells before they can grow and produce cancer. Decreased numbers of NK cells have been linked to the development and progression of cancer, as well as chronic and acute viral infections and other deficiencies of the immune system.

**Macrophages:** Macrophages are a form of white blood cell (originally produced in the bone marrow and called monocytes) that can literally swallow germs and foreign proteins, then release an enzyme that chemically damages, kills, or neutralizes whatever is ingested. The name means "big" (macro) "swallower" or "eater" (phage). Macrophages are the vacuum cleaners and filter feeders of the immune system, ingesting everything that is not normal, healthy tissue—even old body cells or cancer cells.

**Neutrophil:** A neutrophil is a mature white blood cell formed in the bone marrow and released into the blood; there it represents 54% to 65% of the total number of leukocytes. Leukocytes are white blood cells divided into six types (neutrophils, basophils, eosinophils, monocytes, B lymphocytes, and T lymphocytes) and two groups, according to the shape of the nucleus and the presence or absence of granules within the cell; one group includes primarily neutrophils, the other includes lymphocytes. The principal activity of the neutrophil is to ingest foreign particles, especially virulent bacteria and fungi.

**Interferon:** Interferon, familiar to many as a cancer treatment, is a natural protein produced by cells in response to a virus or other foreign substance. Vitamin C and certain herbs can also stimulate its production.

**Interleukin:** Interleukin is a class of proteins with various immune functions, including T-cell activation.

Natural Killer Cell

Nucleus

Cytoplasm

Lymphocyte

Macrophage

"As a rule, integrative medicine techniques tend to be more natural, with one of the fundamental principles being that treatments should actually augment the body's own abilities to heal itself," Dr. Kotsanis explains. "We have adopted the philosophy that supporting the body's own healing faculties is a wiser course for the best long-term results. This type of medicine is also called functional, because it addresses the body's natural functioning processes rather than addressing only the symptoms."

In Dr. Kotsanis's view, the approach benefits the patients by giving them far more choices in health care than those of conventional formats. "Sometimes you choose surgery, but sometimes you choose acupuncture," he observes. "You do whatever you need to do to alleviate the symptoms and improve the quality of life for that patient." Dr. Kotsanis's personal road to integrative medicine, including his firsthand experience with the miseries of chronic illness, has equipped him with both the compassion and medical insight to help many patients with long-term, seemingly immedicable conditions. The following case from his patient files makes this clear.

### Success Story: Reversing Immune System Breakdown

Millicent, 33, poses an all-too-common case of a person with entrenched, debilitating symptoms who consulted many doctors and ended up trusting none—that is, until she met Dr. Kotsanis. Millicent had a long history of chronic conditions, including fatigue, sinusitis, multiple infections, bronchitis, and pain, none of which were improved by repeated rounds of antibiotics or any other drugs or therapies offered.

At one point in her two years of "bouncing around" among physicians, Millicent went to a clinic specializing in environmental medicine. They tested her for allergies to multiple substances and determined that she was reactive to certain chemicals. Millicent received allergy desensitization injections, nutritional supplements, saunas, and dietary advice, but rather than experiencing improvement, her condition continued to deteriorate.

When Millicent first consulted Dr. Kotsanis, she was debilitated to the point that she could no longer maintain her former high-stress, demanding job. She couldn't sleep at night, but often fell asleep during the daylight hours. She was highly frustrated and a bit despondent about the seeming intractability of her condition.

"The core of her problem was a breakdown of her immune system," Dr. Kotsanis says. "It had become hyperactive trying to deal with the multiple infections and allergies; then the antibiotics injured her digestive system and this contributed to her fatigue." A newlywed, Millicent had lost all interest in sex as a consequence of her illness, and her marriage was at risk. "She was in a state of hopelessness—a young woman with no hope, no desire to do anything."

Initially, Millicent "tested" Dr. Kotsanis by agreeing to some acupuncture treatment. Millicent soon moved away, however, and did not return to the area for a year. Feeling only marginally better than when she left, Millicent again consulted Dr. Kotsanis.

Calling on the services of a consulting acupuncturist, Dr. Kotsanis had Millicent tested for heavy metal toxicity; he was concerned about the potential mercury leakage from her eight amalgam dental fillings. Using electrodermal screening (SEE QUICK DEFINITION), the acupuncturist determined that Millicent did have significant toxicity in her body owing to mercury leakage. An analysis of Millicent's urine confirmed the mercury diagnosis.

Over the next six months, Millicent had her mercury fillings carefully removed. To assure the elimination of mercury residues from her body once the fillings were out, Millicent had infusions of a special nontoxic chemical called DMPS (SEE QUICK DEFINITION) to chelate, or bind up, the heavy metal and prepare it for excretion from the body. After six DMPS infusions over a space of three months, Dr. Kotsanis assessed that the mercury had been removed from her body. Prior to the DMPS infusions, Millicent had worn a surgical mask all the time to filter out allergens and toxic materials from the air she breathed. Once the mercury toxicity was eliminated, she no longer required this mask, Dr. Kotsanis notes.

Concurrent with administering the DMPS, Dr. Kotsanis made nutritional and dietary recommendations for Millicent. These included flaxseed oil (two tablespoons daily); extra-virgin olive oil (for cooking and in salads) to help the liver; raw flaxseeds (two teaspoons daily); organic foods; lean meats, such as organically raised chicken, venison, or lamb; and unusual grains such as quinoa, amaranth, and teff.

**Electrodermal screening** is a form of computerized information gathering, based on physics, not chemistry. A blunt, noninvasive electric probe is placed at specific points on the patient's hands, face, or feet, corresponding to acupuncture points at the beginning or end of energy meridians. Minute electrical discharges from these points serve as information signals about the condition of the body's organs and systems, useful for the physician in evaluation and developing a treatment plan.

**DMPS** (2,3-dimercaptopropane-1-sulfonate) is the chelating (binding-up) agent of choice for the removal of elemental mercury from the human body. It can be given orally, intravenously, or intramuscularly and is useful for people who have been exposed to mercury amalgam through their dental fillings or for those who show evidence or suspicion of heavy metal toxicity from other sources.

The more common grains, such as wheat and corn, as well as soybeans, have been far too genetically manipulated and, in Dr. Kotsanis's view, are best avoided by the chronically ill. Organic brown rice and oats were acceptable. Millicent was also instructed to avoid dairy products, red meats (for antibiotic and hormonal residues), and fish (for potential mercury contamination). She was advised to drink 3/4 to 1 gallon of pure water every day to help her system flush out toxins.

As a further aid in detoxifying, Dr. Kotsanis prescribed three products from Metagenics, taken in sequence: UltraClear-Plus®, UltraClear®, and Ultra-Clear Sustain®. UltraClear and UltraClear Plus are metabolic liver detoxification programs in powder form for food-based clearing, made primarily from high-protein white rice and safflower oil. UltraClear Sustain provides nutritional support for patients with gastrointestinal dysbiosis and impaired mucosa. These were to be taken in powder form, at the rate of two scoops daily, mixed with juice or water.

To complement this daily regimen, Millicent took Metagenics' multivitamin (without iron) in a dosage of one tablet, two times daily. "Nutritional problems account for perhaps 50% of the problem in patients with chronic disease," says Dr. Kotsanis.

But Millicent still had discomfort and fatigue and was subject to bouts of crying and serious depression. "Millicent was steadily getting better, but still dragging herself around. She was going through a lot of emotional distress," says Dr. Kotsanis. "I decided she should do some emotional detoxification, because everyone who has a chronic disease needs this."

**Constantine A. Kotsanis, M.D.**: MindBody Health Center International, Baylor Medical Plaza, 1600 West College Street, Suite 260, Grapevine, TX 76051; tel: (817) 481-6342. For more information about **gluten-free and casein-free products**, contact: Feingold Association, 127 East Main, Riverhead, NY 11901; tel: (800) 321-3287. Website: www.feingold.org.

*Emotional Detoxification:* To Dr. Kotsanis, it is important not only to detoxify the internal organs—such as the liver, pancreas, and intestines—of toxic materials, but also to purge the often repressed emotions of pain, grief, and unresolved trauma, in order to achieve a lasting cure.

Dr. Kotsanis worked with psychologist Stephen Vasquez, Ph.D., of Bedford, Texas, who employed a combination of skillful psychological questioning and a form of strobic light therapy to elicit buried emotions. Up to 12 different colored lights are emitted from a device and, after being registered by the eyes, can provoke emotional reactions from a patient. As the lights provoke emotional memories, the patient may begin regressing slowly backward in time as the psychologist asks them questions about their condition.

In Millicent's case, it was revealed that she came from a dysfunctional family. As a child, she was treated like a soldier by her father (a military man) and she felt abandoned by her mother, who suffered from a debilitating illness. Millicent said that she had also been sexually abused by relatives. As an adult, she married a man much like her authoritative father. "These difficult emotional memories can contribute to an already debilitating condition and need to be acknowledged by the patient," says Dr. Kotsanis. "The light therapy approach allows your brain to regress to the point where the affliction formed," he adds. "Once you relive the original problem, you completely cleanse yourself of it." Typically, there are 15 color treatments, each lasting one hour, administered once daily for five days per week. "What psychotherapy takes three years to achieve, this approach can produce in three weeks," Dr. Kotsanis says. The light therapy moved Millicent a couple of steps closer to recovery, he adds.

After these steps—mercury amalgam removal, DMPS, dietary changes, nutritional supplements, detoxification, and light therapy—Millicent was about 60% improved. To complete the recovery, Dr. Kotsanis analyzed Millicent's hormone levels. Using the Adrenal Stress Index (ASI) saliva test, Dr. Kotsanis was able to examine the rhythm

 For more information about the **Adrenal Stress Index**, see chapter 2, Testing. For more about **hypothyroidism**, see chapter 6, Reversing Hidden Thyroid Problems. For more on **psychological factors** underlying CFS, see chapter 11, Healing Psychological and Emotional Factors.

and secretory activity of Millicent's adrenal glands. He learned that Millicent's cortisol levels (an adrenal gland secretion indicative of stress) were exceptionally high, which is often the case in CFS. This meant her adrenal glands were virtually exhausted; hence, her chronic fatigue. In addition, Dr. Kotsanis determined that Millicent's thyroid was mildly underactive, indicating hypothyroidism, which is characterized by symptoms that match many of Millicent's.

Instead of supplementing the adrenal glands or thyroid, Dr. Kotsanis prescribed a formula that would correct the balance of neurotransmitters (SEE QUICK DEFINITION) that directly affect the adrenal glands. He had Millicent take a formula (three times daily) containing brain nutrients, including phosphatidylserine and phosphatidylcholine (both derived from lecithin). Dr. Kotsanis says that had he attempted to correct the brain chemical axis controlling the adrenal glands before removing Millicent's mercury fillings and flushing out residual mercury with DMPS, the treatment would have failed. "The adrenal glands and most of the endocrine system would have been shut down by the mercury," he explains.

 A **neurotransmitter** is a brain chemical with the specific function of enabling communications to happen between brain cells. Chief among the 100 identified to date are acetylcholine, gamma-aminobutyric acid (GABA), serotonin, dopamine, and norepinephrine. Acetylcholine is required for short-term memory and all muscle contractions. GABA works to stop excess nerve signals and thus keeps brain firings from getting out of control; serotonin does the same and helps produce sleep, regulate pain, and influence mood, although too much serotonin can produce depression. Norepinephrine is an excitatory neurotransmitter.

After ten days on this supplement, the brain chemicals in effect realigned themselves and "her whole life turned around—Millicent's energy level skyrocketed," says Dr. Kotsanis. "She was happy and began telling everyone how wonderful she felt." Millicent's self-esteem soared, her vitality returned to normal, and for the first time in many months, she was glad that she was alive again. Her sexual drive, absent for years, returned. Typically this is the last to return when you are chronically ill, according to Dr. Kotsanis. Millicent's husband was delighted. "I have my wife back," he told people. About one month later, Millicent became pregnant and felt herself to be "the happiest woman in town."

This case illustrates Dr. Kotsanis's principle of illness causation and health restoration. "Many factors in Millicent's life led to a gradual breakdown of her immune system. To reverse this, you must clean out the system, starting with the basics: clean the colon, liver, and spleen; remove the heavy metals and toxins; resolve the emotional issues; and put the good nutrition back." It is "extremely essential" to know how the body's detoxification system works. You also must understand that if the immune system is perpetually occupied with inflammation, allergies, and detoxification, it will not have the time or resources to do anything else, such as promote a lasting recovery, Dr. Kotsanis explains. "Everything we do here supports the immune system."

The patient is like a house with three stories, including body, mind, and spirit, says Dr. Kotsanis. "You must keep all three floors clean if you're going to call yourself a holistic physician." Dr. Kotsanis cautions that it's prudent to expect lasting recovery from a complex case of chronic fatigue to take at least 9 to 12 months.

"This case reflects what I call a comeback from hell," Dr. Kotsanis comments. "Two years ago, Millicent was imprisoned in her own home by long-standing environmental toxins, and her family was on the verge of disintegrating. Remember, the average chronic fatigue patient trusts nobody, but they also tend to jump on the bandwagon any time someone promises good results. This case taught me how frustrated a patient can be and how a physician must be patient and thorough in his approach." In retrospect, reflects Dr. Kotsanis, this was one of his most gratifying cases. "After a long journey, Millicent came all the way back to be a vibrant, healthy, and happy person. This is my greatest reward as a physician."

## Building Up the Immune System

As Millicent's case illustrates, restoring a depleted immune system is one key to reversing a chronic illness. Dr. Kotsanis employed dietary recommendations, nutritional supplements, and a variety of detoxification methods to accomplish this. Among the array of other immune-building techniques, immunomodulators and traditional Chinese medicine are also highly successful. An immunomodulator is a substance that can tune, adjust, regulate, or focus—modulate—the activities of the immune system to reverse illnesses. Homeopathic remedies, herbs, hormones, amino acids and other nutritional supplements, and specific dietary changes can all operate as immunomodulators. In the following section, Jesse Stoff, M.D., describes the immunomodulators he uses to rebuild a depleted immune system.

### Immunomodulators for Immune Health

Knowledge of how an individual's immune system is working can be used to precisely direct immune function and restore health. Running standard blood tests (such as the T- and B-cell and NK-cell function tests) to establish the state of the patient's biochemistry and immune function provides the needed information. My focus is on the structure and function of the immune system. It is essential to address both components, because a person's immune system can be structurally intact yet not functioning well. By analogy, this is like having an expensive, perfectly crafted Swiss clock that you forgot to wind; it could keep excellent time, but it isn't even functioning. The test results tell me specifically which areas are malfunctioning or weak; then I can apply the appropriate immunomodulators as treatment. During treatment, I regularly monitor immune status with blood tests so I can track the progress and make changes in treatment as needed.

One example of an immunomodulator is an oral form of transfer factor called NK Daily. Transfer factor is an immunological term indicat-

> It's important to note that if the natural killer cells lack the biochemical support (from nutrients) they need to work appropriately, stimulating them will get you nowhere. You have to provide the key nutrients to stabilize the biochemistry, thereby freeing the immune system to function efficiently.
>
> — *Jesse Stoff, M.D.*

ing a way of passively transferring immunity from one organism to another, thereby stimulating the NK cells. This product uses purified colostrum (first mother's milk after birth) from cows. By stimulating the NK cells, NK Daily gently but thoroughly stimulates immune function.

Another immunomodulator I frequently use is NK Support, a natural immune-building compound that, among other things, contains arabino-galactan, or Larix. Larix is a powdered concentrate of complex carbohydrates derived from the Western larch tree (*Larix occidentalis*). It has been proven to stimulate the activity of NK cells and macrophages (immune cells that "eat" germs). I often prescribe Larix for people with chronic infections—such as chronic fatigue syndrome, pneumonia, or HIV—if their NK function is not at a desirable level of activity. Combining NK Support with vitamin C and iodine activates an immune enzyme needed to dissolve the cell membranes of foreign proteins (such as bacteria or cancer cells) already targeted by NK cells.

In other words, with this simple combination of substances, we can activate a fairly large component of the immune system. Specifically, I typically use ten drops of iodine, three times daily, for four to six weeks; the iodine is in the form of a super-saturated solution of potassium iodide known clinically as SSKI. For vitamin C, I prescribe 1,000 mg, three times daily; for NK Support, one tablespoon in water or juice, three times daily.

It's important to note that if the natural killer cells lack the biochemical support (from nutrients) they need to work appropriately, stimulating them will get you nowhere. You have to provide the key nutrients to stabilize the biochemistry, thereby freeing the immune system to function efficiently. For example, the amino acid (SEE QUICK DEFINITION) L-arginine is helpful to NK cell function; similarly, maintaining the correct ratio of L-arginine and lysine, another amino acid, is also critical. Among dietary sources, L-arginine is available in high amounts in peanuts, almonds, garbanzo beans, soy protein isolate, sunflower seeds, cashews, and other nuts. Lysine-rich foods include cottage cheese, chicken, tuna, turkey, yogurt, steak, and other meat and dairy products.

There are approaches for selectively stimulating B or T immune cells. For B cells, a formula called Immune Boosters is effective, as it supports the nutrient needs of these cells throughout the 24-hour (circadian) cycle. A homeopathic remedy called Stibium can aid the T cells and help reorganize the troubled, chaotic immune system.

The adrenal hormone precursor DHEA (SEE QUICK DEFINITION) is also effective in activating T4 cells. The DHEA that I prescribe is in a long-acting base form, 100 mg daily. The advantage of using a long-acting, slow-releasing form is that you avoid the risk of getting a spike of DHEA into the blood—a sudden hormone increase that could depress the brain's pituitary gland. The amino acid L-glutamine (one teaspoonful in juice or water, three times daily) can help maintain white blood cell populations and certain T-cell production at desirable levels. This amino acid provides nitrogen needed for white blood cell function and the health of the

small intestines, which is why L-glutamine is considered essential for intestinal health during times of stress and critical illness.

Removing the toxic load from the liver is another way to assist the immune system. The liver is the body's main filter of toxins. When the amount of toxins circulating becomes too high and overwhelms the liver, the immune system must then deal with the toxins that ordinarily would have been eliminated from the body. I use an herbal extract called *Carduus marianus* (milk thistle) as an aid for liver detoxification. An individualized formula of Chinese herbs is also useful for liver cleansing.

To focus on the nutrient deficiency side of immune system dysfunction, I employ a daily intravenous nutritional product called Metbal®.

Described as a cellular metabolic enhancer or "super vitamin," this natural product pumps nutrients into the cells in very high concentrations in a short time period. Originally developed in the 1970s to increase the ability of cells to absorb critically needed nutrients, Metbal is made from four natural agents: ribose (150 mg), vitamins B3 (20 mg) and C (75 mg), and the amino acid alanine (15 mg). The product is infused intravenously for five to ten minutes. Metbal appears to trigger the immune system, correct DNA damage by supplying nutrients essential for repairs and rebuilding, and increase the ability of cells to assimilate nutrients. An alkaline diet also supports the assimilation of nutrients. A good alkaline diet would include a variety of fruits, vegetables, beans, and nuts; persimmons, seaweed, lentils, and pumpkin seeds are excellent alkaline foods.

 **Jesse Stoff, M.D.**, is medical director of Immune Therapies, International. From 1985 to 1991 Dr. Stoff was editor of the *Journal of Anthroposophic Medicine* and from 1986 to 1991 he was vice president of the Physicians' Association for Anthroposophic Medicine. Dr. Stoff is co-author of *Chronic Fatigue Syndrome: The Hidden Epidemic* (HarperCollins, 1992). To contact Jesse Stoff, M.D.: Immune Therapies International, Southwest Professional Plaza, 2122 North Craycroft Road, Tuscon, AZ 85712; tel: (866) 937-3450. Website: www.drstoff .com.

EDITOR'S NOTE

*Beta-1,3-Glucan:* Ever since the 1940s, scientists have been honing their knowledge of the remarkable abilities of beta-1,3-glucan as an immunomodulator. It effectively stimulates and activates the immune system and works therapeutically in cases of infection, cancer, ulcers, radiation exposure, and trauma. Beta-1,3-glucan, a simple sugar derived from the cell wall of a common yeast called *Saccharomyces cerevisiae* (baker's yeast), is now available in a supplement form as MacroForce. Macro-Force's beta-1,3-glucan is a purified isolate and does not contain any yeast proteins that would otherwise provoke allergic reactions in sensitive individuals, according to Leonid Ber, M.D., vice president of research and development for ImmuDyne, Inc., of Houston, Texas, the makers of MacroForce.

The research supporting the claims for beta-1,3-glucan as an immune system activator has been building steadily in recent decades. In 1996 alone, 144 scientific studies were published on the medical uses of beta-1,3-glucan. One fact has consistently emerged from these studies: beta-1,3-glucan produces its multiple broad-scale immune effects because it is a nonspecific immune stimulator. This means it causes a response capable of being directed at many conditions—perhaps all.

Research at Harvard University in the 1980s showed that the macrophage—a key immune system white blood cell that "eats" unwanted, foreign microbes—has a specific receptor for beta-1,3-glucan. In nontechnical terms, we might say the yeast talks directly to the immune cell. When the macrophage is activated by this contact, it starts a "cascade of events turning the cells into 'an arsenal of defense,'" explains Donald J. Carrow, M.D., a physician based in Tampa, Florida, who has used beta-1,3-glucan successfully with many patients.

Dr. Carrow further notes that the specificity of this macrophage receptor site may explain why beta-1,3-glucan "is one of the most potent stimulators of the immune response." Dr. Carrow says that "there is now evidence to show that beta-1,3-glucan is, from an evolutionary point of view, the most widely and most commonly observed macrophage activator in nature."[1]

Myra D. Patchen, M.D., of the U.S. Armed Forces Radiobiology Research Institute, suggests that beta-1,3-glucan appears to work as a free-radical scavenger. She believes it may even protect the macrophages from damage by radiation, toxins, heavy metals, invading microbes, and other poisons (collectively called free radicals) in the body. Beta-1,3-glucan's capabilities for resisting infections are well documented.

Scientists at the State University of São Paulo, in Brazil, tested beta-1,3-glucan's ability to stimulate the immune system against a fungal skin infection. Nine patients with serious fungal infections were given beta-1,3-glucan intravenously once weekly for one month, followed by monthly doses for 11 months. They also received a conventional antifungal drug. There was only one case of relapse among these patients,

To contact **Donald J. Carrow, M.D.:** Florida Institute of Health, 4908 Creekside Drive, Suite A, Clearwater, FL 33760; tel: (727) 573-3775. Website: www.alternativemedicine.com/donaldcarrow.

Research at Harvard University in the 1980s showed that the macrophage—a key immune system white blood cell that "eats" unwanted, foreign microbes—has a specific receptor for beta-1,3-glucan. In nontechnical terms, we might say the yeast talks directly to the immune cell.

while another group of eight infected patients who were treated only with the antifungal drug had five relapses. The researchers also observed that the nine patients in the first group had far lower residual traces of the fungal infection in their blood chemistry, concluding that "the patients who received beta-1, 3-glucan, in spite of being more seriously ill, had a stronger and more favorable response to therapy."[2]

Evidence from animal studies demonstrates that beta-1,3-glucan can reduce the amount of conventional antibiotics required to treat infectious conditions such as peritonitis (inflammation of the membrane lining of the abdominal and pelvic cavities). In mice infected with a bacteria to produce peritonitis, a combination of beta-1,3-glucan and a standard antibiotic increased their long-term survival by 56%. Bacterial counts were noticeably down within eight hours of the injection and the numbers of key immune cells were markedly higher. "Clinical use of immunomodulators may alter conventional use and dosage of antibiotics," suggested study director William Browder, M.D., of Tulane University in New Orleans.[3]

**Resetting the Immune System's Thermostat with Thymus Protein:** Located behind the sternum in the chest, the thymus gland is part of the body's endocrine and lymphatic systems. It grows during childhood, reaches its maximum size at puberty, and then begins to gradually shrink for the rest of one's life. This is unfortunate, because one of the thymus gland's principal tasks in the body is to release specialized proteins that stimulate white blood cells—the immune system's prime defense molecules—to resist and resolve infections. With age, then, as the thymus

> The thymus is like an immune system thermostat, and it regulates the immune system at an optimal point.
>
> — *Terry Beardsley, Ph.D.*

gland becomes smaller, there is often a corresponding gradual reduction in the immune system's potency in protecting the body against infections, illnesses, and disease.

The immune system continues to function, of course, because pre-programmed T cells (a type of white blood cell) are still circulating in the body, but at a reduced level. It's the thymus's job to keep the body supplied with fresh, vigorous T cells. "The thymus is like an immune system thermostat, and it regulates the immune system at an optimal point," says Terry Beardsley, Ph.D., of the University of California at San Diego, who in the 1980s conducted research that led to developing a thymic protein supplement (derived from calf thymus cells) called Bio-Pro Protein A to address the problem of thymic insufficiency.

As early as the 1960s, researchers sought to develop an extract of thymus protein capable of stimulating the immune system and the T lymphocytes. But the extracts they came up with contained only small fragments of the targeted thymus protein; Thymosin had 13 amino acids and Thymopoetin had only 5 amino acids. While these fragment extracts showed some immune-stimulating effects, they were not particularly useful in programming T4 lymphocytes. Then, in 1983, Dr. Beardsley successfully isolated the complete thymic protein (containing 500 amino acids, or protein building blocks) that activates the T4 helper cells (*Proceedings of the National Academy of Sciences*, 1983). BioPro Protein A is derived from calf thymus cells; these live cells are then cloned (copied) in the laboratory, after which the protein is extracted and purified.

Dr. Beardsley's innovation was in preserving an intact, activated protein in the same complete form as would be produced by the human thymus itself. As a result of being a complete protein, BioPro Protein A is effective at programming T4 helper cells to release interleukin 2 (one of the immune system's activators of "killer T cells"). The substance both increases the numbers of these critical white blood cells and enhances their activity. Dr. Beardsley was able to show that thymus cells can be transplanted between species without being rejected and that the extracts remain biologically active, producing a stimulatory effect on the immune system.

As a commercial product, BioPro Protein A comes in single-dose packets (4 mcg) containing 12 trillion biologically active protein molecules in maltodextrin powder. The recommended dose is typically one to three packets per day, depending on your particular needs. If you are not ill, a maintenance dose of one packet every day or two should be sufficient. The extract should be slowly dissolved under the tongue (where it is absorbed directly into the bloodstream), as stomach acids will destroy the fragile structure of the protein.

Another study showed that thymus extract has a beneficial effect on cancer, specifically for four patients with non-Hodgkin's lymphoma, three with Hodgkin's disease, and one with myeloma (Blut, 1983). After three months on thymus extract, "the total number and the percentage of T cells increased significantly," stated the researchers. They concluded that treatment with thymus extract was "effective in restoring immunocompetence in patients with T-cell deficiency."

According to certified nutritionist Gayle Black, Ph.D., of New York City, the daily use of thymic protein fortified her immune system as she underwent chemotherapy for breast cancer. Normally, chemotherapy drastically reduces white blood cell counts, thereby dangerously weakening immune competence, but in Dr. Black's experience, during the six months of chemotherapy, her white blood cell count never dropped below 2,500, a relatively healthy level. Even better, her levels of CD4-helper and CD8-killer white blood cells increased.

A similarly favorable report comes from licensed nutritionist and registered radiology technologist Terri Clark, L.N.C., of Miami, Florida. Clark was diagnosed with breast cancer, which soon spread to her bones and lungs, requiring twice-monthly drainage of one to two quarts of liquid from her lungs. Clark attributes her successful recovery from this otherwise life-threatening cancer to her use of 8 to 12 mcg daily of thymic protein over an 11-month period. Clark's cancer markers (blood substances indicating cancer, determined by laboratory tests) fell dramatically: her CEA went from 354 to 5, while her CA15-3 dropped from 900 to 85. "At this time, my lungs are completely free of any signs of disease," states Clark.

Studies with patients using thymus extracts have shown positive results. A small clinical trial involving patients with Epstein-Barr virus (associated with mononucleosis and chronic fatigue syndrome) also shows the strong therapeutic effect of BioPro Protein A. Six participants took 4 mcg of BioPro Protein A, three times daily, for 60 days. After treatment, the Epstein-Barr virus levels for four of the six patients were reduced, in one case by 75%. All patients reported a reduction in symptoms and no adverse side effects. Five said they had increased energy levels and needed less sleep; others said their "energy level increased dramatically— probably 50% or more" and that they had "less tiredness during the day."[4]

***Immunocal: Immune Nutrient from Milk Protein:*** One of the most important substances required by the immune system for optimal functioning is an amino acid complex called glutathione. However, supplementation is made difficult by the complexity of the body's system for delivering glutathione to cells. Canadian researchers figured out a way to deliver glutathione effectively in the form of a natural milk protein supplement called Immunocal; early research suggests it has benefits for chronic fatigue syndrome, cancer, AIDS, hepatitis, and age-related conditions such as Alzheimer's, Parkinson's, and arteriosclerosis.

thymus gland

The thymus gland activates bone marrow or stem cells to respond to foreign or abnormal cells (bacteria, toxins, tumor cells, or transplanted tissue). Once activated, these cells develop into T lymphocytes (the "T" stands for "thymus-derived"), the "workers" of the cell-mediated immune system that responds to antigens (foreign substances), but not to the body's own tissues.

Glutathione is a tripeptide, a small protein consisting of three amino acids (glutamic acid, cysteine, and glycine) bound together. The substance functions as a principal antioxidant, scavenging free radicals and toxins such as lipid peroxides that would otherwise damage, even destroy, cells. It accomplishes this valuable task by working with an enzyme called glutathione peroxidase. Further, glutathione regulates the activities of other antioxidants such as vitamins A, C, and E. However, when the body is suffering from oxidative stress, supplies of glutathione become depleted. Oxidative stress is a condition in which the body is unable to detoxify itself completely and is overrun by free radicals because antioxidants are depleted. Oxidative stress affects the nervous, immune, and endocrine systems, and it may underlie many of the symptoms associated with chronic fatigue.

Glutathione exerts another protective and scavenging role in concert with the liver, the body's primary organ of detoxification and internal cleansing. In the liver, glutathione combines with toxins, carcinogens, and waste products as a way of more effectively securing their elimination from the body. In addition, glutathione helps red blood cell membranes and other cellular proteins maintain their structure, and aids the production of leukotrienes, immune system cells crucial for working against inflammation.

But glutathione also has an important role in supporting the activity of white blood cells called lymphocytes (the key players in the body's immune response) as well as antibodies (specialized immune defense cells). In fact, for lymphocytes to do their job, glutathione must be present. The tricky fact about glutathione is that you can't simply take in more glutathione as a supplement; it must be made inside the cells. In other words, glutathione doesn't enter cells directly; rather, it must be made within them by precursors.

Recognizing this biochemical fact, Canadian researchers developed Immunocal in 1993 to deliver to the cells the necessary precursors for glutathione. In the course of researching dietary protein sources capable of boosting the immune system, Gustavo Bounous, M.D., of McGill University in Montreal, Quebec, discovered the substance that later became Immunocal. Today, Dr. Bounous serves as the medical director of Immunotec Research, the manufacturers of Immunocal, located in Vaudreuil-Dorion, Quebec, Canada.

Immunocal is a natural food supplement consisting of concentrated milk protein powder containing unusually high amounts of glutathione precursors, according to Immunotec Research. "Immunocal promotes optimal functioning of the immune system by sustaining normal levels of glutathione and glutathione precursors in the lymphocytes. Glutathione, acting as the cellular antioxidant, allows for a full immune response," says Immunotec literature. Immunocal contains concentrates of three substances in the whey portion of milk (serum albumin, alpha-lactalbumin, and lactoferrin). These contain a large quantity of cystine, an amino acid breakdown product that is a more usable form of cysteine (the amino acid precursor of glutathione). Studies have shown that cysteine levels tend to be the rate-limiting factor (the biochemical bottleneck) in maintaining the ideal level of glutathione.

For more information about **Immunocal**, visit the website: www.immunocal.com.

The problem with cysteine (both a protein building block and an antioxidant) is that it is found in only trace amounts in a limited number of foods, including raw egg whites, milk, and meats. If the body is under immune stress, as happens with a viral infection, dietary sources may not be sufficient to produce enough glutathione. If you isolate cysteine and take it in large quantities, however, it can be toxic. Rapidly metabolized (that is, burned up, digested by the body), cysteine is unusable as a dietary supplement. Immunocal solves this problem because it contains cystine—cysteine in a more practical form. This form is readily released during digestion and transported to target cells, where it can be broken down into cysteine. Once in the cells, cysteine can then be used as raw material for the synthesis of glutathione, the goal of all this biochemistry. For example, proper amounts of glutathione enable white blood cells (lymphocytes such as T cells, B cells, and natural killer cells) to reproduce in order to make antibodies or to attack foreign substances directly.

Five hundred liters of fresh, raw cow's milk are necessary to produce one kilogram of Immunocal, according to Immunotec. It is produced using a gentle process and low temperatures to preserve the biological activity of the proteins. Recommended dosage is one pouch (10 g) of Immunocal daily. You add the powder to 4 to 6 ounces of milk, water, or juice and shake gently to mix. There are no reported side effects from using Immunocal, says Immunotec.[5]

## Traditional Chinese Medicine

William M. Cargile, B.S., D.C., F.I.A.C.A., former chairman of research for the American Association of Oriental Medicine, has treated CFS patients using acupuncture alone, concentrating specifically on building the immune system. Dr. Cargile treats CFS using the acupuncture points that relate to autoimmunity and clearing all the meridians (SEE QUICK DEFINITION) in the body. He also strongly advises patients to undergo allergy testing before acupuncture treatment so they can rid their diets of allergens that may jeopardize treatment.

Dr. Cargile notes that the immune system uses 60% of the body's energy storage compound, called ATP (adenosine triphosphate—SEE QUICK DEFINITION), which manufactures proteins to make immune antibodies. "You don't have enough energy because your im-

**Acupuncture meridians** are specific pathways in the human body for the flow of life force or subtle energy, known as *qi* (pronounced "chee"). In most cases, these energy pathways run up and down both sides of the body, and correspond to individual organs or organ systems, designated as Lung, Small Intestine, Heart, and so on. There are twelve principal meridians and eight secondary channels. Numerous points of heightened energy, or *qi*, exist on the body's surface along the meridians; these are called acupoints. There are more than 1,000 acupoints, each of which is potentially a place for acupuncture treatment.

> People with CFS have a compromised immune system that is weak and at the same time hyperactive. My objective is to strengthen and simultaneously desensitize, normalize, and regulate the immune system.
>
> — *Maoshing Ni, D.O.M., Ph.D., L.Ac.*

mune system is using all the ATP for the production of antibodies, until there is none left. That is why you feel so bad," he explains.

One of Dr. Cargile's patients, Emily, a 54-year-old woman with chronic fatigue syndrome, was diagnosed with idiopathic chronic fatigue, meaning her condition did not have a known cause such as cancer or thyroid or endocrine abnormalities. "She had a thirteen-year history, with no relief, and a continuous worsening of the condition," says Dr. Cargile. "She literally did not have the motivation to walk to the kitchen more than once a day." Dr. Cargile used acupuncture to stimulate both Emily's immune system and the production of ATP in her body. Within five treatments, Emily, who previously had spent up to 20 hours a day in bed, was walking three miles daily, with her energy level restored.

Maoshing Ni, D.O.M., Ph.D., L.Ac., of Marina del Rey, California, also reports successful treatment of chronic fatigue syndrome with traditional Chinese medicine. "The people who come to see me have been bounced from one internist to another," he says. "They've been through the mill and been rejected by the Western medical establishment." He concurs with Dr. Cargile that the key to CFS is in improving immune function. "People with CFS have a compromised immune system that is weak and at the same time hyperactive. My objective is to strengthen and simultaneously desensitize, normalize, and regulate the immune system," he explains.

 **ATP** stands for adenosine triphosphate, a substance found in all cells—particularly muscle—and responsible for energy. When enzymes split ATP, energy is released (12,000 calories/mole of ATP) from the high-energy phosphate bonds. This bond can be instantly split on demand whenever energy is required to run cellular functions—ATP then becomes ADP. When energy is returned, it becomes ATP again. ATP is often called the cell's energy currency because it can be continually spent and remade again in a matter of minutes.

 To find **acupuncture and TCM practitioners** in your area, see the Yellow Page Practitioner Directory at www.alternativemedicine.com.

To accomplish this, Dr. Ni uses a combination of acupuncture, Chinese herbs, and lifestyle changes, including diet, exercise, rest, and meditation. He explains, "Herbs are used to support immune functions. They are easily assimilated and adapted by the body. I also implement a low-stress diet. Up to thirty to forty percent of the body's energy goes to digestion, so we want to conserve that energy as much as possible." Patients reportedly experience a 65% to 80% relief of symptoms after the treatment period (generally, three months) and are then able to return to a normal life. After a three-month follow-up treatment, Dr. Ni reports that 90% to 95% of his patients have recovered from CFS. "Acupuncture reprograms the body and the herbs support that reprogramming," states Dr. Ni.

# five

# Detoxifying the Body

Alternative medicine physicians working with chronic fatigue know that removing toxins from the body is an essential phase in restoring their patients to health and vitality. Every year, people are exposed to thousands of toxic chemicals and pollutants in air, water, food, and soil. People living today carry within their bodies a "chemical cocktail" made up of industrial chemicals, pesticides, food additives, heavy metals, general anesthetics, and the residues of conventional pharmaceuticals, as well as of legal (alcohol, tobacco, caffeine) and illegal (heroin, cocaine, marijuana) drugs.

Today, people are exposed to chemicals in far greater concentrations than were previous generations. For example, over 70 million Americans live in areas that exceed smog standards, and most municipal drinking water contains over 700 chemicals, including excessive levels of lead. Some 3,000 chemicals are added to the food supply, and as many as 10,000 chemicals—in the form of solvents, emulsifiers, and preservatives—are used in food processing and storage. These can remain in the body for years.[1]

To make matters worse, food and product labels do not always list every ingredient. When people consume these foods—especially seafood, meat, and poultry—they ingest all the chemicals and pesticides that have remained as accumulated contaminants in the food chain. These pollutants lodge in the body—loading it up with poisons—and manifest in a variety of symptoms, including decreased immune function, nerve cell toxicity, hormonal dysfunction, and psychological disturbances.

Serafina Corsello, M.D.

Dr. Corsello stresses that if you don't take care of the intestines, eliminate its toxic load, and rebalance its bacterial population, "no immune disorder will ever truly get relieved."

## The Loading Theory of Toxicity

The "loading theory" of toxicity—according to its formulator, Serafina Corsello, M.D., director of the Corsello Centers for Nutritional Complementary Medicine in New York City and Huntington, New York—states that no single factor causes a disease, such as exposure to infectious agents or psychological traumas that lower immune resistance. Rather, the cumulative load of multiple poisons creates an illness. You don't suddenly get sick; it takes a long time for the body to break down. This is compounded of layers of toxicity, malnutrition, and dysfunction, she notes. No single factor alone can cause chronic fatigue. People don't get a disease—they develop it, Dr. Corsello explains. "I touch a lot of my chronic fatigue patients. I embrace them. I take care of them. I'm exposed to the virus—but I don't get chronic fatigue from them."

The loading theory outlines a process of many factors acting together in the creation of illnesses. Over time, these multiple factors weigh down the immune system and eventually throw it out of balance. Among the typical multiple stressors are toxic metals (mercury leaching from fillings, aluminum), petrochemical residues (pesticides and fertilizers), chemical pollutants (in the water and air), electromagnetic pollution (power lines), undiagnosed food allergies, nutritional deficiencies, biochemical imbalances, insufficient exercise, and emotional stress (family, job, and personal).

All these factors impinge on the immune system's natural ability to resist the downhill slide into illness, says Dr. Corsello. "These factors interact and compound each other to break down the immune system. In fact, these stressors may be accumulating for years, over a lifetime, before they send the system into disregulation." The loading theory of illness is the cornerstone of the Corsello Center's approach to patients, from the moment they first call for an appointment.

Increasingly, toxicity is being identified as the predisposing factor in a long list of acute and chronic illnesses, including environmental illness and chronic fatigue, degenerative diseases, and cancer. "The current level of chemicals in the food and water supply and the indoor and outdoor environment has lowered our threshold of resistance to disease and has altered our body's metabolism, causing enzyme dysfunction, nutritional deficiencies, and hormonal imbalances," says Marshall Mandell, M.D., a pioneer of environmental medicine based in Norwalk, Connecticut.

Where do all the toxins come from? They come from a polluted environment (air, water, and food), lack of water, overconsumption of food, a faulty, nutritionally inadequate diet, lack of exercise, accumulated stress, excess antibiotic use, and chronic constipation and poor elimination. Bioaccumulation (a buildup in the body of foreign substances) seriously compromises physiological and psychological health. Since 1985, hundreds of studies have demonstrated the dangers to health from toxic bioaccumulation.[2] Since 1945, toxins have accumulated in the human system faster than they can be naturally eliminated, which means the body now needs assistance in detoxifying.

Detoxifying the body is another important component in promoting the health of the immune system and addressing other factors that may be contributing to your chronic fatigue. As our environment and food are increasingly saturated with chemicals, the body's mechanisms for elimination of toxins cannot keep up with the chemical deluge. The constant circulation of toxins in the body taxes the immune system, which must continually strive to destroy them.

When combined with multiple infections and nutritional deficiencies, this toxic overload may be the proverbial last straw in the development of CFS. Given that many people with CFS have chemical allergies and that environmental illness is a disease reaction to twentieth-century chemicals, it is advisable to take measures to remove the toxins stored in the body.

### The Immune Vigilance of the Intestines

Intestinal toxicity is also intimately related to immune dysfunction. The large and small intestines are actually part of the immune system. In fact, "the intestinal mucosa and some of its submucosal structures constitute the largest immunological system of the body," states Dr. Corsello. The intestines' mucus layers trap debris and pathogens and represent the

A healthy intestine is immunologically vigilant against undesirable pathogens and toxins. One that is overburdened and
compromised fails to perform its immune defensive role and
may start contributing to the emergence of an autoimmune illness or other chronic disease.

active front of immune function. The large and small intestines, at 25
feet long, comprise the body's largest internal organ and represent a key
part of the body's immune system, says Dr. Corsello, accounting for perhaps 80% of the body's lymphatic-immune resources. "The digestive system is one of the first screening systems against the daily load of contact with bacteria, viruses, and parasites, which, if left unchecked, would
constitute a grave threat to our entire immune system."

A healthy intestine is immunologically vigilant against undesirable
pathogens and toxins. One that is overburdened and compromised fails
to perform its immune defensive role and may start contributing to the
emergence of an autoimmune illness or other chronic disease. "A large
onslaught of infective agents can overcome the immune vigilance of most
people, even in the presence of so-called 'normal' immune systems," Dr.
Corsello notes.

The intestines contain a complex and delicately balanced population
of mixed microflora in which the friendly, beneficial bacteria should out-
number the harmful ones. But this ecology is easily upset, says Dr.
Corsello, leading to a condition of imbalance called dysbiosis. "At the
Center, we have observed an almost immediate relationship between
stressful events and the exponential growth of dysbiotic organisms such
as *Candida albicans* and other pathogens."

Another factor that upsets intestinal ecology is parasites, as discussed
in chapter 3. These enter the body (or the numbers of resident ones
increase) from contaminated water and food supplies (both domestic and
from foreign travel) and/or repeated courses of antibiotics that diminish the proportion of friendly intestinal bacteria. Despite this, "there is
an overwhelming lack of awareness of this by Western physicians, especially American-trained physicians, who refuse to acknowledge that par-
asitosis [parasite infestation] is a major factor in systemic illness."

Dr. Corsello notes that physicians at her center have observed a strong
correlation in their patients between having intestinal parasites and a

range of chronic conditions such as arthritis, respiratory problems, heightened allergies, menstrual disorders, and prolonged bowel disorders. Such people with chronic, untreated parasitic states are highly prone to develop autoimmune disorders. "I've yet to see a menopausal woman with severe symptoms who doesn't have parasites."

An imbalance among the intestinal microflora can lead to food allergies, both acute and delayed, Dr. Corsello says. You might eat a food today and experience an allergic reaction to it 24 to 36 hours later, yet fail to make the connection—but your body always does. "Dysbiosis and delayed food allergies are almost universally present in people with autoimmune disorders."

Otherwise healthy foods become branded as foreign and undesirable by the intestine's immune guards; these foods do not get properly digested and, enwrapped by immune system proteins, they may pass inappropriately into the blood circulation as an immune complex (SEE QUICK DEFINITION). This is the increasingly common condition called leaky gut syndrome. Undigested foods then become part of the overall suppressive load on the immune system.

If the intestines are unbalanced (dysbiotic) and "leaky," bacteria and parasites "can overcome the defensive intestinal barrier and, through the circulatory system—both the lymph and the blood—invade organs. The circulating immune complexes can then trigger a variety of diseases affecting the connective tissue (collagen) layer of the body, such as arthritis and lupus," Dr. Corsello says. She stresses that if you don't take care of the intestines, eliminate its toxic load, and rebalance its bacterial population, "no immune disorder will ever truly get relieved."

 **Serafina Corsello, M.D.:** The Corsello Centers for Nutritional Complementary Medicine, 175 East Main Street, Huntington, NY 11743; (516) 271-0222. The Corsello Centers for Nutritional Complementary Medicine, 119 West 23rd Street, Suite 400, New York, NY 10011; tel: (212) 727-3600. Website: www.corsello.com.

 **Circulating immune complexes (CICs)** form in the body when poor digestion results in undigested food proteins "leaking" through the intestinal wall and into the bloodstream. The immune system treats these foreign substances or antigens as invaders, causing antibodies to form and couple with them. This antigen and antibody combination is known as a CIC. In a healthy person, CICs are neutralized, but in someone with a compromised immune system, they tend to accumulate in the blood, where they burden the detoxification pathways or initiate an allergic reaction. If too many CICs accumulate, the kidneys cannot excrete enough of them via the urine. The CICs are then stored in soft tissues, causing inflammation and bringing stress to the immune system. The overload can lead to a variety of chronic health conditions.

# Surviving Toxic Immune Syndrome

With these general observations about toxicity established, we move deeper into the subject with the clinical recommendations of William R. Kellas, Ph.D., and Andrea S. Dworkin, N.D., of the Center for Advanced Medicine, in Encinitas, California, authors of *Surviving the Toxic Crisis* (1996) and *Thriving in a Toxic World* (1996). Here are the recommendations of Drs. Kellas and Dworkin for surviving what they call "the toxic immune syndrome":

At the Center for Advanced Medicine, our focus is to help our patients get their lives back on track by getting to the root causes of their illness. The idea for this approach evolved out of the medical problems I (William Kellas) faced in the early 1970s when I developed a crippling autoimmune disease called ankylosing spondylitis in my twenties. At the time, my doctors told me I would probably remain in a wheelchair for the rest of my life. I refused to accept this verdict and immediately started to search for answers. I had all my mercury amalgam fillings removed; I flushed all the parasites out of my intestines; I did chelation therapy to remove the mercury from my system; I had my dental bite balanced; I had whiplash and nose injury problems corrected. It took me about ten years to regain my health, but that's because I had to piece it all together on my own. Now that we know what's required, we can produce the same results in our patients in less than a year.

It was my study of healing methods for myself that led me to the philosophy of our clinic: always look for the root, underlying cause of any illness. Along the way, I met other practitioners with health problems who were similarly searching for alternative methods of healing. "We fit in where our patients want to be, because all of our doctors or their families were also once patients," says Gary Shima, M.D., our former medical director.

Our clinic serves patients who prefer a more natural alternative to health and healing, supported by sound medical principles. We offer the best of technology and natural healing methods, including immunotherapy, ten different kinds of intravenous therapy, colonics, acupuncture, allergy therapy, clinical nutrition, massage, craniopathy, naturopathy, chiropractic, and Feldenkrais bodywork.

Our guiding principle is this: *what you don't see may be sinking your ship*. This ship, of course, is your body and health. Disease occurs after your immune system breaks down; this happens as the result of an

William R. Kellas, Ph.D.

> There are many steps in a patient's road to bad health. We call these cumulative steps "primary toxic suppressors." They include such factors as mercury dental amalgams, chemical toxins, surgeries, electromagnetic radiation, poor nutrition, structural problems, and others.
>
> — *Dr. William Kellas*

onslaught of toxic suppressors and the accumulation of biochemical deficiencies, all of which allow unwanted microorganisms to invade and flourish in the body. The result is chronic illness, which we define as a health problem you've had for 120 days or more.

Have you already been to doctors and heard them say, "You're not really sick," yet you know you're not well? Most chronic patients we see have consulted at least ten physicians and still haven't received lasting help. Getting to the root causes rather than just aiming for relief of symptoms is the main characteristic of comprehensive health care and the only way to get real help.

There are many steps in a patient's road to bad health. We call these cumulative steps "primary toxic suppressors." They include such factors as mercury dental amalgams, chemical toxins, surgeries, electromagnetic radiation, poor nutrition, structural problems, and others. These, in turn, adversely affect the immune system—the key to your body's optimal functioning—and produce what we call the toxic immune syndrome. This is a multifaceted condition of weakness and susceptibility that sets up a domino effect of poor health.

Here's how it works. Let's say you have a structural problem with your back, spine, neck, or overall posture. This restricts the nerve supply to your organs and digestive system; the result of this is poor digestion, which can lead to putrefaction of food materials in your intestines. From this, you might develop food sensitivities as the healthy food becomes toxic. Add to this the negative influence of antibiotics from dental work, surgery, or medications, and you begin knocking out the beneficial bacteria in your system that should be screening out harmful influences.

You may experience symptoms such as pain, stiffness, fatigue, infection, weight gain, allergies, or headaches. These symptoms may vary according to your weakest genetic link or vulnerability. Now you are open to microbial invasion and long-term internal infections. This can then throw your hormonal system out of balance, blocking the smooth action of your digestive and lymph systems. As a result, toxins overload your body's natural filters and you are unable to detoxify. In effect, your body becomes poisoned from within and begins to develop illnesses in the various organs, such as jaundice in the liver, urinary infection in the bladder, and constipation in the intestines.

Your body is now more vulnerable to petrochemicals in your foods and environment, leading to, for example, chronic fatigue, reduced sperm count, or infertility. Following this, your tissues become inflamed and more deeply set illnesses develop, such as cancer, fibromyalgia, and edema. All of this then feeds back to your brain, producing contractions in the membranes covering your brain and spinal cord, which then misalign the vertebrae and skull.

Dental problems, produced by mercury amalgam fillings, electrical charges from dental work, and misalignments in the jaw are major players in a surprising number of health conditions. Other dental-related problems that contribute to this negative domino effect include whiplash, which can imbalance the bite; cranial sutures out of alignment; patient sensitivity to dental materials; bite imbalance; and infected, toxic root canals. Here the medical and dental branches should work together on diagnosis (medical) and treatment (dental) of these problems.

**William R. Kellas, Ph.D.**, and **Andrea S. Dworkin, N.D.**: The Center for Advanced Medicine, 4403 Manchester Avenue, Suite 107, Encinitas, CA 92024; tel: (760) 632-9042. Website: www.ctradvmed.com.

The good news about this circle of ill effects is that it also shows us how to regain health by way of reversing the stages in the toxic loop, although you'll need to take several steps at once to see improvement. When you clear up one problem, this enables the other parts of the interrelated system to function better, which in turn helps to clear up further problems all the way around the circle. To be effective, a clinic must help stop the influx of toxins, remove the toxins from all the body systems, and support the body nutritionally and biochemically in healing disease.

The U.S. Centers for Disease Control and Prevention (CDC) divide the causes of illness into these categories: heredity, 18%; environment, 19%; medical intervention, 10%; and lifestyle, 53%. This means that 82% of the causes of disease are within your control: improving your environment, avoiding medical interventions, and changing how you live.

## Dr. Kellas's Six Steps to Detoxification and Healing

1. **Eliminate intake of toxins and cleanse all toxic suppressors from the body.**

   First, you must stop bombing your body with more toxins. Toxic suppressors can include heavy metals (mercury, aluminum, cadmium, copper, lead, arsenic, nickel), chemicals (carcinogens, fluoride, chlorine, food additives), and radiation (electromagnetic, microwave, nuclear, solar, X rays, computer monitors). They can also include ingested hormones, steroids, drugs, alcohol, toxic water, caffeine, processed foods, inhaled or absorbed pesticides, perfume, smog, nicotine from cigarettes, noise, and stress. The toxic suppressors must be eliminated before medications and other natural approaches will have permanent effect.

2. **Detoxify the body and unblock detoxification pathways.**

   Even though you have reduced the entry of new toxins into your body, old toxins are still in your bloodstream, lymph nodes, and organs. Our treatments involve chelation therapy to remove metals from the blood, intravenous vitamin C (to detoxify the blood), sauna (to remove chemicals), and detoxification diets (to remove allergens and yeast-supporting conditions). We also prescribe fasting, organ flushes, enzymes, amino acids, physical therapy, lymph drainage, constitutional water therapy (to cleanse the lymph system), exercise, and colonics, and we provide counseling for the patient's emotional and spiritual issues.

3. **Provide the body with biochemical and nutritional support.**

   Now that the cleansing is completed, it's time to support your body's natural restoration and defense. To support the body's biochemistry, we prescribe minerals, enzymes, vitamins, pure water, oxygen therapy, amino acids, herbs, and essential fatty acids.

That 82% is the focus of our treatments at the clinic. Our philosophy is that chronic degenerative disease, which takes years to develop and show its effects, is best prevented and treated by comprehensive health care, along the lines I've outlined above. Our patient care is coordinated with all our different practitioners, who share a similar philosophy of healing and have equal access to the patient charts and test results. Our staff meets regularly to discuss the best way to work together for the patient's health.

Comprehensive health care removes the obstacles to the body's natural healing processes, but it's important to remember that healing usually occurs as a series of "baby steps." As it took a long time to reach your present state of ill health, it will probably take some months, possibly years, to restore it as completely as possible. Even so, we are get-

4. **Align and rebalance all body structures.**

We use chiropractic, osteopathy, and dental work to rebalance the nervous system; trigger points to realign the electrical system; gamma globulin, cyclic AMP, transfer factor, allergy antigens, and low-dosage immunotherapy to support the immune system; and Feldenkrais, soft tissue and lymph manipulation, and craniosacral work to rebalance the muscles and their movements. When you rebalance the bite and remove the toxins from the mouth you have already won 60% of the detoxification battle.

5. **Eliminate harmful microorganisms and disease-producing parasites from the body.**

Once the primary suppressors and toxins are removed from your environment and your body, it's time to go after the secondary suppressors, or opportunistic microorganisms. Harmful microbial organisms within your system—such as bacteria, worms, protozoans, mycoplasmas, fungus, parasites, and viruses— must be flushed out. We've found that certain conventional drugs (Flagyl and Fasigyn) work best, in conjunction with tetracycline, acidophilus, and sometimes an herbal formula and/or bismuth gel, over a 21-day intensive program. In addition, you must kill the parasites outside the body, in the skin, under the nails, and in the hair; for this we use iodine baths every five days.

6. **Rebuild, restore, and regenerate the health of the body's interrelated systems.**

The key to achieving this step is to strengthen the immune system. Here we use "probiotics" (beneficial microorganisms) such as *L. acidophilus* and *L. bifidus*. We also provide emotional counseling to help fortify the patient's psychological attitude during the process, to accept the healing, and to rework a new way of looking at themselves and life.

ting dramatic improvements in people with fibromyalgia, chronic fatigue, and multiple sclerosis in less than a year.

## Detoxification Therapy

"A body with a healthy immune system, efficient organs of elimination and detoxification, and sound circulatory and nervous systems can handle a great deal of toxicity," states Leon Chaitow, N.D., D.O., of London, England. "But if a person's immune system has been damaged from chronic exposure to environmental pollutants, restoring these functions, organs, and systems can be accomplished only through detoxification therapies, including fasting, chelation, and nutritional, herbal, and homeopathic methods, which accelerate the body's own natural cleansing processes." Intestinal detoxification is also an important method of removing toxins from the body and, as discussed earlier, the intestines are in themselves an essential part of the immune system.

Most alternative medicine physicians agree that detoxification is essential and that it brings many benefits to the person undertaking it. One of the most important and longest-lasting effects of detoxification therapy is the reduction of stress on the immune system, says Elson Haas, M.D., director of the Preventive Medical Center of Marin in San Rafael, California. Other benefits can include increased vitality, reduced blood pressure and blood fats (cholesterol and triglycerides), improved assimilation of vitamins and minerals, and mental clarity.

**CAUTION** Any effort at detoxifying should always be planned and executed under direct supervision of a physician. Recovering alcohol or other substance abusers, diabetics, people with eating disorders, and those who are underweight or physically weak or who have a hypothyroid or hypoglycemic condition should not detoxify without strict medical supervision.

Everyone has a natural, specific level of tolerance for toxins that cannot be exceeded if good health is to be maintained. When the body gets overwhelmed with toxins, the immune system mechanisms malfunction, and fatigue, confusion, aggression, or mental disorder may occur. Other symptoms indicating that you may need detoxification are headaches, joint pain, recurrent respiratory problems, back pain, inhalant allergy symptoms (nasal or sinus), insomnia, mood changes, food allergies, and digestive ailments.

### Scrubbing and Repopulating the Intestines

Taking care of a patient's intestinal system is the first order of business in the Corsello Center's treatment plan, explains Dr. Corsello. Their intestinal cleansing plan consists of a blend of 80% insoluble and 20% soluble fiber from flaxseed and fruit pectin mixed with vitamin C powder and fruit juices. This formula begins to disinfect and scrub the intestines, removing layers of yeast, bacteria, and parasites.

The next step is to repopulate the intestines with more friendly bacteria (SEE QUICK DEFINITION), or probiotics, such as *Lactobacillus acidophilus* and *Bifidobacterium*. Repopulating causes a "gentle war" in your intestines, says Dr. Corsello. The unwanted yeasts and bacteria are killed off and the probiotics establish themselves as the predominant species. Research has proven that giving probiotics to rebalance the intestinal immune defenses reduces inflammation of the intestinal lining and is helpful in both treating and preventing food allergies, notes Dr. Corsello.

"Since gut immune suppression is often responsible for systemic immune suppression, this approach may have life-or-death repercussions." To aid this process, Dr. Corsello prescribes a salad dressing made from flaxseed oil and extra-virgin cold-pressed olive oils mixed with vitamin E and garlic. This supplies the intestines with needed essential fatty acids (both omega-3s and omega-6s) and it helps to heal the damaged mucosal layers.

The third step in restoring intestinal efficiency is to give the patient injections or slow-drip intravenous infusions of B vitamins, selenium, zinc, manganese, and liver-protecting substances (taurine, glutathione). If your intestines are in dysbiosis and you take B vitamins orally, they become food for all the infective agents resident in the intestines; but if you inject them, the B vitamins bypass intestinal barriers and enter the bloodstream directly, says Dr. Corsello. "Most people who are ill suffer from malabsorption," she adds. Nutrient infusions maximize absorption and produce quicker results; the infective agents eventually starve to death.

The fourth step involves major dietary changes. "If patients are eating junk foods, then no matter what I do, their dietary choices will harm the process of restoring their intestines." The dietary plan is based on three factors: first, eliminate all foods known to produce allergic reactions in the patient; second, match the diet to the patient's blood type; and third, match the diet with the biochemistry of the specific disease process. "Our nutritional interventions have a precise biochemical knowledge behind them and are very specifically tailored."

**Friendly bacteria**, or probiotics, refers to beneficial microbes inhabiting the human gastrointestinal tract that are essential for proper nutrient assimilation. The human body contains an estimated several trillion beneficial bacteria comprising over 400 species, all necessary for health. Among the more well known of these are *Lactobacillus acidophilus* and *Bifidobacterium bifidum*. Overly acidic bodily conditions, chronic constipation or diarrhea, dietary imbalances, consumption of highly processed foods, and excessive use of antibiotics and hormonal drugs can interfere with probiotic function and even reduce the number of microbes, setting up conditions for illness.

## How to Soak Out Your Toxins with Detoxifying Baths

In this section, Joseph Dispenza, director of the Parcells Center in Santa Fe, New Mexico, explains the benefits and techniques of using therapeutic bathing as a way of cleansing and healing:

The skin is the largest organ of the body and 65% of body cleansing is accomplished through it. Cleansing the skin with detoxifying baths is a science, according to the late naturopathic pioneer Hazel Parcells,

Determining how efficiently the body can detoxify itself is especially useful for CFS sufferers. Here are two laboratory tests that can help.

**Detoxification Profile:** If your liver is unable to adequately detoxify your body's store of toxins and waste products, this situation may contribute significantly to the emergence and continuation of your chronic fatigue. Excess free radicals and by-products of incomplete metabolism resulting from poor detoxification (called "toxic intermediate metabolism") can create problems in the cells. Specifically, these toxins can interfere with the movement of substances across the cell membrane and induce damage to the mitochondria, the cells' "energy factories." The Detoxification Profile helps to identify places where your system is impaired in its ability to detoxify.

**Oxidative Stress Profile:** When your ability to detoxify is impaired and/or you are deficient in antioxidants, free radicals run unchallenged throughout the body, damaging cells. They tend to affect the immune, endocrine, and nervous systems, damaging mitochondria, interrupting communication among cells, and depleting key nutrients and antioxidants. This is called oxidative stress. The Oxidative Stress Profile assesses the degree of free radical damage in the body and measures the body's level of glutathione, an amino-acid complex central to detoxification.

 For information about the **Detoxification Profile** and **Oxidative Stress Profile**, contact: Great Smokies Diagnostic Laboratory, 63 Zillicoa Street, Asheville, NC 28801; tel: (800) 522-4762. Website: www.gsdl.com.

 For more on **glutathione and detoxification**, see chapter 4, Restoring Immune Vitality.

---

N.D., D.C., Ph.D. Her therapy of detoxifying baths was developed over a period of 50 years of clinical observation and application. With a program of good nutrition, they stand as proven methods to help the body regain and remain in good health.

"Cleanse the body, give it the right building materials, and nature will heal and build," said Dr. Parcells. She also said: "If you want to be healthy, you have to trade your wishbone for a backbone and get to work." The principle of Dr. Parcells's therapeutic baths is based on the chemical axiom that "the weak will draw from the strong." In this case, cool water will draw toxins out of a

 **EDITOR'S NOTE** **Joseph Dispenza**, director of the Parcells Center and the author of ten previous books, is the author of Live Better Longer: The Parcells Center Seven-Step Plan for Health and Longevity (HarperSanFrancisco, 1997). Hazel Parcells practiced naturopathic medicine for nearly 60 years, until her death at the age of 106 in January 1996.

> "Cleanse the body, give it the right building materials, and nature will heal and build," said Dr. Parcells. She also said: "If you want to be healthy, you have to trade your wishbone for a backbone and get to work."

Hazel Parcells, N.D., Ph.D., D.C.

heated body. The hot water solution draws toxins out of the body to the surface of the skin. Then, as the water cools, the toxins are pulled from the surface of the skin by the change in temperature and go into the water. Specifically, here are Dr. Parcells's bath formulas:

*Formula #1: Environmental Radiation or X Rays:* Do this bath if you have been exposed to environmental radiation or X rays. Air travel, for instance, will increase levels of radiation in your body; dental X rays will leave deposits in the body that interfere with healthy functioning. This bath is indicated if you have been feeling general muscular aches, mild nausea, fatigue, headaches, slight dizziness, or a disturbance in equilibrium.

Dissolve one pound of sea salt or rock salt and one pound of baking soda in a tub of water as hot as can be tolerated. Mix salt and soda thoroughly with the water, then stay in the bath until the water has cooled.

*Formula #2: Heavy Metal Exposure:* (Note: If you are sensitive to chlorine, don't do this bath.) If you have been exposed to heavy metals (such as aluminum), carbon monoxide or unburned carbons, or pesticide sprays, this bath can help detoxify your body of these substances. Cooking with aluminum will bring on symptoms; frequent airplane commuters absorb carbon monoxide through the skin, which then gets inside the body; eating foods that have not been cleaned of pesticide contamination can lead to an accumulation of pesticides in the cells. This bath is indicated if you are experiencing decreased energy, shortness of breath, lightheadedness, impaired equilibrium, or a general feeling of being "out of sorts."

Add one cup of regular brand Clorox® bleach (with the blue-and-white label) to a full tub of water as hot as can be tolerated. Mix thoroughly with the water. Stay in the bath until the water has cooled; do not shower for at least four hours following the bath. The bath can, and will, remove toxins with utmost effectiveness. You'll feel the difference.

*Formula #3: Low-Grade Radioactive Materials:* If you have been exposed to low-grade radioactive materials in the atmosphere or have consumed food irradiated by cobalt 60, this bath will be useful. It is prudent to assume that residues of cobalt 60 are found in a wide range of foods, from fresh fruits and vegetables to grains and packaged meats; don't expect to find them labeled as such. Conditions that would benefit from this bath include soreness of the gums or mouth, swollen glands, sore throat, and indigestion (an inability to treat food comfortably in the stomach).

Dissolve two pounds of baking soda in a tub of water as hot as can be tolerated; mix thoroughly. Stay in the bath until the water has cooled; do not shower for at least four hours following the bath.

*Formula #4: General Toxicity:* Try this general detoxifying bath if you are suffering from general muscle aches and pains, or fatigue brought about by physical exertion or mental or emotional stress. It is particularly useful to raise the acid level in the body to help build immunity and to ward off a feeling that you are about to be ill.

Add two cups of apple cider vinegar (pure, not the "flavored" variety) to a tub of water as hot as can be tolerated; mix thoroughly. Stay in the bath until the water has cooled. Do not shower for at least four hours following the bath.

*General Tips on Detoxifying Baths:* Therapeutic bathing is most effective when done before bedtime, because the body detoxifies during sleep. Use only one bathing formula per evening. Do not mix ingredients from different formulas; each bath is recommended only for specific indications, as described. The baths can be continued without harm until relief from symptoms is noticed. If redness, dryness, or roughness of the skin develops, it is an indication that the body is working to remove toxins. These aspects of cleansing are not uncommon.

 For more information about **detoxification**, contact: Parcells Method of Healing, P.O. Box 50010, Albuquerque, NM 87181; tel: (505) 293-3771. Website: www.parcellscenter.com.

To minimize discomfort, rub a little olive oil or almond oil or non-petroleum-based baby lotion on your skin after bathing. If you feel you have a need for all the baths, alternate them on different evenings. If these baths are in any way too rigorous or unpleasant, cut back on your use of them, or discontinue.

## More Detoxification Baths with Salts and Herbs

Jacqueline Krohn, M.D., M.P.H., who practices medicine in Los Alamos, New Mexico, offers the following techniques for using hot herbal baths as an effective way to detoxify the body. The hot water stimulates blood flow near the skin surface, opens pores, and increases perspiration, thereby supporting the faster release of toxins, Dr. Krohn explains in her book, *The Whole Way to Natural Detoxification*. She suggests starting with a trial series of plain-water hot soaks as a preparation because, depending on one's toxic load, detoxification baths "can make you feel very ill" as the toxins move out of your body.

Dr. Krohn advises an initial five-minute immersion in water as hot as you can tolerate, then building in five-minute increments to a thirty-minute soak. Before taking the bath, shower and scrub your body thoroughly using soap and a loofah sponge, and take another cleansing shower after the soak; follow the same procedure for the detoxification baths, described below. Always use extreme care when stepping out of a hot bath, as standing up abruptly may cause temporary dizziness.

Dr. Krohn cautions that if you experience dizziness, headache, exhaustion, fatigue, nausea, or weakness, stop the bath and wait a few days before resuming the program. If you experience none of these symptoms, then proceed with three detoxification baths per week. Dr. Krohn recommends taking some vitamin C before and after each bath (to help remove toxins) and drinking an eight-ounce glass of pure water during each bath (to encourage sweating). Dr. Krohn suggests using only one of the following protocols per bath; each substance has a different detoxifying benefit.

- **Epsom Salts.** Start with 1/4 cup of Epsom salts added to the bath water, and build gradually to four cups per bath.

- **Apple Cider Vinegar.** Start with 1/4 cup added to the water, then increase gradually to one cup.

- **Hydrogen Peroxide.** Add up to eight ounces of food-grade 35% hydrogen peroxide to a tub half full of warm water.

- **Baking Soda.** Eight ounces of baking soda (sodium bicarbonate) may be used; alternatively, mix equal amounts of baking soda and sea salt, gradually increasing to one pound of each.

- **Ginger Root.** Peel and slice a small piece of fresh ginger root into numerous pieces, boil in water, then steep for 30 minutes and strain. Add the resulting herbal broth to your bath water.

- **Clay.** Although clay is traditionally used for a facial cleansing pack, it can also detoxify when 1/2 cup is added to a tub of hot water.

- **Burdock Root.** Slice a handful of burdock root into small pieces. Boil it in two quarts of water for 30 minutes, strain the liquid, then add it to the bath.

- **Oatstraw.** Add a heaping handful of this herb to two quarts of water and boil for 25 minutes; strain and pour it into the bath.

- **Herbal Teas.** Herbs such as catnip, yarrow, peppermint, boneset, blessed thistle, pleurisy root, chamomile, blue vervain, and horsetail may also work as detoxifiers when added to your bath, Dr. Krohn says. She advises mixing one cup of a single brewed herb tea (boiled, simmered, and filtered) to the bath; use only one herb at a time, she adds.

### How to Do a Natural Liver Flush

The healthy and efficient functioning of the liver is central to well-being and disease prevention, which explains why it's advisable to periodically flush the organ clean using natural substances, says master herbalist and acupuncturist Christopher Hobbs, L.Ac., author of *Healing with Herbs and Foods*. The liver is the body's chief detoxification organ, so it must be kept in optimal condition. "Liver flushes are used to stimulate elimination of wastes from the body, to open and cool the liver, to increase bile flow, and to improve overall liver functioning," says Dr. Hobbs. "I have taken liver flushes for many years now and can heartily recommend them." Here are Dr. Hobbs's instructions for preparing and administering a liver flush:

- **Citrus Juice.** Squeeze enough fresh lemons or limes to produce one cup of juice. A small amount of distilled or spring water may be added to dilute the juice, but the more sour it tastes, the better it will perform as a liver cleanser. Orange and grapefruit juices may also be used, provided they are blended with some lemon or lime juice.

- **Garlic and Ginger.** To the citrus juice mixture add the juice of one or two cloves of garlic, freshly squeezed in a garlic press, and a small amount of freshly grated raw ginger juice. Grate the raw ginger on a cheese or vegetable grater, then put the shreds into a garlic press and squeeze out the juice.

- **Olive Oil.** Add one tablespoon of high-quality olive oil (such as extra-virgin) to the citrus, garlic, and ginger juice. Either blend or shake the ingredients to guarantee complete mixing.

- **Taking the Flush.** The liver flush is best taken in the morning, preferably after some muscle stretches and breathing exercises, says Dr. Hobbs. Do not eat any foods for one hour following the flush, he adds.

## Lead Poisoning and Chronic Fatigue

Undiagnosed lead exposure may be a contributing cause of chronic fatigue syndrome. A woman, 47, was admitted to the hospital with confusion and headaches and a ten-year history of constipation, fatigue, and weight loss. Her blood lead level was ten times above what is considered "safe." Further investigation revealed that for 28 years she had used water from a hot water heater contaminated with deteriorated lead solder, according to *The Lancet* (April 27, 1996).

- **Cleansing Herbal Tea.** After an hour has elapsed, Dr. Hobbs recommends taking two cups of an herbal blend he calls "Polari Tea." It consists of dry portions of fennel (one part), flax (one part), burdock (1/4 part), fenugreek (one part), licorice (1/4 part), and peppermint (one part). Simmer the herbs (excepting the peppermint) for 20 minutes, then add the peppermint and allow to steep for ten minutes. For convenience, you may prepare several quarts of the tea in advance.

- **Continuing the Flush.** Dr. Hobbs suggests doing the liver flush twice yearly, in the spring and fall, for two full cycles each. A cycle consists of ten consecutive days of taking the flush ingredients, followed by three days off, then another ten days on. "I have never seen anyone experience negative side effects from this procedure."

- **Detoxification Phases.** In cleansing the liver there are two phases, known as Phase I and Phase II. These refer to the natural two-step process the liver conducts to rid the body of toxins. During Phase I, the liver converts toxic compounds into intermediate toxins. In Phase II, the liver converts these intermediate toxins into substances that can be eliminated from the body, delivering them to the colon (via the gallbladder) or bladder for excretion.

Christopher Hobbs, L.Ac.

"I have taken liver flushes for many years now and can heartily recommend them," says Christopher Hobbs, L.Ac. "I have never seen anyone experience negative side effects from this procedure."

## Seven Steps to Promote Detoxification

W. Lee Cowden, M.D., of Fort Worth, Texas, suggests the following seven steps that anyone can adopt to assist their body in eliminating toxins and to promote immune and digestive health:

***1. Make Dietary Changes.*** Start eating a diet that is high in fiber and fresh raw vegetables and fruits and very low in mucus-producing foods. It would be preferable to completely stop eating all milk products from cows and all refined white flour products, such as pastas, breads, and baked goods. At least for the duration of this program, it is also advisable to reduce your intake of sugar, eggs, meats, fowl, most fish, nuts, seeds, and unsprouted beans and grains.

***2. Reduce Your Stress Load.*** Practice stress-reduction techniques before each meal. These might include muscle relaxation, deep breathing, or the visualization of a favorite natural setting. Listening to a stress-reduction audiotape before the meal can be helpful. It is also advisable to eat in a calm, pleasant environment, either by yourself or with a companion whose presence does not produce stress or discomfort in you.

***3. Practice Lymphatic Drainage.*** It is important to take steps to clean out your lymphatic system, especially the lymph vessels that attach to the intestines. You can do this by gently bouncing on a mini-trampoline or rebounder for 5 to 15 minutes once daily. This will stimulate the numerous lymph nodes in your neck, chest, and groin to start draining toxins into the bloodstream for removal from the body.

***4. Brush Your Skin.*** In the early morning, soon after you get up, take a wooden brush with stiff natural bristles and lightly brush your skin.

Move the brush across the skin toward the center end of each collarbone, as important lymph drainage sites are located here. Spend eight to ten minutes dry brushing your entire body. This procedure will mechanically aid your lymph system in its detoxification efforts. Do the dry brushing before taking a bath, but be aware that skin brushing just before bedtime can make it difficult to fall asleep. As a variation on skin brushing, use a loofah sponge to brush your skin.

**5. Do Ozonated Bathing.** Many of the toxins that build up in the body are fat soluble and gather in the fatty tissues. If you immerse yourself in a tub of warm ozonated water for 30 minutes once daily for two to three weeks, this will aid in removal of the toxins from your body. Ozone ($O^3$, a form of oxygen) purifies the bath water by killing living viruses, bacteria, fungi, and parasites. It will also oxidize the water-insoluble toxins on the skin, turning them into water-soluble toxins. Once water soluble, they may be flushed from the system.

Purify the tap water by running it through a KDF solid charcoal showerhead filter as you fill the tub. A KDF solid charcoal showerhead filter can remove up to 99% of the toxic substances found in tap water. Next, bubble ozone into the water, using an ultraviolet ozone generator and an ozone-diffusing bath bubbler. (Do not use an electric-spark ozonating system; this produces more nitrates and other

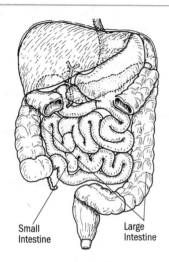

Small Intestine          Large Intestine

The small and large intestines.

The lymph nodes are part of the lymphatic system, the body's master "filtration system." These clusters of immune tissue act like spongy filter bags, detect foreign and potentially harmful substances in the lymph fluid. While the body has many dozens of lymph nodes, they are mostly clustered in the neck, armpits, chest, groin, and abdomen. Lymph fluid (one to two quarts) accounts for 1% to 3% of body weight. Exercise can increase lymph flow by 15 times.

harmful chemical substances.) This converts the ozone that is accumulating in the air above the bubbling water back into oxygen so that it is not irritating to the lungs. Bubble the ozone for 15 minutes before you get into the tub and also during your 30-minute soak. During the 30-minute soak, scrub your entire skin surface three times with a loofah sponge or natural fiber brush.

**6. Fortify Yourself with Nutrients.** It is important to take at least 400 IU of vitamin E, 25,000 IU of beta carotene and/or mixed carotenoids, 2,000 mg of vitamin C, and 100 mg of grape seed extract (pycnogenol) either 30 to 40 minutes before your ozonated bath or 10 to 15 minutes after it.

**7. Use Special Supplements.** Before each bath, take one lozenge of superoxide dismutase (SOD) and 100 mg of L-glutathione powder. Dissolve both substances under your tongue; this enables them to be absorbed faster and more completely. These nutrients will facilitate toxin removal from your system. SOD is an antioxidant enzyme that protects the system against free-radical damage from chemicals or radiation. L-glutathione is a sulfur-containing peptide (made of amino acids, which are protein building blocks) and antioxidant essential to the body's toxic-waste disposal system.

 All protocols are for adult dosage only and are generalized; that is, dosages and conditions will vary with the individual. Before beginning any treatment, consult a qualified health-care professional. This is especially important if you are pregnant or nursing children. Listen to your body; build up the dosage slowly and carefully and only go at a rate you can tolerate.

### Additional Internal Cleansing Programs

In addition to the commercial products mentioned above, there are several others available over the counter, enabling anyone to start a self-care detoxification program to cleanse not only the intestines, but other organs as well. However, people with CFS are cautioned to do so only under the guidance of a physician.

**A.M./P.M. Ultimate Cleanse™** "When was the last time you cleaned your liver, your heart, your lungs, or your body's sewage system?" asks nutritionist Lindsey Duncan, C.N. Duncan offers a practical way to accomplish this, using a series of inner detoxification products, including Super Cleanse, Ultimate Fiber, and A.M./P.M. Ultimate Cleanse.

The A.M./P.M. Ultimate Cleanse program is set up as a two-part vegetarian detoxification formula. It involves 29 cleansing herbs, amino acids, antioxidants, digestive enzymes, vitamins, and minerals, and five kinds of fiber. Both Multi-Herb and Multi-Fiber formulas (components in the program) are taken in the morning and evening, in gradually increasing dosages, for several weeks. Positive signs that the detoxification program is working include flu-like sensations, runny nose, transient pimples, headaches, "brain fog," or fatigue, all of which will pass in one or two days.

"The goal is to stimulate, feed, and detoxify the complete internal body, not just the bowel," states Duncan. "My objective was to address all five channels of elimination, as well as all of the vital organs and tissues in the body." By the end of the program, a person should be having two to three bowel movements every day. Once the internal system is cleaned out, nutrient absorption can proceed much more efficiently. The key to the effectiveness of the Ultimate Multi formula, Duncan explains, is the timing: the morning formula stimulates, the evening formula relaxes. Following your body's natural digestive and cleansing cycles is the key to proper detoxification and supplementation, says Duncan, who adds that the entire line of A.M/P.M. products are available in most health food stores.

***Cleanse Thyself™: The Arise & Shine Program:*** One of the cardinal principles of alternative medicine is that a healthy colon is the key to lasting wellness and vitality. While food is meant to pass through the colon in about 14 hours (called "transit time"), poor diet, lack of fiber intake, stress, excessive antibiotics, and other factors can slow matters almost to a standstill, allowing only a small portion of waste matter to be actually eliminated from the body. It may be shocking to know that autopsies have found 20 to 30 pounds of old fecal matter still lodged in the myriad intricate folds of the small and large intestine.

Fecal matter that remains for long-term storage in the colon becomes the seedbed for many illnesses; this is why periodic colon cleansing is widely recommended by alternative medicine practitioners, including naturopath Richard Anderson, N.D., N.M.D. In 1986, he introduced the Cleanse Thyself self-care colon cleansing program. The program enables you to "clean your entire alimentary canal from your tongue to your stomach, to your organs, all the way down to your colon," says Dr. Ander-

 For more information about the **Cleanse Thyself** program, visit the website: www.ariseandshine.com, or call (800) 688-2444.

son, whose Arise & Shine company, makers of Cleanse Thyself, is based in Mount Shasta, California.

**How the Colon Gets Clogged and Toxic:** One of the prime places to see the effects of inappropriate choices in diet over the years is in the state of the colon. Many people continually eat high levels of acid-forming foods such as sugars, processed grains, eggs, and meat, says Dr. Anderson. These foods deplete the body of electrolytes (SEE QUICK DEFINITION), which in turn make the bile—the intestinal fluid that helps digestion—more acidic. Bile that is acidic cannot digest food normally, and this causes the buildup of mucoid plaque, an abnormal fecal substance, on the inner wall of the intestines. This plaque (also known as false mucoid lining) can diminish digestive performance and cause a buildup of toxins in the intestines and liver. The process then feeds on itself, as the formation of plaque further inhibits normal digestion, which causes toxins and disease-causing organisms to be absorbed by the body through the intestines rather than eliminated.

As digestion becomes less efficient, the body is not able to produce sufficient amounts of helpful substances needed for functioning, which leads to still higher levels of toxins in the bowel, explains Dr. Anderson. Liver function becomes compromised, no longer efficiently filtering out toxins, and the body's immune defenses are taxed by this toxic overload and become less competent at resisting illness.

 **Electrolytes** are substances in the blood, tissue fluids, intracellular fluids, or urine, which conduct an electrical charge, either plus or minus. Examples of electrolytes include acids, bases, and salts, such as potassium, magnesium, phosphate, sulfate, bicarbonate, sodium, chloride, and calcium. Electrolytes provide inorganic chemicals for cellular reactions and control mechanisms such as the conduction of electrochemical impulses to nerves and muscles. Electrolytes are also needed for key enzymatic reactions involved in metabolism (the release of energy from food).

There is a psychological dimension to colon toxicity, too, says Dr. Anderson. Negativity and heavy emotions get "stuck" in the body, as if anchored by the old mass in the intestines. The result can be the propagation of outmoded feelings, attitudes, and thoughts—"negative thought patterns," says Dr. Anderson—all of which can negatively influence one's health. "If we do not cleanse our bowels and replenish the electrolyte reserves, our body's ability to heal itself is greatly diminished."

**Cleaning Out Your System:** The Cleanse Thyself program embodies the principles of naturopathic detoxification. Dr. Anderson recommends that the prospective user first test both saliva and urine for pH (SEE

Negativity and heavy emotions get "stuck" in the body, as if anchored by the old mass in the intestines. The result can be the propagation of outmoded feelings, attitudes, and thoughts—"negative thought patterns," says Dr. Anderson—all of which can negatively influence one's health.

QUICK DEFINITION) balance, using pH tester papers included in the kit. The pH is the degree of acidity and alkalinity of a solution, measured on a scale of 1 (acidic) to 14 (alkaline). The results of the pH test, which indicate your body's electrolyte levels, determine which level of the Cleanse Thyself program should be used, from the Mildest Phase to the Master Phase. Dr. Anderson explains that the Mildest Phase of the Cleanse Thyself program is designed for those whose bodies are weaker or chronically or severely ill, or those who are elderly enough that they need a very gentle approach to cleansing.

"Persons who use the mildest phase generally show a severely over-acidic condition prior to preparing for cleansing. For such a person, the first step before beginning to cleanse must be to begin to alkalinize so that the body has enough resources to handle cleansing in a positive manner." The Master Phase of the cleanse involves fasting from solid foods while taking the supplements along with fresh juices. "The Master Phase should only be attempted by persons whose bodies have already attained an adequate reservoir of electrolytes and strength to handle this powerful level of cleansing," says Dr. Anderson.

 The term **pH**, which means "potential hydrogen," represents a scale for the relative acidity or alkalinity of a solution. Acidity is measured as a pH of 0.1 to 6.9, and alkalinity is 7.1 to 14; a pH of 7.0 is considered neutral. The numbers refer to how many hydrogen atoms are present compared to an ideal or standard solution. Normally, blood is slightly alkaline, at 7.35 to 7.45; urine pH can range from 4.8 to 7.5, although normal is closer to 7.0.

For example, those starting on the Mildest Phase should have a breakfast that consists of fresh fruit, while their lunch and dinner should emphasize alkaline-forming foods, such as salad greens, raw vegetables, potatoes, and more fresh fruits. The user on this phase also consumes two Cleanse Thyself Shakes, consisting of liquid bentonite (a purifying clay), psyllium husk powder (a fibrous bulking agent), and pure water. The Mildest Phase is well suited both for people who can't take the time off from work for a more demanding clean-out and for those who are too toxic and weak to handle a stronger regimen, says Dr. Anderson.

To soften and break up toxic waste material while detoxifying cells, the program provides two customized elements, called Chomper and Herbal Nutrition. Chomper is an herbal laxative (in tablet form) containing plantain, *Cascara sagrada*, barberry, peppermint, sheep sorrel, fennel seed, ginger root, myrrh gum, red raspberry, rhubarb root, goldenseal, and lobelia. Herbal Nutrition is a vitamin supplement (containing alfalfa, dandelion, shavegrass, chickweed, marshmallow root, yellow dock, rosehips, hawthorne, licorice root, Irish moss, kelp, amylase, and cellulase) that helps strengthen and nourish the body during the detoxification process. Both Chomper and Herbal Nutrition are taken daily, says Dr. Anderson.

Each successive stage in the Cleanse Thyself program involves stricter dietary controls, a higher intake of program supplements, and a correspondingly deeper cleansing. Typically, the overall cleansing program takes four weeks, in which three are devoted to the Pre-Cleanse, and one week to the Power or Master Phase. The Pre-Cleanse is essential, Dr. Anderson says, because it allows the herbs enough time to prepare the mucoid plaque for removal and to start neutralizing stored intestinal toxins such as pesticides, drugs, and heavy metals.

Mucoid plaque tends to be anywhere from 1/64 to one inch thick, with a texture from stiff and hard to soft, flexible, or gooey. It is often blackish green in color and somewhat resembles rubber or leather, says Dr. Anderson. It is the strange product of many years of inappropriate diet, malabsorption, and colonic stagnation. "It is not uncommon for pieces to come out more than 2-4 feet long, but the average is 6-18 inches," Dr. Anderson says. Based on figures obtained from customer testimonials, out of a total user base of about 70,000 people, Dr. Anderson estimates that about 95% of the program's users have eliminated mucoid plaque.

**Intensifying the Detoxification:** The Gentle Phase, also called Pre-Cleanse, is the step most commonly used, says Dr. Anderson. Even if you are continuing with the other two phases (Power and Master), Dr. Anderson recommends staying on this phase for at least one week and up to three weeks to prepare your system for the more demanding cleansing ahead. "What took months, years, or a lifetime to create cannot be cleaned up in a week's time," he says. This phase prepares the mucoid plaque in the intestine for removal and reduces the stress on your liver by giving it time to process more waste.

The second step, called Power Phase, is appropriate only for those who have completed the Pre-Cleanse, cautions Dr. Anderson. Here "you are likely to remove many feet of toxic mucoid plaque and pounds of toxic waste." In this stage, a new component called Flora Grow is added to replenish beneficial intestinal bacteria depleted by antibiotics and years of poor eating habits, says Dr. Anderson.

The third step, called Master Phase, produces the most powerful detoxification. No meals are allowed in this phase, but it includes five Cleanse Thyself Shakes, five doses of Chomper and Herbal Nutrition, one dose of Flora Grow, and an enema twice daily. If you have cleansing reactions when starting this phase, you are not ready to begin the Master Phase and should go back to the Gentle Phase, Dr. Anderson cautions.

"As you begin to cleanse your digestive system, other parts of your body will respond as well," says Dr. Anderson. "You'll not only rid yourself of toxic, pathogenic waste, you'll also release toxic feelings and emotions." A common refrain from users new to colon cleansing is "I eliminated more than I ever thought I had in me." According to a testimonial from a user in Australia, "The main improvements I have noticed are energy levels, vision, hair, skin, mental attitude, ability to cope with stress situations—generally I'm a much happier and healthier person." Other benefits cited by users include cessation of menstrual pain, migraines, and joint pain; fewer colds;

 It is common to have physical reactions to the detoxification process, such as headaches, vomiting, diarrhea, fatigue, or dizziness, says Dr. Anderson. For all the discomfort, this is actually a sign that the process is working and that you are eliminating toxins from your body. If these symptoms occur, don't move on to either of the higher phases before your body has a chance to recover, cautions Dr. Anderson. He recommends that users wait to progress to the next phase until they have been without these symptoms for at least three days.

resolution of lifelong sinus congestion, itching, ulcers, and a breast cyst; weight loss; and better concentration, among many others.

**Probiotics for the Intestines:** The human body contains an estimated several trillion beneficial bacteria comprising over 400 species, all necessary for health. Many of these "friendly" bacteria, also called probiotics, reside in the intestines, where they are essential for proper nutrient assimilation. Among the more well-known of these are *Lactobacillus acidophilus* and *Bifidobacterium bifidium*.

Prior to 1945 and the introduction of mass-market foods and chemicalized agriculture, Westerners normally obtained adequate amounts of probiotics from fresh vegetables. Friendly bacteria are actually soil-based organisms that are incorporated into plants and then eaten by humans. However, overly acidic bodily conditions, chronic constipation or diarrhea, dietary imbalances, consumption of overly processed foods, and the excessive use of antibiotics and hormonal drugs can interfere with probiotic function and even reduce their numbers in the body. When the body's probiotic population drops, conditions are set for illness, unless steps are taken to replenish them.

In general, probiotic supplements are useful both for maintaining good health and for gaining relief from chronic health conditions such as acne, skin problems, allergies, arthritis, high cholesterol, yeast infections, and intestinal disturbances. In 1996, researchers at the University of Washington School of Medicine reported that microorganisms with therapeutic properties (probiotics) can be used successfully to treat and prevent selected vaginal, urinary tract, and intestinal infections, such as diarrhea associated with antibiotics, infantile diarrhea, and candidiasis. Probiotics, formerly a "neglected" modality, now "may offer an alternative to conventional antimicrobials to which many pathogenic microorganisms eventually develop resistance," stated Gary W. Elmer, Ph.D., author of the research report.[3]

***FOS: Health Food for Friendly Bacteria:*** Alternative medicine physicians have long recognized the benefit of supplementing with "friendly" bacteria, or probiotics, to restore the balance of flora in the intestines and thus promote intestinal health. Probiotics are especially important after an intestinal detoxification program.

A new approach to restoring the balance of intestinal flora was developed in Japan in the mid-1980s. Called prebiotics, it involves introducing nutrients that directly feed the beneficial bacteria already in place in a person's large intestine, most typically *Bifidobacteria* and *Lactobacilli*. Japanese researchers determined that a naturally occurring form of carbohydrate called fructo-oligosaccharides (FOS), found in certain foods in minute amounts, could be a perfect food for *Bifidobacteria*.

FOS acts like an intestinal "fertilizer," selectively feeding the friendly microflora in the large intestine so that their numbers can usefully increase. *Bifidobacteria* work to lower the pH in the large intestine to a slightly more acidic condition; this discourages the growth of unfriendly bacteria. Feeding the friendly bacteria is a crucial step in maintaining the correct balance of intestinal microflora; when they are out of balance (dysbiosis), intestinal function is compromised.

Studies have demonstrated that taking ¼ teaspoon (1 g) of FOS powder daily for four weeks led to a fivefold increase in the total count of beneficial bacteria. A Japanese study found that when 23 hospital patients, 50 to 90 years old, took 8 g of FOS daily for two weeks, their *Bifidobacteria* levels increased by ten times. Benefits from increasing *Bifidobacteria* levels include, among others, relief of constipation or diarrhea, promotion of regularity, serum cholesterol reduction, control of blood sugar levels, immune function enhancement, improved calcium absorption and B vitamin synthesis, better digestion of milk proteins, and a reduction of the detoxification load on the liver.

While FOS is found in garlic, honey, Jerusalem artichokes, soybeans, burdock, chicory root, asparagus, banana, rye, barley, tomato, onion, and triticale, according to nutrition expert Robert Crayhon, M.S., C.N.: "There is not enough FOS in foods in the average diet to get an optimal or therapeutically significant dose."

Technically, you would have to eat 429 garlic cloves to get the amount of FOS in one teaspoon of FOS powder. That's why FOS is synthesized using a natural process that optimizes the yield. Recognizing this, in Japan today over 500 commercially prepared foods contain FOS (known there as "neosugar"), with the endorsement of Japan's minister of health. FOS, which

 For more about **detoxification methods**, see chapter 9, Addressing the Allergy Connection.

is made by fermenting sucrose with a fungus called *Aspergillus niger* (*Aspergillus oryzae* is used to make miso and soy sauce), is about 30% as sweet as sucrose.[4]

## Toxicity and the Health of the Cells

Francine, age 10, was diagnosed with a mysterious, severe neurological disorder. She was tired all the time, had chronic muscle pains, couldn't walk or stand easily, and wasn't able to concentrate at school. For convenience, her doctors called it fibromyalgia. They gave Francine antibiotics to treat bacteria that they discovered in her system, but this was not the cause, says Thomas Rau, M.D., director of the Paracelsus Clinic in Lustmühle, Switzerland. "It was only a secondary infection, which the antibiotics made worse." Soon she developed colitis and was eventually brought to Paracelsus by ambulance.

There, she was helped by an approach called biological medicine, which involves looking at the condition of the body's cells. This information will lead to an understanding of why the body is sick. When cells become imbalanced, conditions are set for infection, illness, or chronic disease to begin; when cells are rebalanced, conditions are set for healing and a return to health. "As we see it, sickness is not caused by bacteria, but the bacteria come with the sickness," Dr. Rau says. "This is biological thinking. Bacteria, viruses, or fungi can only change form and flourish if they have the suitable cellular conditions. They develop from within the organism; they do not invade it from without."

Correcting the cellular imbalance is at the core of biological medicine, a concept founded by the Clinic's namesake, Paracelsus, a sixteenth-century alchemist, physician, and medical troublemaker. The idea is that knowing the biochemistry of the cells—the pH balance of acidity and alkalinity, the oxidation-reduction (SEE QUICK DEFINITION) potential—is of paramount importance to the physician's treatment plan. Biochemical changes can be the result of outside influences, such as faulty diet, inadequate nutrition, chemical or heavy metal exposure, chronic organ toxicity, stress, or trauma.

As the first stage in Francine's treatment, Dr. Rau put her on a detoxification program to flush the toxins, including mercury, out of her body. He used a combination of DMPS (SEE QUICK DEFINITION) and sodium bicarbonate infusions (an alkalinizing preparation) to remove mercury from Francine's body and to reduce the extreme acidity of her cells. Although her blood pH was 7.38 and thus alkaline, Francine's urine

**Oxidation-reduction** refers to a basic chemical mechanism in the cell by which energy is produced from foods. Electrons (negatively charged particles in an atom) are removed from one atom, resulting in "oxidation" of this first atom, and then are added or transferred to another atom, resulting in "reduction" of this second atom. The molecules that give up their electrons are referred to as oxidized; the molecules that accept electrons are referred to as oxidants. This continual process of energy metabolism is actually a flow of electrons, or a minute electrical current within the cell.

**DMPS** (2,3-dimercaptopropane-1-sulfonate) is the chelating (binding-up) agent of choice for the removal of elemental mercury from the human body. It can be given orally, intravenously, or intramuscularly and is useful for people who have been exposed to mercury amalgam through their dental fillings or those who show evidence or suspicion of heavy metal toxicity from other sources.

**SANUM remedies**, developed by Guenther Enderlein, M.D., Ph.D. (1872–1968), are produced by SANUM-Kehlbeck GmbH & Co. KG, D-2812 Hoya, Germany. The line includes about 100 preparations of benign microorganisms or protein particles identified by pleomorphic practice. For example, "Mucokehl" is *Mucor racemosus*, a fungus that regulates microorganisms affecting the thickness of the blood. These remedies, injected around the tumor site, adjust the pH and cellular terrain and help the pathogenic microorganisms revert back to harmless forms. In effect, the SANUM remedies help the body restore the optimal cellular terrain for health.

had a pH fluctuating between 4.0 and 5.0, which is very acidic. The pH norm for urine is about 6.8, says Dr. Rau.

In addition, Dr. Rau's team gave Francine daily intravenous infusions of vitamins B, C, and E, plus magnesium and other trace elements. They prescribed a specific diet and administered both homeopathic and Enderlein (SANUM—SEE QUICK DEFINITION) remedies, all in an effort to improve the acid-base conditions of her cells. After about three weeks on this program, Francine was able to walk and speak normally again. After four weeks, she was able to ride a bicycle; and six months after beginning treatment, she was in school again as a normal, healthy child, after having been seriously ill for 18 months prior to seeing Dr. Rau.

 To contact **Thomas Rau, M.D.**: Paracelsus Clinic, CH-9062, Lustmühle bei St. Gallen, Switzerland; tel: 41-71-335-71-71. Website: www.paracelsus.ch.

Reversing neurological problems specific to children is a specialty at Paracelsus Clinic. Tourette's syndrome, attention deficit disorder, and hyperactivity often have a strong toxicity factor involved, says Dr. Rau. Frequently, aluminum toxicity is the cause. Poor nutrition, a diet based on highly processed foods, and sodas containing phosphoric acid lead to a deficiency in trace elements. This, in turn, upsets the cellular terrain—making it too acidic—and enables aluminum to enter the tissues and wreak havoc. "Aluminum only gets into your body if the terrain is acid," says Dr. Rau. Once again, whether you're concerned with diagnosis or healing, the terrain is everything.

# six

# Reversing Hidden Thyroid Problems

A major and often overlooked cause of chronic fatigue syndrome is an underactive thyroid gland, a condition known as hypothyroidism. Many people with CFS have not been properly tested for thyroid problems—in large part because, according to conventional medicine, hypothyroidism is a separate illness from CFS and a diagnosis of one precludes a diagnosis of the other.

Putting each illness into its own category does not serve the interests of the patient. Since thyroid hormones are integral to maintaining optimal body energy levels and are required for proper immune system function and nearly all aspects of body function, hypothyroidism can be central among the multiple factors involved in creating CFS. If that is the case, successfully reversing the syndrome will require discovering the hidden thyroid imbalance along with all the other contributing factors.

Knowledge of the importance of the thyroid to human health has been known by Western doctors since the 1950s, but most have chosen to ignore it. It was Broda O. Barnes, M.D., Ph.D.—a pioneer in thyroid research and the author of 100 medical articles on this gland—who made the remarkable claim that was ignored by the medical establishment then and is still not sufficiently heeded today. Dr. Barnes stated that untreated thyroid problems are responsible for 64 common medical ailments suffered by about 40% of the population. Many alternative medicine physicians agree with Dr. Barnes and believe that, given the increasing preva-

> Broda O. Barnes, M.D., Ph.D., stated that untreated thyroid problems are responsible for 64 common medical ailments suffered by about 40% of the population.

lence of chronic and degenerative illness, we need to pay more attention to Dr. Barnes's conclusions.

Thyroid problems may be on the rise due to the increasingly toxic environment in which we live. Radiation is probably the greatest environmental cause of hypothyroidism and other thyroid problems, including tumors and thyroid cancer, states Lita Lee, Ph.D., an enzyme therapist based in Lowell, Oregon, who frequently treats thyroid-generated problems. As of November 1995 the incidence of childhood thyroid cancer had increased 100 times in those areas of Ukraine, Belarus, and Russia most directly exposed to the Chernobyl nuclear accident in April 1986, according to experts from the United Nations. Childhood thyroid cancer is the fastest way in which the impact of radiation exposure shows up in the body.

Mercury toxicity can also produce hypothyroidism, according to Dr. Lee. This heavy metal, comprising up to 50% of mercury amalgam dental fillings (SEE QUICK DEFINITION), poisons an enzyme critical in converting T4—the inactive form of the thyroid hormone—into T3, the active form. Other thyroid inhibitors include fluoride (common in water, foods, and toothpaste); synthetic and genetically engineered hormones (such as estrogen) in meat, dairy products, poultry, and eggs; excess polyunsaturated fats such as soybean, safflower, canola, corn, and flaxseed oils; and excess iodine.

In this chapter, you will learn how hypothyroidism and other thyroid disorders can contribute to CFS and how

 **Mercury fillings**, or amalgams, have been used in dentistry since the 1820s, but not until 1988 did the routine use of mercury raise questions serious enough for the Environmental Protection Agency (EPA) to declare scrap dental amalgam a hazardous waste. Evidence now shows that mercury amalgams are the major source of mercury exposure for the general public, at rates six times higher than that found in fish and seafood. Studies by the World Health Organization show that a single amalgam can release 3 to 17 mcg of mercury per day. A Danish study of a random sample of 100 men and 100 women showed that increased blood mercury levels were related to the presence of more than four amalgam fillings in the teeth. Mercury toxicity has been shown to have destructive contributory effects on kidney function, in cardiovascular disease, neuropsychological dysfunction, reproductive disorders, and birth defects, to name a few. Symptoms of mercury toxicity make a very long list: anorexia, depression, fatigue, insomnia, arthritis, multiple sclerosis, moodiness, irritability, memory loss, nausea, diarrhea, gum disease, swollen glands, headaches, and many more.

## The Thyroid Gland

The **thyroid gland**, the largest of the body's seven endocrine glands, is located just below the larynx in the throat and has interconnecting lobes on either side of the trachea. The thyroid is the body's metabolic thermostat, controlling body temperature, energy use, and, for children, the body's growth rate. The thyroid controls the rate at which organs function and the speed with which the body uses food; it affects the operation of all body processes and organs. Of the hormones synthesized in and released by the thyroid, T3 (tri-iodothyronine) represents 7% and T4 (thyroxine) accounts for almost 93% of the thyroid's hormones active in all of the body's processes. Iodine is essential to forming normal amounts of thyroxine. The secretion of both these hormones is regulated by thyroid-stimulating hormone, or TSH, secreted by the pituitary gland in the brain. The thyroid also secretes calcitonin, a hormone required for calcium metabolism.

**Hypothyroidism** is a condition of low or underactive thyroid gland function that can produce numerous symptoms. Among the 47 clinically recognized symptoms are fatigue, depression, lethargy, weakness, weight gain, low body temperature, chills, cold extremities, general oversensitivity to cold, infertility, rheumatic pain, menstrual disorders (excessive flow, cramps), repeated infections, colds, upper respiratory infections, skin problems (itching; eczema; psoriasis; acne; dry, coarse, scaly skin; skin pallor), memory disturbances, concentration difficulties, paranoia, migraines, oversleep, "laziness," muscle aches and weakness, hearing disturbances, burning/prickling sensations, anemia, slow reaction time and mental sluggishness, swelling of the eyelids, constipation, labored difficult breathing, hoarseness, brittle nails, and poor vision.

thyroid

they can be reversed with alternative medicine. In the section that follows, Stephen E. Langer, M.D., of Berkeley, California, co-author of *Solved: The Riddle of Illness*, discusses the effects of thyroid dysfunction and relates two medical case histories, one of CFS and the other of Hashimoto's autoimmune thyroiditis (HAIT), which shares many of the symptoms of CFS.

## The Thyroid and Chronic Fatigue

There is a hidden reason why chronic fatigue, muscle pain, depression, weight problems, and other conditions are so hard to diagnose. It's called the thyroid gland. The thyroid is the largest of the body's seven endocrine glands, and its role in all aspects of healthy body functioning is paramount, yet it is also probably the most overlooked factor in a great many health problems, from chronic fatigue to obesity, depression to skin problems. Since I began medical practice in 1967, the single most important element in my approach has been attention to the thyroid gland and two hormones it secretes. The thyroid controls how fast energy is burned in every cell, a process called metabolic activity. The healthy functioning of the thyroid is central to everything else in the body and, as Dr. Barnes said, problems here can contribute to numerous medical conditions.

Yet the "cure" is surprisingly simple: nothing has so low a toxicity level and is as easy and inexpensive to use as thyroid hormone, correctly administered by a physician. There is much more room for therapeutic intervention with thyroid-based health conditions than with other glandular problems because, while the thyroid is central to so many body functions, hormonal adjustments can be made with minimal disturbance of the overall system.

## *The Whole Body Becomes Underactive*

The list of thyroid-related health problems is long and disturbing. (See sidebar, "The Thyroid Gland.") When the thyroid is underactive, everything in the body gradually becomes hypoactive as well, from circulation to libido. But here's the problem: it's my estimation that a large number of clinically severe

 **Stephen Langer, M.D.**: 3011 Telegraph Avenue, Suite 230, Berkeley, CA 94705; tel: (510) 548-7384. *Solved: The Riddle of Illness*, which he co-authored with James F. Scheer, was published by Keats Publishing in 1995.

thyroid conditions go undetected for long periods of time and some, regrettably, are never picked up. In addition, people are often erroneously treated for chronic health conditions that are really based on the thyroid and that would respond well and quickly to a small dose of thyroid hormone.

Take skin problems, for example. One of the first things the body does when the thyroid is underactive is reduce the blood supply to the skin to conserve energy. As a result, a person with this problem will perspire less, bacteria can flourish on the skin, and acne lesions can develop. If you aggressively treat the acne and ignore the thyroid, you won't see much permanent change.

> There is a hidden reason why chronic fatigue, muscle pain, depression, weight problems, and other conditions are so hard to diagnose. It's called the thyroid gland.
>
> — *Stephen Langer, M.D*

As another example, consider depression. I treated a patient who had been depressed for 60 years; yet when he took thyroid hormone, his depression was gone within a month. Whatever his previous physicians prescribed focused on his depression but missed the underlying thyroid cause, so he was miserable for most of his lifetime. Incidentally, although medical research and statistics suggest that an underactive thyroid is more common in women, I contend there is as much underactive thyroid and thyroiditis (inflamed thyroid) in men as in women.

### Success Story: Reversing Ten Years of Hypothyroidism

When Frank, 47, first came to my office, he had near-total body failure—in other words, he was almost permanently bedridden. He had chronic fatigue, intermittent headaches, light sensitivity, multiple chemical sensitivities, heart palpitations, mood swings, and anxiety fluctuating with depression. Frank was cold all the time, his appetite was poor, his mental abilities were sluggish, and he'd been sick for most of the previous ten years. He was also on prescription antidepressants.

I ordered standard laboratory tests for Frank's thyroid function, to evaluate the status of his T3, T4, TSH, and FTI (free thyroxine index, to see how much thyroxine was actually active). Some physicians only look at T4 levels. Taken alone, this is pointless. TSH is the most sensitive indicator of thyroid function, but the whole thyroid panel should be run. Of the four, Frank's TSH levels were elevated; the normal range is 0.35 to 5.5, but his was 10.6. Any elevation of TSH means the thyroid gland is failing functionally, because it has had to compensate in order to sustain the body's multiple functions.

Frank started taking ¼ grain daily of natural thyroid hormone derived from animals. Over the next three months, I gradually increased the dosage to almost two grains per day. My preference was to run a series of allergy sensitivity tests, but Frank's budget didn't allow for this. As a way of working around this, he began a low-fat diet that was high in complex carbohydrates and low in glycemic foods, which means foods whose carbohydrate (or simple sugar) composition is absorbed too rapidly into the bloodstream.

Frank tracked his diet to see which foods provoked problems, and identified wheat, corn, and dairy as allergenic foods to be eliminated. In addition, he took a high-potency multivitamin/mineral supplement and about 1,000 mg total of the essential fatty acids omega-3 and omega-6 (SEE QUICK DEFINITION). These were in the form of gamma-linolenic acid (GLA) from borage oil (240 mg, twice daily) and eicosapentaenoic acid (EPA; 240 mg, twice daily). Frank also took daily doses of Ester C (a form of vitamin C; 500 mg), calcium (125 mg), and magnesium (65 mg). I increased his dietary protein intake so that more amino acids (the building blocks of proteins) would be available to his brain where they could help offset the biochemical aspect of his depression.

Over the three months Frank took the thyroid hormone, I watched his condition steadily improve. His stamina, energy, digestion, muscular function, and mood got progressively

 **Omega-3 and omega-6 oils** are the two principal types of essential fatty acids, which are unsaturated fats required in the diet. The digits "3" and "6" refer to differences in the oil's chemical structure with respect to its chain of carbon atoms and where they are bonded. A balance of these oils in the diet is required for good health. The primary omega-3 oil, alpha-linolenic acid (ALA), is found in flaxseed (58%), canola, pumpkin seeds, walnuts, and soybeans. Fish oils, such as salmon, cod, and mackerel, contain the other important omega-3 oils, DHA (docosahexaenoic acid) and EPA (eicosapentaenoic acid). Omega-3 oils help reduce the risk of heart disease. Linoleic acid or cis-linoleic acid is the main omega-6 oil and is found in most plant and vegetable oils, including safflower (73%), corn, peanut, and sesame. The most therapeutic form of omega-6 oil is gamma-linolenic acid (GLA), found in evening primrose, black currant, and borage oils. Once in the body, omega-3 and omega-6 are converted to prostaglandins: hormone-like substances that regulate many metabolic functions, particularly inflammatory processes.

better. All of his systems had been operating at suboptimal levels; restoring the correct level of thyroid hormone was like stoking the flames in all his cells. Frank was a classic "basket case" before taking the thyroid hormone, but now he is a functional human being, doing a world better than he was before. He's able to fend for himself, prepare his own meals, and exercise regularly without being drugged to the eyeballs on conventional medications that gave him practically every side effect possible. In fact, Frank's mental processes improved so much with the thyroid hormone that he was able to stop taking all his prescription drugs.

# The Thyroid and Its Hormones

The thyroid has four principal hormones: T1, T2, T3, and T4. Thyroid hormones are stored in the thyroid and released to the body as needed. T1 (mono-iodothyronine) and T2 (di-iodothyronine) are not considered especially active. T4 (thyroxine) contains iodine, is produced exclusively in the thyroid gland, and accounts for almost 93% of the thyroid's hormones active in all of the body's processes; its chief function is to increase the speed of cell metabolism, or energy conversion.

Iodine and the amino acid tyrosine are essential to forming normal amounts of T4. When the body requires more T3, T4 can give up its iodine to form T3 which, while representing only about 7% of the thyroid hormone complement, has a greater biological activity by a factor of three to four times. About 80% of the body's T3 comes from converting T4, typically in the liver and kidneys. When T4 conversion runs smoothly—that is, the enzyme cascade (sequencing of enzymes in chemical reactions) is correct—normal body temperature and metabolic rates are maintained.

If the thyroid is functioning poorly, however, T4 breaks down to form reverse tri-iodothyronine, or rT3 (a different chemical version of T3). Stress, fasting, illness, or elevated cortisol (from the adrenal glands) can contribute to the occurrence of this faulty conversion. As rT3 levels increase, metabolism and body temperature decrease, and various enzymes fail to function properly. In addition, as rT3 levels build, levels of T3 decrease, leading to low T3 syndrome, thyroid dysfunction, and a skewed ratio of T3 to rT3. This condition of elevated rT3 is known as Wilson's Syndrome.

Total blood levels of T3 and T4 consist of only 1% biologically active components (called the free levels), while 99% is the metabolically inactive portion bound to proteins. In a healthy person, total T4 levels as indicated in a blood test (or thyroid panel) are 4.5 to 12.5, but for someone with hypothyroidism (underactive thyroid), those values will be less than 4.5. For Free-T4, the normal range is 0.9 to 2; hypothyroid, less

than 0.9. For Free-T3, normal is 80 to 220; hypothyroid, less than 80. TSH is normally 0.3 to 6; for hypothyroid, greater than 6.

The formation and secretion of T3 and T4 are regulated by a complex sequence of hormonal causes and effects, set off by the brain's hypothalamus gland. The hypothalamus secretes a substance called thyrotropin-releasing hormone (TRH), which in turn directs the pituitary gland to produce thyroid-stimulating hormone, or TSH (thyrotropin). Because TSH has a direct effect on the production of T4 and T3, TSH blood levels are conventionally taken as the best index for thyroid dysfunction, both hypo and hyper (overactive). When thyroid function is low, TSH levels normally go up.

## Success Story: Ending Three Years of Painful Thyroiditis

A second major health problem relating to an underactive thyroid is Hashimoto's autoimmune thyroiditis (SEE QUICK DEFINITION), known as HAIT or simply thyroiditis. Here the thyroid gland is enlarged, though usually without pain. However, the autoimmune factor is involved because the body releases antibodies against its own thyroid as if it were a foreign object in the body. HAIT seems to run in families, with most patients being between the ages of 13 and 40. Typical symptoms include fatigue, memory loss, depression, and a sense of nervousness that can range from mild anxiety to serious panic attack. You can also have allergies, irregular heartbeat or palpitations, muscle and joint pain, sleep disturbances in which you wake up with your mind racing and heart beating fast, reduced sexual interest, menstrual irregularities, headaches, digestive disorders, and intestinal problems from diarrhea to constipation. Also, you are likely to have the sensation of a lump in your throat; this is actually your inflamed, slightly swollen thyroid gland.

When I am confronted with this symptom picture, I routinely have the patient's thyroid antibodies (SEE QUICK DEFINITION) checked. For example, a person's thyroid hormone levels (such as T4) may be normal but their thyroid antibodies are elevated. Many physicians miss this; in my opinion, thyroid antibody tests should be run routinely on anyone with a chronic health problem. If a patient has a low elevation of thyroid antibodies, I will start this person on a low dose of thyroid hormone even if their thyroid hormone levels are supposedly normal. Let me explain this by presenting a case.

 **Hashimoto's autoimmune thyroiditis (HAIT)** is a disease in which the body releases antibodies that attack the thyroid gland as if it were a foreign enemy. Characterized by an enlarged thyroid, other symptoms of HAIT include deep fatigue, memory loss, depression, anxiety, digestive disorders, sleep disturbances, muscle and joint pain, and allergies, among others. HAIT strikes predominantly women between the ages of 13 and 40. Most sufferers gradually develop hypothyroidism.

An **antibody** is a protein molecule containing about 20,000 atoms, made from amino acids by B lymphocyte cells in the lymph tissue and set in motion by the immune system against a specific foreign protein (antigen). An antibody, also referred to as an immunoglobulin, may be found in the blood, lymph, saliva, and the gastrointestinal and urinary tracts, usually within three days after the first encounter with an antigen. The antibody binds tightly with the antigen as a preliminary for removing it from the system or destroying it.

Theodora, 43, came to me with multiple symptoms. She had chronic fatigue, joint and muscle pain, headaches, insomnia, numerous infections, frequent sore throats, and nasal congestion; she was always on the verge of having a cold. She also had intermittent heart palpitations, irregular periods, intestinal gas, indigestion, constipation, and diarrhea. Her muscle pain was so widespread she felt that every muscle in her body hurt.

Testing revealed that while her thyroid hormone levels were normal, her level of thyroid antibodies was sky-high. I started her on a low dose of thyroid hormone, at ¼ of a grain (15 mg) per day, then gradually increased this to three grains over the next year. My HAIT patients often ask me if they must remain on thyroid hormone indefinitely. I have been able to wean many of my HAIT patients from a thyroid supplement in a relatively short time—within three to six months—by bolstering their immune system nutritionally. A lab test indicated Theodora was deficient in three amino acids, as well as vitamin B5, inositol, and zinc. Rather than prescribing amino-acid supplements, I had her increase her dietary protein intake. To address the other deficiencies, I started Theodora on a high-potency multivitamin/mineral.

Another test indicated that Theodora had elevated *Candida albicans* yeast in her intestines. To address this, Theodora started a high complex carbohydrate diet and avoided refined sugars, sweets, and fruits. She began rotating her foods so that her system was not constantly having to process the same foods. Through food allergy testing, I determined that Theodora was sensitive to a long list of foods, including kidney beans, rye grain, cheddar cheese, egg yolk, wheat, almonds, figs, kale, and others. I also gave her grapefruit seed extract (500 mg, three times daily) to help detoxify her intestines; *L. acidophilus* capsules (two capsules, three times daily) to recolonize her intestines with the appropriate "friendly" bacteria; and high-potency garlic (one tablet, twice daily). All of this helped to remedy her intestinal problems. In general, people with thyroid problems tend to have sluggish intestines.

 For more on **nutritional supplements for CFS**, see chapter 10, Ending Nutritional Deficiencies with Supplements.

 Patients with preexisting heart problems should not take high doses of thyroid hormone (more than two grains/day) except under a physician's careful supervision.

After about six months on this program, many of Theodora's symptoms were much reduced, and after a total of 12 months, she was about 75% improved. Her muscle pains were greatly diminished, her energy level was much better, all signs of flu and cold were gone, she was able to exercise comfortably, and all her digestive processes were practically normal.

# Thyroid Problems and Nutritional Deficiencies in CFS

As Dr. Langer has demonstrated, diagnosing an underactive thyroid is crucial in successfully reversing a chronic illness such as CFS. Addressing nutritional deficiencies is equally vital. We have seen in cases throughout this book that deficiencies of this type are usually a feature in CFS. Raphael Kellman, M.D., founder and medical director of the Center for Progressive Medicine in New York City, describes how he addresses these factors. He also explains his four-point program for reversing CFS and discusses the impact of the psychological component, which he calls "the meaning dimension":

From my clinical experience, it seems clear that two key factors in chronic fatigue syndrome are often overlooked as contributing causes. These are an underactive thyroid gland and undiagnosed nutrient deficiencies. About 40% of the patients I see in my practice who have chronic fatigue are actually suffering from hypothyroidism. Nutrient tests reveal that many chronic fatigue syndrome patients have numerous vitamin deficiencies, notably vitamin C and the B complex vitamins. Knowing about these two hidden factors enables me to use thyroid hormones and precise nutrient prescribing to help reverse the symptoms of chronic fatigue syndrome.

## Success Story: Fatigued from an Underactive Thyroid

The case of Kristi, 34, excellently illustrates how an underactive thyroid gland can contribute to many of the symptoms associated with chronic fatigue syndrome and, for Kristi, to an unusual and highly premature stroke for which she had to be admitted to the hospital. When she consulted me, Kristi was able to work, but needed about 11 hours of sleep every night and was still deeply tired all the time. She reported that she had been overweight much of her life and that in recent months she had developed various gastrointestinal problems, including constipation and abdominal pain.

Kristi's conventional doctors were unable to account for her stroke nor could they explain (or treat) her fatigue. Kristi also suffered from allergies, rashes, and occasional hair loss, had difficulty concentrating, and often felt unaccountably cold. Most of these symptoms are straightforward markers for a thyroid deficiency, which means the thyroid gland is not producing enough hormones to sustain its multiple functions.

However, to determine whether the thyroid is underperforming, you need to use the right thyroid test.

Although my clinical experience shows that a significant number of chronic fatigue patients have underlying hypothyroidism, this fact is often not picked up in the standard thyroid hormone tests. I often correlate TSH results with the patient's body temperature (less than 97.8° F suggests a thyroid problem) and the results of a thyroid sonogram, which indicates if the thyroid is enlarged. Clinically, the bottom line is that when we treat many chronically fatigued people, basing treatment on the assumption of an underactive thyroid, they get much better, thereby confirming the diagnosis.

 For more information about **thyroid testing**, see chapter 2, Testing. For more about **magnesium and CFS**, see chapter 10, Ending Nutritional Deficiencies with Supplements.

 The TRH stimulation test is inexpensive (about $100) and is performed by most laboratories.

In Kristi's case, according to a TRH (thyrotropin releasing hormone) stimulation test, her TSH level was at 25, way above normal. Armed with this information, I put Kristi on the synthetic thyroid supplement Synthroid, starting at a dosage of 0.125 mcg daily. To complement this, I gave her an animal-derived glandular called Thyrosine Complex (containing pancreas, spleen, and liver extracts). Kristi took this three times daily. Tyrosine (which she also took as an additional supplement at 1,000 mg daily) is a precursor to the T4 thyroid hormone. It is likely that Kristi's underactive thyroid was the predisposing factor in her stroke, a link that Dr. Barnes first proposed in the 1950s.

A vitamin and nutrient status blood test indicated that Kristi was deficient in vitamins C and B complex. For patients with hypothyroidism and poor gastrointestinal function and nutrient absorption, I supply nutrients by intravenous infusion rather than through oral supplements. Once weekly, for about six weeks, Kristi received an IV infusion of B complex and magnesium (4 cc each), and 6 to 10 g of vitamin C. At the same time I gave her grape seed extract (200 to 300 mg daily), and a bioflavonoid (SEE QUICK DEFINITION) that enhances the concentration of vitamin C between cells. It also helps the cells pick up, absorb, and retain the vitamin C, thereby saturating the tissues, rather than having it excreted into the urine.

In addition to the IV intake, Kristi took oral vitamin C at 500 mg, six times daily, along with a complete vitamin B complex (125 mg) and

## Is Your Thyroid Underactive? Two Simple Tests Will Tell You

Broda Barnes, M.D., in his classic work *Hypothyroidism: The Unsuspected Illness* (New York: Harper & Row, 1976), introduced the axillary (under the armpit) temperature test as an easy way to determine adequate thyroid function. Dr. Barnes said that a resting body temperature below 97.8° F indicates hypothyroidism; menstruating women should take the underarm temperature only on the second and third days of menstruation. However, according to Lita Lee, Ph.D., a different approach might be better.

"From clinical experience, I believe the oral temperature is much more accurate than the axillary temperature. The oral temperature should be 98° F in the morning before you become active and should increase to 98.6° F to 99° F for at least ten hours daily. The best time to do this test is about 20 minutes after lunch, because that's when the temperature and pulse are at their optimum levels. Women should do this during their menstrual periods to ensure missing the rise of temperature during ovulation."

Another way to tell if you are hypothyroid is to measure your resting pulse, advises Dr. Lee. The healthy resting pulse should be about 85 beats per minute (the national average is around 72); but if your pulse is less than 80, you may have an underactive thyroid. Babies have a pulse greater than 100 until around the age of eight years when the pulse slows down to around 85.

"The idea of a slow pulse being healthy is folklore," Dr. Lee explains. "Studies of healthy people who have no heart disease were found to have an average pulse of 85 beats per minute. Studies of the smartest high school students showed a pulse of 85 versus a pulse of 70 in below-average students. On the other hand, some low-thyroid people have a high pulse of over 100 beats per minute. These are people who literally run on adrenaline."

magnesium (1,000 mg daily in two divided doses)—patients with chronic fatigue often have low levels of magnesium in their red blood cells. As a further boost to her energy levels and to support her immune system, Kristi started taking the Chinese herb astragalus (500 mg, twice daily). Astragalus is a tonic for strengthening the immune system, enabling it to better resist disease and infection.

On this program, Kristi noticed some improvement immediately; within four weeks she felt a significant difference. After four months, she was 100% better. She had lost 45 pounds, her hair had grown back, and she felt "vital" for the first time in her life. Today, eight months later, Kristi feels like a "new" person. This case shows how the TRH test made all the difference in outcome. Had Kristi undergone this test some years earlier, it is possible the stroke and obesity could have been prevented.

## Is Thyroid Disease Due to an Excess of Conventional Drugs?

One of the major contributing causes of thyroid disease may be an excess of conventional drugs and environmental substances, says medical researcher Lynne McTaggart.

For example, lithium, taken for manic-depressive disorder, can produce hypothyroidism in up to 33% of long-term users, while the heart drug Cordarone can produce either an overactive or underactive thyroid condition that cannot be detected for 18 months, at which point it is well established. The long-term use of interferon-alpha for hepatitis can also generate either form of thyroid imbalance; certain drugs for lowering cholesterol have rendered a thyroid underactive. Research shows that other drugs, such as cough mixtures, antiseptics, and radiographic contrast agents, can render the thyroid either hypo or hyper.

Some evidence exists linking smoking with depressed thyroid function, while most illnesses and surgical procedures can upset the thyroid's function. The thyroid is particularly sensitive to events carrying a strong emotional charge, such as a death or divorce. One of the "greatest culprits," says McTaggart, is the widespread use of iodized salt. In the industrialized nations, some populations may consume too much iodine, because some regions have sufficient natural iodine in the soil and diet. An excess of only a few milligrams daily can unbalance the thyroid.

*Source:* McTaggart, Lynne, and Harald Gaier. "Thyroid Disease: Overactive Medicine." *What Your Doctors Don't Tell You* 7:7 (October 1996), 2–5. Available from: WYDDTY, 4 Wallace Road, London N1 2PG; tel: 0171-354-4592.

## *Success Story: Fatigued from Nutrient Deficiencies*

In perhaps 40% to 50% of my CFS patients, an underlying thyroid problem is the root cause, while a nutritional deficiency or central nervous system imbalance may be the source of the rest of the symptoms. The latter was the case with Tonya. Tonya, 31, had suffered from mild but chronic depression for almost four years and required at least ten hours of sleep a night. During the day, she usually felt tired, which led to her missing many days of work. There were week-long stretches when her fatigue worsened. In her case, the TRH stimulation test came out negative, which meant she did not have an underactive thyroid. But a vitamin and essential nutrient test indicated deficiencies. I started Tonya on the same IV and oral nutrient program I used with Kristi, but without thyroid hormones or glandular extracts (SEE QUICK DEFINITION). At the same time, I implemented a four-part regimen that I often use for CFS patients.

*1. Gastrointestinal.* Addressing gastrointestinal function is a basic step in reversing nutrient deficiencies. If you're not absorbing nutrients, no matter what supplements you take, they will not have the intended effect. Though some of the recommendations here may be obvious, they are crucial to eliminating deficiencies. Eat about 50% less food and do not eat "garbage" foods—processed foods devoid of nutrients—

which overwhelm and toxify the intestines. Eat whole grains, organically raised fresh fruits and vegetables, beans, and small amounts of fish, chicken, or turkey. These high-fiber dietary changes alone will do much to start cleansing the bowel of toxins and impacted matter.

Specific supplements can improve intestinal function and nutrient absorption. I often prescribe betaine hydrochloric acid (the stomach's primary digestive "juice") and digestive enzymes to enhance digestion. B complex vitamins (125 mg daily) and *Lactobacillus acidophilus* and other "friendly" bacteria aid the gastrointestinal tract in absorbing nutrients, as does consuming at least ten glasses of pure water daily. Once you've established better intestinal function, then it's far more likely that nutrients taken as supplements will be more completely absorbed.

**2. Circulation.** You have to ensure that blood circulation is working efficiently because blood flow is what heals, delivering essential nutrients and removing toxins. Often CFS patients are overweight, which means there is stagnation and poor circulation. I often use the herb hawthorn (250 mg, three times daily) to improve blood circulation to the extremities (legs, feet, arms, hands). The herb *Ginkgo biloba* (120 mg, twice daily) enhances blood circulation to the brain and thereby improves memory. Regular exercise should be encouraged, too, as it stimulates circulation and, despite a patient's tiredness, the exertion will ultimately help them feel better.

A **bioflavonoid** is a pigment within plants and fruits that acts as an antioxidant to protect against damage from free radicals and excess oxygen. In the body, bioflavonoids enhance the beneficial activities of vitamin C, and are often formulated with this vitamin in supplement form. Originally called vitamin P until 1950, bioflavonoids include citrin, hesperidin, rutin, quercitin, epicatechin, flavones, and flavonols. When taken with vitamin C, bioflavonoids increase the absorption of vitamin C into the liver, kidneys, and adrenal glands. Acting as antioxidants, they also protect vitamin C from destruction by free radicals.

A **glandular extract** is a purified nutritional and therapeutic product derived from one of several animal glands, including the adrenal, thymus, thyroid, ovaries, testes, pancreas, pineal, and pituitary. It is prescribed by a physician for a person whose corresponding gland is underfunctioning and not producing enough of its own hormone. The various glands are part of the endocrine system, which, along with the nervous system, coordinates the functioning of all of the body's systems.

**3. Immune System.** You need to support the immune system, but it's tunnel vision to assume that it is only the immune system that has anything to do with healing. The immune system is not separate from the body's other systems and the body itself does not know of an "immune" system distinct from all its other operations. They are interconnected.

> Clinically, the bottom line is that when we treat many chronically fatigued people, basing treatment on the assumption of an underactive thyroid, they get much better, thereby confirming the diagnosis.
> — *Raphael Kellman, M.D.*

As discussed above, astragalus (500 mg, twice daily) and vitamin C (500 mg, four times daily) with grape seed extract (200 mg daily) are indicated as excellent immune supporters. In addition, Siberian ginseng (500 mg daily) combined with a liver extract has been shown to enhance the activity of T lymphocytes (white blood cells). To gain this advantage, Tonya took Aqueous Liver Extract (which contains vitamin B12), Siberian ginseng extract, and 11,000 mg of raw liver (but free of fat or cholesterol) in each capsule. Also helpful and regular features of my program are echinacea (250 mg, four times daily), coenzyme Q10, and, on occasion, garlic.

**4. Central Nervous System.** This approach to supporting the central nervous system is sometimes called neurotransmitter precursor therapy. Neurotransmitters (SEE QUICK DEFINITION) are key brain chemicals that convey important functional "messages," while precursors are substances—often amino acids (protein building blocks)—necessary for synthesizing the brain chemicals. There are clinical grounds for suggesting that in some chronic fatigue patients a neurotransmitter deficiency is a contributing factor.

Specifically, I find chronic fatigue patients deficient in norepinephrine, serotonin, and dopamine. This helps explain the problems in mental functioning and processing often encountered in these patients. It's common for such patients to have trouble concentrating and remembering. They sometimes feel mentally bombarded by external noises and cannot filter out extraneous sounds from essential ones

 **QUICK DEFINITION**

A **neurotransmitter** is a brain chemical with the specific function of enabling communications to happen between brain cells. Chief among the 100 identified to date are acetylcholine, gamma-aminobutyric acid (GABA), serotonin, dopamine, and norepinephrine. Acetylcholine is required for short-term memory and all muscle contractions. GABA works to stop excess nerve signals and thus keeps brain firings from getting out of control; serotonin does the same and helps produce sleep, regulate pain, and influence mood, although too much serotonin can produce depression. Norepinephrine is an excitatory neurotransmitter.

## Some Key Supplements in Tonya's Nutritional Program

**N-acetyl cysteine (NAC)** is an antioxidant made from the amino acid cysteine that works against cellular damage caused by toxins and free radicals; specifically, NAC can protect the liver from toxicity derived from drugs and chemical exposures.

**DMAE (dimethyl amino ethanol)** is a mind-enhancing, nervous system-restoring nutrient normally present in small amounts in the human brain and abundant in sardines and anchovies. It is believed to help elevate mood, improve memory, concentration, and learning, aid sleeping at night, and increase daytime energy.

**Milk thistle (silymarin)** is often suggested for cases of chronic hepatitis and drug-induced liver disease. As a potent antioxidant, it protects the liver, which is the second largest organ in the body and is responsible for processing all nutrients, toxins, and drugs.

**Lecithin** (found in grains, beans, and egg yolks) is an excellent source of choline, which is needed to make the brain chemical acetylcholine and to help metabolize fats; if there is insufficient choline in the body, fats get trapped in the liver and block metabolism.

**Inositol** (a fiber component) is considered a B vitamin; it works closely with choline—especially in cases of liver disorders, diabetes, and depression—and helps remove fats from the liver, preventing stagnation of liver fats and bile.

**Phosphatidylcholine** (a combination of two fatty acids, choline and phosphate) is needed to maintain cell membranes and to help reduce multiple liver symptoms from hepatitis and cirrhosis, and fatty liver from alcohol or diabetes.

(such as a human voice). This, in turn, increases their stress and anxiety levels.

When you increase the levels of precursors required to make the key brain chemicals, this increases the patient's brain energy levels and general cognitive abilities. The amino acids tyrosine (which I give at 500 to 2,000 mg daily) and phenylalanine (500 to 1,000 mg daily) are precursors to dopamine and norepinephrine. When giving these amino acids, you must also provide vitamin B6 and vitamin C, which are needed for the body to convert the precursors to neurotransmitters.

When patients respond to this form of treatment, it confirms our diagnosis and also shows that, for them at least, the source of chronic fatigue is in the brain. Patients with reduced libido respond especially well to enhancing dopamine levels, while memory and cognitive problems seem associated with deficiencies of either norepinephrine or acetylcholine. To boost mental performance, acetylcholine, choline, lecithin, DMAE (300 to 500 mg daily), and N-acetyl cysteine (100 to 400 mg daily) are helpful.

Some chronic fatigue patients also have a problem with their liver, called fatty infiltration, which means too much fat is deposited in the liver. Often patients with this problem are overweight because they can't metabolize fat. Nutrients helpful in reversing this are milk thistle (70 to 140 mg, three times daily), lecithin (12 mg, three times daily), inositol (600 mg daily), and phosphatidylcholine (1,200 mg, four times daily).

So this was Tonya's complete program, which I introduced in stages. She responded excellently at the point we added the central nervous system component. That made a big difference. After six weeks, she was about 80% improved. After about four months on the program, Tonya was completely recovered. Her successful outcome, joined with that of many other patients, convinces me that a broader theory of health is emerging to embrace the idea that a web of causes leads people to illness—and that we need a web of treatments to achieve wellness.

### "The Meaning Dimension"

In some cases, a patient's response to treatment is not as good as it could be. There seems to be something preventing their body from responding better. Often, I discover that the source is what I call "the meaning dimension." When people have a decreased sense of meaning in their lives, that lack of meaning can be a prime cause of the physical problem and interfere with treatment. This is a clear demonstration of the interrelatedness of the body, mind, and spirit. It is difficult to reverse a chronic illness without restoring health on all three levels, as Katerina's case shows.

Katerina, 54, complained of chronic fatigue. I put her on our nutritional and detoxification program, yet she did not respond well to the treatment, even after several months. Although Katerina did not complain of depression, I sensed that she felt her life was virtually meaningless. To provoke a strong emotional response as a basis for finding meaning in her life, I suggested she watch Steven Spielberg's movie *Schindler's List*, which is about Holocaust victims in 1940s Europe. At first, Katerina thought this would depress her, but the morning after watching the film, she woke feeling energized. She had rediscovered the meaning dimension.

Nobody complains of fatigue when they have just won the lottery. Similarly, you don't feel fatigued in moments of compassion, joy, laughter, or grief—moments in which life feels meaningful. Katerina saw that she did not have enough of these moments in her life, but that she could if she chose to. Katerina eventually changed her job but, in the short term, she began experiencing life differently, with a new attitude, and it was this attitude shift and the emergence of personal meaning in her life that made all the difference in Katerina's recovery. Within three months, she was free from fatigue. Mere recognition of the lack of meaning—bringing the problem to the forefront—is often sufficient to release the hold on the body and allow it to respond to treatment.

## The Importance of Pinpointing Thyroid Dysfunction

The following two cases show how pinpointing thyroid dysfunction can lead to a successful reversal of all the patient's symptoms. The first case, from Raphael Kellman, M.D., shows the importance of using the correct test to prove thyroid dysfunction.

### Year-Long Extreme Fatigue

Mona, 42, had suffered with extreme fatigue for a year. Waking in the morning, after eight to ten hours of sleep, she would feel more tired than when she went to bed, and during the day she often needed a nap. While she ate relatively little, Mona was steadily gaining weight, and she also experienced bloating, constipation, and occasional abdominal pains; her skin was dry; her hair was thinning; her menstruation was irregular and was preceded by PMS. Mona also reported that she had difficulty concentrating, was forgetful, and felt depressed, even though she had no strong psychological or emotional reasons for it.

When Mona's conventional physician performed a routine thyroid hormone test (for T3 and T4 levels), the results came back "normal." Although, on the basis of these results, she was advised to "rest and not worry," Mona thought otherwise, and sought a different thyroid test to measure TSH levels. But this test yielded "normal" results, too. Mona's

### Iodine, the Thyroid, and the Goiter Belt

Iodine is essential to forming normal amounts of thyroxine (T4); as long as one consumes roughly the U.S. RDA of 150 mcg of iodine, the thyroid gland should be able to make all the T4 it needs. In the early 1970s, U.S. health authorities referred to the "goiter belt," meaning those regions in the U.S., mostly in the Midwest, in which the incidence of goiter (enlarged thyroid gland) was unusually high. This problem was later traced to iodine deficiency.

Since that time, most people in the U.S. have used iodized table salt, from which they obtain the minuscule amount of iodine needed to keep their thyroid gland theoretically healthy and functional. Yet today there is still a high incidence of thyroid problems, or "hidden hypothyroidism," despite dietary fortification with iodized salt. For a variety of reasons, the thyroid gland of an increasing number of people is becoming dangerously underactive, upsetting systems throughout the body and mind.

doctor, noticing her anxiety and depression, wrote her a prescription for Prozac.

"Her life seemed to be spiraling downward," comments Dr. Kellman. "Her depression subsided a little on the Prozac, but her fatigue, weight, and other problems got worse." Dr. Kellman immediately ran the TRH thyroid test on Mona; her TSH level was 22 after stimulation, objectively indicating an underactive thyroid. He started Mona on Synthroid (a synthetic form of T4) and Thyrostim (a natural supplement containing amino acids, vitamins, and thyroid extract) to convert T4 to T3.

In addition, Mona began a nutritional program to help her body regain normal thyroid function. Dr. Kellman observes, "It's not enough to replace the low T4 with synthetics. The underlying causes of the underactive thyroid must be addressed as well." Many of these causes—including nutrient deficiencies, overload of toxins and free radicals, hormonal imbalances (such as high cortisol), and mental and physical stress—benefit from improvements in diet and nutrition. By adding the nutritional program, Dr. Kellman was able to gradually lower Mona's doses of Synthroid and eventually stop the medication altogether.

 **Raphael Kellman, M.D.**, is an internist who blends conventional and holistic/alternative medicine, a fusion he calls "post-modern medicine." He also holds a degree in philosophy. He can be contacted at the Kellman Center for Progressive Medicine, 124 East 36th Street, New York, NY 10016; tel: (866) 432-5123. Website: www.kellmancenter.com.

EDITOR'S NOTE

"Within two weeks Mona began to feel more energy and more alive," notes Dr. Kellman. "A few weeks later, her brain fog began to lift and her attention span was significantly better. In no time, she was back to her old self and began noticing weight loss and thicker, fuller hair, and her skin was normal again. Soon her periods were more regular and her PMS became tolerable, and in six weeks, Mona's mood was much better and her energy level was, in her words, 'The best I can ever remember.'"

### Burgeoning Fatigue Following Pregnancy

The second case involving an underactive thyroid comes from Martin Feldman, M.D., who practices in New York City.

Mara, 32, gave birth after an untroubled pregnancy, but three weeks after delivery, she began to notice a drop in her energy. By mid-afternoon every day, Mara needed a nap, and she had to rest again in the early evening; in addition, she developed an intolerance to cold. The energy drain progressed steadily for the next three months, at which point she consulted Dr. Feldman. Mara told him that prior to her pregnancy, she had not experienced any of these symptoms.

Routine blood tests for Mara's thyroid function (T3, T4, and TSH) came back "normal." This is a common problem, observes Dr. Feldman. "The blood levels are fine, but the thyroid is not right." To refine his diagnostic picture of Mara's thyroid function, Dr. Feldman ran an antimicrosomal antibody test and an antithyroglobulin antibody test, but these also yielded supposedly normal results. Both of these tests measure the body's possible autoimmune response to its own thyroglobulin (a protein present in the thyroid gland), thereby indicating a thyroid imbalance.

Finally, Dr. Feldman had Mara do the basal body temperature test for thyroid function by placing a thermometer under her arm as soon as she woke up in the morning and before getting out of bed. Her temperature was lower than the norm for this test (97.7° F), thereby confirming some degree of thyroid sluggishness. As a corollary, Dr. Feldman ran Mara through the Ragland Postural Blood Pressure test. For this, you rest horizontally for five minutes and your blood pressure is recorded, explains Dr. Feldman. Then you stand up and your blood pressure is recorded again. In a healthy person, the values increase slightly, or remain constant. In Mara's case, her blood systolic pressure (measured when the heart contracts, as opposed to diastolic, when the heart rests and fills with more blood) dropped slightly, indicating that her adrenal gland function was suboptimal.

Knowing that both thyroid and adrenals were underfunctioning, Dr. Feldman recommended certain key "repair ingredients to allow the thyroid to put itself back into optimal function." His preference, which he achieves in two thirds of his cases, is to avoid giving the external pharmaceutical form of thyroid hormone because the drug does the natural work of the thyroid and the thyroid will shut down. The body then becomes dependent on the pharmaceutical thyroid hormone.

To start his thyroid revival program, Dr. Feldman prescribed a liquid herbal blend called #8THY, containing skullcap, parsley, uva ursi, and dulse. As a starting dose, Dr. Feldman advised Mara to put five drops of the tincture in very warm but not boiling water, then let it sit for perhaps ten minutes for the alcohol in the tincture to evaporate. Mara took this blend at the rate of five drops, three times daily, then progressed to ten and eventually 15 drops, three times daily.

Next, Dr. Feldman gave Mara the mineral selenium (200 mcg daily

> If Mara had been on conventional drugs, she might have felt
> some improvement, but no permanent improvement, because
> it wouldn't have addressed "the root cause—an underactive
> thyroid."                                    —Martin Feldman, M.D.

to start, building to 400 mcg) to enhance the conversion of T4 to T3. Glutathione is an amino acid that also helps in this conversion of thyroid hormone, although the dosage must be determined individually, says Dr. Feldman. He also gave Mara zinc picolinate (22 mg to start, then increasing) because zinc is part of the thyroid formation system; riboflavin, or vitamin B2 (75 mg daily), as it also helps convert T4 to T3; the amino acid L-tyrosine (500 mg daily, building to 1,000 mg), because it's needed to produce thyroid hormone; the mineral rubidium (80 mcg daily in four divided doses) to help the L-tyrosine; and glutamic acid (variable dosage) to help the glutathione.

The third element of Dr. Feldman's thyroid revival program was a homeopathic sarcode called Thyroid Plus. A sarcode is a homeopathic preparation made from animal tissue or secretions—in this case, from an animal's thyroid. Thyroid Plus, which contains 11 different homeopathically prepared substances, comes in drop form and must be taken directly in the mouth, not mixed with water, says Dr. Feldman. Mara took this at the rate of 5 drops, three times daily, building to 10 drops, then to 15 drops.

Dr. Feldman's fourth element involved glandular supplements. He gave Mara Thytrophin PMG, which is thyroid hormone from cows

**Martin Feldman, M.D.:** 132 East 76th Street, New York, NY 10021; tel: (212) 744-4413.

processed to remove its thyroxine, making it a food, not a hormone, he says. Mara took four tablets daily, then increased to six (each containing 45 mg). Dr. Feldman emphasizes that the dosage and even the selection of a thyroid glandular is highly specific to the individual patient. Finally, to reset the adrenal glands, Dr. Feldman started Mara on an adrenal supplement.

Progress came quickly for Mara. After ten weeks on this multifaceted program, her energy had returned to normal and her basal body temperature was within the normal range. If Mara had been on conventional drugs, she might have felt some improvement, but no permanent improvement because it wouldn't have addressed "the root cause—an underactive thyroid," says Dr. Feldman.

## Reversing a Case of CFS Linked with Hypothyroidism

Clark, 53, enjoyed an active lifestyle—jogging, playing golf, and lifting weights—until chronic fatigue syndrome brought his fitness regimen to a halt. Over the course of a few months, Clark developed severe fatigue, headaches, night sweats, sensitivity to light and cold, low body temperature, short-term memory loss, and disorganized thought processes. He received a diagnosis of CFS. Clark sought the help of Jesse Stoff, M.D., of Tucson, Arizona, co-author of *Chronic Fatigue Syndrome: The Hidden Epidemic* (Dr. Stoff's protocols were the subject of chapter 1). "After I read his book," Clark says, "I felt that he was the doctor to help me fight and eventually beat this disease." In fact, Clark was so impressed with Dr. Stoff's writings on the subject that he moved from Washington state to Tucson to undergo his treatment.

To determine the cause of Clark's CFS, Dr. Stoff ran extensive blood tests. The tests showed that Clark had numerous vitamin and mineral deficiencies, in addition to hypothyroidism and candidiasis. Based on this information, Dr. Stoff prescribed a treatment plan that combined thyroid hormone, herbal remedies, vitamin supplements, diet, and stress reduction. After two years with Dr. Stoff, Clark's fatigue had been reduced considerably, but he still experienced constant symptoms. Not satisfied with only partial recovery, Dr. Stoff referred Clark to John Dommisse, M.D., another Tucson physician who has had success in treating CFS.

Dr. Dommisse determined that, while Clark's T3 level had improved under Dr. Stoff's care, his T4 was still low. Adding T4 supplements to Clark's treatment was "one of the main contributions I was able to make to Clark's recovery," Dr. Dommisse observes. He also identified and corrected a few remaining vitamin and mineral deficiencies. Following these final adjustments in treatment, Clark was able to go back to jogging, playing golf, and lifting weights several times a week. "I give total credit for my full recovery to Doctors Stoff and Dommisse," Clark says. "I feel positive that this disease has been beaten and that my future will be CFS free."[1]

## Testing "Normal" but Still Feeling Exhausted

Bette, 47, felt drained of energy all the time. Her body temperature registered subnormal (95° F to 96° F) in the morning and even though she ate a low-fat diet and exercised six times weekly, she was unable to lose weight—both are typical signs of hypothyroidism. At 188 pounds, which was far too much weight for her height, Bette was troubled with constantly sore feet. In addition, she suffered from a chronic infection, skin problems, and depression.

Bette's physician ran a TSH test to check her thyroid, but the results came back "normal." In his mind, this resolved the question of hypothyroidism. Instead of testing further, he suggested she try Weight Watchers and put her on a conventional weight-loss drug. The drug lowered her blood pressure to dangerous levels (78/57; an average healthy reading is 120/80).

Consultation with John Dommisse, M.D., set Bette on a different course. "I would never use the TSH blood level as the sole test for screening for hypothyroidism or monitoring its treatment," says Dr. Dommisse. He reports that he usually treats for hypothyroidism if the TSH results are even in the middle of the normal range (greater than 2 mIU) and that, provided the thyroid treatment is not excessive, he "always sees a definite clinical advantage to this approach." Dr. Dommisse ran three thyroid tests (Free-T3, Free-T4, and 3rd-Generation TSH) on Bette to more accurately assess the state of her thyroid. While the results for Free-T4 and 3rd-Generation TSH were in the normal range, Bette's Free-T3 was below normal. Tests on vitamin and mineral status revealed that Bette was deficient in zinc, manganese, vitamin B12, and chromium, but had an excess of copper.

Dr. Dommisse started Bette on supplements to redress her nutrient deficiencies. He advised her not to drink her tap water or use it in cooking because the copper plumbing in her house was the likely source of the excess copper in her body. For thyroid imbalances, Dr. Dommisse typically relies on combinations of T4 (Levoxyl, Synthroid), T3 (Cyto-mel), and Armour Thyroid (natural desiccated hog thyroid). He finds these effective, especially when the Free-T3 level is lower than the Free-T4, as in Bette's case.

Within a few months of starting Dr. Dommisse's program, Bette's

 **John V. Dommisse, M.D.:** 1840 East River Road, Suite 210, Cambric Corporate Center, Tucson, AZ 85718; tel: (520) 577-1940. Website: www.johndommissemd.com. **Leonard Haimes, M.D.:** Haimes Centre Clinic, 7300 North Federal Highway, Suite #100, Boca Raton, FL 35487; tel: (561) 995-8484. For **doctors knowledgeable in HGH therapy**, contact: The American Academy of Anti-Aging Medicine, 1510 West Montana Street, Chicago, IL 60614; tel: (773) 528-1000. Website: www.worldhealth.net.

fatigue disappeared, her infection and skin problems cleared up, her depression lifted, she lost 50 pounds, and her feet no longer hurt.[2]

## Human Growth Hormone in the Treatment of CFS

The proper balance of hormones is vital to health. An underactive thyroid can lead to a hormonal imbalance or deficiency that can, in turn, lead to CFS. But CFS patients who suffer from an underactive thyroid may find relief in a new technique that is starting to catch on with physicians nationwide: human growth hormone (HGH) therapy. According to Leonard Haimes, M.D., medical director of the Haimes Centre Clinic in Boca Raton, Florida, who devoted six months to a thorough review of the research on HGH, recent research shows an expanding range of conditions for which HGH appears effective, including thyroid problems and chronic fatigue.

Adults who have an underactive thyroid gland appear to be deficient in growth hormone, says Dr. Haimes. When such patients are given adequate

## What Is Human Growth Hormone?

Human growth hormone (HGH), naturally secreted by the pituitary gland in the brain, is a small protein-like hormone similar to insulin. HGH is secreted in very brief pulses during the early hours of sleep and remains in circulation for only a few minutes. During adolescence, when growth is most rapid, production of HGH is high. After age 20, HGH production declines progressively at an average rate of about 14% per decade; by age 60, it is not uncommon to measure a growth hormone loss of 75% or more.

Originally, growth hormone, which consists of 191 amino acids (protein building blocks), was used in the early 1980s to correct disturbances in normal growth; later it was synthesized for adult use. Benefits from HGH include increased muscle mass, improved physical strength, reduced fatigue, decreased fat (especially abdominal fat), increased bone strength, revitalization of liver, kidney, spleen, and brain functions, increased exercise capacity, improved kidney blood flow and efficiency, improved cardiac function, reduced risk from cardiovascular problems, and a general enhancement in the sense of well-being.

HGH, they show gains in energy, muscle strength and mass, mental abilities, and psychological attitude. For those CFS sufferers who have been diagnosed with an underactive thyroid, HGH therapy can replace the growth hormone they've lost as a result, thereby restoring energy and stamina to their bodies. The short-term therapeutic effects of HGH (foremost among which is its ability to stabilize the immune system) are impressive, says Dr. Haimes. One of his patients, a 33-year-old man, had suffered from chronic fatigue syndrome for three years, yet after only 20 days of HGH therapy (about ten injections), he was able to return to work, his symptoms alleviated.

HGH is not an altered product, such as a bioengineered tomato in which the genetic structure has been changed, Dr. Haimes explains. Rather, it is grown or duplicated from the "genetic blueprint" of the naturally occurring hormone found in the human pituitary gland; thus, it is identical to it. HGH therapy is expensive (it can cost $250 a week), but there are many who regard this investment in health as well worth the money.

# seven

# Eliminating Heavy Metal Toxicity

*Your Mercury Fillings May Be Fatiguing You*

The cases discussed in previous chapters show how mercury toxicity contributes to chronic fatigue, immune breakdown, and hypothyroidism. These are just a few of the health disorders associated with dental mercury amalgam, yet the amalgam is still widely used in the United States to fill cavities in teeth. Euphemistically called "silver" fillings, mercury amalgam fillings are actually only 35% silver. Mercury, a heavy metal, makes up 50% of the mix, with tin (9%), copper (6%), and a trace of zinc comprising the rest. Mercury amalgams have been used in dentistry since the 1820s; every year, more than 100 million mercury amalgam fillings are put into the mouths of U.S. dental patients, despite the fact that, in 1988, the Environmental Protection Agency (EPA) declared scrap dental amalgam a hazardous waste.

Even the American Dental Association (ADA), which has so far refused to ban amalgams, now instructs dentists to "know the potential hazards and symptoms of mercury exposure such as the development of sensitivity and neuropathy," to use a no-touch technique for handling the amalgam, and to store it under liquid, preferably glycerin or radiographic fixer solution, in unbreakable, tightly sealed containers.[1]

Evidence now shows that mercury amalgams are the major source of mercury exposure for the general public, at rates six times higher than mercury from fish and seafood. Studies by the World Health Organization show that a single amalgam can release 3 to 17 mcg of mercury per day. A Danish study of a random sample of 100 men and 100 women showed that increased blood mercury levels were related to the presence of more than four amalgam fillings in the teeth.

Mercury toxicity has been shown to have destructive contributory effects on kidney function and in cardiovascular disease, neuropsychological dysfunction, reproductive disorders, and birth defects, to name a few. Symptoms of mercury toxicity make a very long list: anorexia, depression, fatigue, insomnia, arthritis, multiple sclerosis, moodiness, irritability, memory loss, nausea, diarrhea, gum disease, swollen glands, headaches, and many more. Following are a few highly revealing case presentations in which mercury toxicity played a major role in the development of chronic fatigue.

## Success Stories: CFS Reversed by Mercury Amalgam Removal

The following are clinical accounts of people whose chronic fatigue syndrome was dramatically reversed after they had their mercury amalgam dental fillings removed.

### All Symptoms Gone

After he underwent a root canal procedure at the age of 15, Earl suffered severe fatigue and anxiety. At 28, he had a nervous breakdown. At the age of 32, suffering from fatigue, anger, anxiety, back problems, low blood sugar, nervousness, ringing in his ears, concentration loss, and prematurely graying hair, he consulted acupuncturist David J. Nickel, O.M.D., L.Ac., of Santa Monica, California. Dr. Nickel performed a mercury vapor analysis on Earl's teeth and found that the level of toxic fumes from Earl's six mercury amalgam fillings was 42 times higher than the Environmental Protection Agency's maximum allowable limit. A hair analysis indicated that Earl also had aluminum, copper, and mercury at toxic levels in his tissues and that he had an exceptionally slow metabolic rate.

Dr. Nickel put Earl on a nutritional supplement program, after which there was significant improvement in his metabolic rate and blood sugar levels, but limited improvement in his other symptoms. After Earl had all six mercury amalgams and his root-canal tooth removed, he began to experience major changes, states Dr. Nickel. In a month, his energy level returned to near what he had enjoyed over 15 years earlier and he was able to exercise, work, and play strenuously with no exhaustion. His other symptoms improved as well. "I don't remember when I have ever felt so good," Earl said.

> Almost all my patients who have had their mercury-based fillings removed show moderate to dramatic improvement in their health in usually less than one month.
>
> — *David J. Nickel, O.M.D., L.Ac.*

According to Dr. Nickel, removal of the mercury fillings and root canal filling was responsible for Earl's return to health. "Of the 90% of my patients with amalgam dental fillings, most have a mercury-induced copper toxicity, high calcium levels, and reduced thyroid and adrenal function," states Dr. Nickel. "Mercury is associated with 258 different symptoms and copper with over 100. Almost all my patients who have had their mercury-based fillings removed show moderate to dramatic improvement in their health in usually less than one month."[2]

**David J. Nickel, O.M.D., L.Ac.:** 1530 Lincoln Boulevard, Suite E, Santa Monica, CA 90401; tel: (310) 396-0175. Website: www .primezyme. com. Dr. Nickel is the author of *700+ Quick Fixes, Nutritional Reference Manual* (Santa Monica, CA: Health Acu Press, 1994).

### Reversing Seven Years of Chronic Fatigue

By the time he came to acupuncturist M. M. van Benschoten, O.M.D., of Reseda, California, Albert, age 37, had been beset by chronic fatigue syndrome for seven years. He reported headaches, chest pain, fatigue, lymph node swelling, muscle aches, irritability, and light-headedness. Although Albert had elevated blood levels of Epstein-Barr virus, normally associated with chronic fatigue syndrome, Dr. van Benschoten's analysis of Albert's acupuncture meridians (SEE QUICK DEFINITION) showed several bacterial and viral infections capable of producing his symptoms.

In addition, he found mercury toxicity from dental amalgams to be the fundamental underlying cause of the suppression of Albert's immune system. To arrive at this conclusion, Dr. van Benschoten used a diagnostic technique in an analytical approach called "acupoint biophoton diagnostics." He explains that toxic metals, such as mercury, interfere with the normal energy

**Acupuncture meridians** are specific pathways in the human body for the flow of life force or subtle energy, known as *qi* ("chee"). Typically, meridians run up and down both sides of the body and correspond to individual organs or organ systems. There are twelve major meridian pathways and eight secondary ones. Over a thousand points of heightened *qi* energy, known as acupoints, exist on the body's surface along the meridian pathways.

Toxic metals, such as mercury, interfere with the normal energy patterns in various acupuncture pathways. Harmful energies set up interference patterns ("biophoton" emissions) in the meridians, according to Dr. van Benschoten, shown here testing patients' energy patterns.

patterns in various acupuncture channels; harmful energies set up interference patterns in the meridians.

Dr. van Benschoten prescribed a series of Chinese herbs to clear the bacterial, viral, and heavy metals, including chrysanthemum, angelica dahurica, isatis, bupleurum, cnidium, astragalus, salvia, platycodon, siler, taraxacum, ligustrum lucidum, and fructus lycium. After taking these herbs for six weeks, Albert was headache free and had relief from fatigue and chest pain. The degree to which mercury toxicity was interfering with his energy pathways also was reduced. Three months later, Albert had 14 mercury amalgams removed.

To contact **M. M. van Benschoten, O.M.D.**: 19231 Victory Boulevard, Suite 151, Reseda, CA 91335; tel: (818) 344-9973.

However, on Albert's next visit, Dr. van Benschoten found that the mercury interference had increased. "Overzealous removal of all amalgam fillings can significantly increase the patient's mercury levels if done without adequate precautions during amalgam removal and proper mercury detoxification therapy," notes Dr. van Benschoten. He instructs his patients to wear an oxygen mask during amalgam removal, in addition to having their dentists use a rubber dam and high-speed suction with water.

After mercury amalgam removal, Chinese herbal medicines can successfully detoxify the patient and restore immune function, says Dr. van Benschoten. For Albert, he prescribed a second series of herbs, including moutan, taraxacum, prunella, glycyrrhiza, grifola, ligustrum lucidum, and verbena to clear the mercury from his system. After taking them for several months, Albert reported that he was free from chronic fatigue and had a stronger resistance to infection.[3]

 For those contemplating removal of their mercury dental fillings, extreme care must be taken to protect the body from mercury poisoning during the amalgam removal process. Further, mercury residues throughout the body must be carefully removed through the use of some form of chelating agent—such as garlic, seaweeds, vitamin C, and the like—that will bind with the mercury and help to remove it safely from the body.

## The Toxic Dangers of Mercury Fillings

Some dentists, such as Richard D. Fischer, D.D.S., of Annandale, Virginia, refuse to work with mercury amalgams. Dr. Fischer even had his own silver fillings removed to make the point. "I don't feel comfortable using a substance designated by the Environmental Protection Agency to be a waste-disposal hazard," he says. "I can't throw it in the trash, bury it in the ground, or put it in a landfill, but they say it's okay to put it in people's mouths. That doesn't make sense."

The use of mercury in fillings is banned or severely curtailed in many European countries. According to the German Ministry of Health, "Amalgam is considered a health risk from a medical viewpoint due to the release of mercury vapor."[4] But for a long time, the ADA asserted that the mercury amalgam was a tightly bound chemical complex that would not permit any leakage or release of mercury. This was conclusively proven wrong in 1985 when studies showed that the air inside a mouth with mercury fillings continually contained elemental mercury vapor and that chewing substantially increased this vapor level. Amalgams can also erode and corrode with time (ideally they should be replaced after seven to ten years), adding to their toxic output. Studies by the World Health Organization (WHO) show that a single amalgam can release 3 to 17 micrograms of mercury per day.[5]

Since mercury vapors are continuously released from amalgam fill-

> I don't feel comfortable using a substance designated by the Environmental Protection Agency to be a waste-disposal hazard. I can't throw it in the trash, bury it in the ground, or put it in a landfill, but they say it's okay to put it in people's mouths. That doesn't make sense.  — *Richard D. Fischer, D.D.S.*

ings, as long as you have mercury dental fillings, you inhale mercury vapor 24 hours a day, 365 days a year. The resulting level of mercury in the body has serious health consequences. Research has demonstrated that the body's tissues—especially in the brain, kidneys, jaw, lungs, gastrointestinal tract, and liver—absorb and store mercury. Mercury toxicity has been shown to have destructive effects on kidney function and contribute to cardiovascular disease, neuropsychological dysfunction, reproductive disorders, and birth defects, to name a few. Like other heavy metals, mercury has been shown to cause damage to the lining of arteries. This means that if amalgam fillings are present, your circulatory system is constantly being exposed to the damaging effects of this heavy metal. It's interesting to note that cardiovascular disease has become widespread only since the 1920s, about the time of increased use of heavy metals in dental therapy, but long after humans began consuming eggs, meat, milk, butter, and cheese, which are commonly thought to contribute to heart disease.

According to Edward Arana, D.D.S., president of the American Academy of Biological Dentistry, in Carmel Valley, California, among the other problems caused specifically by mercury amalgam fillings are:

- Chronic fatigue syndrome and lack of energy
- Tendency toward chronic inflammatory changes, including fibromyalgia, rheumatoid arthritis, and phlebitis
- Chronic neurological illnesses, especially when numbness is one of the leading symptoms
- Lowering of the pain threshold
- Disturbances of the immune system

Mercury poisoning can also lead to symptoms such as anxiety, depression, confusion, irritability, and the inability to concentrate, all of which are symptoms of CFS. Such poisoning often goes undetected for years

## Select Symptom Analysis of 1,569 Patients Who Eliminated Mercury Amalgam Fillings

The following represents a summary of 1,569 patients in six different studies evaluating the health effects of replacing mercury-containing dental fillings with non-mercury fillings. The data was derived from the following sources: 762 Patient Adverse Reaction Reports submitted to the U.S. Food and Drug Administration by patients and 807 patients' reports from Sweden, Denmark, Canada, and the U.S.

| % of Total Reporting | Symptom | Number Reporting | Number Improved or Cured | % of Cure or Improvement |
|---|---|---|---|---|
| 14% | Allergy | 221 | 196 | 89% |
| 5 | Anxiety | 86 | 80 | 93 |
| 5 | Bad temper | 81 | 68 | 84 |
| 6 | Bloating | 88 | 70 | 80 |
| 6 | Blood pressure problems | 99 | 53 | 54 |
| 5 | Chest pains | 79 | 69 | 87 |
| 22 | Depression | 347 | 315 | 91 |
| 22 | Dizziness | 343 | 301 | 88 |
| 45 | Fatigue | 705 | 603 | 86 |
| 15 | Intestinal problems | 231 | 192 | 83 |
| 8 | Gum problems | 129 | 121 | 94 |
| 34 | Headaches | 531 | 460 | 87 |
| 12 | Insomnia | 187 | 146 | 78 |
| 10 | Irregular heartbeat | 159 | 139 | 87 |
| 8 | Irritability | 132 | 119 | 90 |
| 17 | Lack of concentration | 270 | 216 | 80 |
| 6 | Lack of energy | 91 | 88 | 97 |
| 17 | Memory loss | 265 | 193 | 73 |
| 17 | Metallic taste | 260 | 247 | 95 |
| 7 | Multiple sclerosis | 113 | 86 | 76 |
| 8 | Muscle tremor | 126 | 104 | 82 |

*Source:* Ziff, S. "Consolidated Symptom Analysis of 1,569 Patients." *Bio-Probe Newsletter* 9:2 (March 1993), 7–8.

because the symptoms presented do not necessarily suggest mercury as the initiating cause.

Charles Gableman, M.D., a former practitioner of environmental medicine, now living in Lake Forest, California, always advised the removal of his patients' amalgam fillings. Patients with chronic fatigue

> Patients with chronic fatigue syndrome or with allergies, thyroid dysfunction, or a lack of resistance to infections all improve after their fillings are properly removed.
>
> — *Charles Gableman, M.D.*

syndrome or with allergies, thyroid dysfunction, or a lack of resistance to infections all improve after their fillings are properly removed, says Dr. Gableman. He believes it is possible that these patients have suffered from basic allergies their entire lives, and that the mercury toxicity from the fillings simply adds to the body's toxic load and "pushes them over the edge," resulting in chronic medical problems.

 **Biological dentistry** stresses the use of nontoxic restoration materials for dental work and focuses on the unrecognized impact that dental toxins and hidden dental infections can have on overall health. Typically, a biological dentist will emphasize the following: the safe removal of mercury amalgams; in many cases, either the avoidance or removal of root canal fillings; the investigation of possible jawbone infections (cavitations) as a "dental focus" or source of body-wide illness centered in the teeth; and the health-injuring role of misalignment of teeth and jaw structures.

Extensive clinical evidence based on patient case histories from many alternative medicine doctors attests to the effects of mercury amalgam toxicity. For example, a patient of biological dentist (SEE QUICK DEFINITION) Hal Huggins, D.D.S., of Colorado Springs, Colorado, had for years endured fatigue, mononucleosis (for which she was hospitalized at age 16), bladder infections, and, eventually, Epstein-Barr virus, candidiasis, food allergies, and muscle spasms. Finally, her own investigation led her to consider the possibility of mercury poisoning and she consulted with Dr. Huggins. He found a tooth with a root canal that had been filled with a dental amalgam. Once the amalgam was removed, her symptoms abated.

### The Domino Effect of Mercury Toxicity

"When I see a patient with mercury fillings, I always think, 'It's the teeth, stupid!'" says Bruce Shelton, M.D., M.D.(H), Di.Hom., director of the Allergy Center in Phoenix, Arizona. "Mercury amalgams are as close as you can get to the center of the illness universe; their use in dentistry has set us up for most of the health problems we see today." In his practice, Dr. Shelton frequently observes a domino effect of illness that begins with mercury toxicity. He reports that 90% of his patients who come in with allergies have an overgrowth of the yeast-like fungus *Candida albi-*

## Exposing the Mercury Hazard in Your Mouth

A Danish dentist has added another valuable piece to the mounting evidence that mercury in dental fillings can be injurious to health.

H. Lichtenberg, D.D.S., of Hilleroed, Denmark, tested 103 of his dental patients, with an average age of 47, for oral mercury vapor emission from their mercury amalgams. Dr. Lichtenberg used a Jerome 413X mercury vapor analyzer (Texas Instruments). On average, each of the patients had at least 14 symptoms associated with mercury poisoning; each patient also had an average of 22 amalgam surfaces.

Dr. Lichtenberg found that the concentration of mercury vapor varied from 3 mcg/cubic meter of air to 329 mcg/m$^3$, with an average of 54.6. Individuals with mercury vapor readings exceeding 50 had an average of 26.8 mercury amalgam surfaces and 1.2 gold and/or porcelain fillings or crowns, while those whose readings were less than 50 had an average of 19.8 amalgam surfaces. In other words, the amount of amalgam surface per mouth is directly related to the amount of mercury vapor likely to be released.

In Denmark, levels up to but not exceeding 50 mcg/m$^3$ of mercury vapor are permitted in a workplace for people working 40 hours a week. Thus, with Dr. Lichtenberg's patients, the mercury exposure not only exceeded Denmark's "safe" amount, but it represented an exposure sustained for 168 hours a week (24 hours a day), indefinitely. Safety levels are relative, however, because Switzerland and Russia allow only 10 mcg/m$^3$; the U.S. allows 100 mcg/m$^3$. A recent Canadian conference proposed a Tolerable Daily Intake (TDI) for mercury of 1.0 mcg for a person weighing about 150 pounds. Dr. Licht-

enberg's patients, on average, were exposed to a TDI that was over 50 times this norm.

Dr. Lichtenberg also reported that more than half of his patients complained of one or more symptoms commonly associated with mercury toxicity, including general fatigue, headaches, irritability, poor memory and concentration, bloating, joint pain, cold hands and feet, and muscle fatigue. As the mercury vapor concentration values increased, so did symptoms of intestinal cramps, irritability, dizziness, and leg cramps, said Dr. Lichtenberg. "It would seem that the number of individual symptoms varies depending on the number of amalgam surfaces present," he stated.

Dr. Lichtenberg further reported that, since about 1976, dentists have tended to use an amalgam with 10% more copper content. However, this type of amalgam can release up to 50 times more mercury and copper vapor than older amalgam types, he says. Dr. Lichtenberg's research also demonstrated that patients with gold fillings or crowns and metal or porcelain crowns experienced a mixing of metals in the mouth that leads to additional corrosion of the mercury fillings, thereby releasing yet more mercury vapor. Summarizing his findings, Dr. Lichtenberg states that "mercury poisoning from the amalgam fillings is widespread throughout the population."

---

*Source:* Lichtenberg, H. "Mercury Vapor in the Oral Cavity in Relation to the Number of Amalgam Surfaces and the Classic Symptoms of Chronic Mercury Poisoning." *Journal of Orthomolecular Medicine* 11:2 (Second Quarter 1996), 87–94.

*cans.* This overgrowth can be due to heavy metals in the body, principally from mercury in the teeth, minute amounts of which continually drain into the body tissues, Dr. Shelton says. "The body is smart and wants to protect itself at all costs. One of the natural absorbers of heavy metal is *Candida*. The body attracts this yeast (and parasites) into the

Mercury amalgams are as close as you can get to the center of the illness universe; their use in dentistry has set us up for most of the health problems we see today.

—*Bruce Shelton, M.D., M.D.(H), Di.Hom.*

Bruce Shelton, M.D.,
M.D.(H), Di.Hom.

intestines to act as a natural sponge for the mercury. The body, in trying to protect itself against mercury, creates another problem—a yeast infestation."

The next stage of the domino effect is that patients in this predicament typically develop leaky gut syndrome. "If we do not totally digest and absorb our foods before they are broken to basic chemicals, then we have a 'leaky gut.' For example, a little piece of fish that is still chemically fish instead of amino acids will trigger an immune reaction." In this way, Dr. Shelton says, leaky gut syndrome leads, in turn, to food allergies. Soon the person becomes a universal reactor, allergic to multiple chemicals—to seemingly everything. Environmental illness is then the end-product of a string of health problems that stem from mercury and build, one upon the other.

"Although dental work tends to be very expensive, if you can get a patient to have their teeth corrected, they will get well," reports Dr. Shelton. Unfortunately, in his experience, only the more serious patients—the ones who have been scared by their illnesses—are generally willing to have the necessary dental work. Those who do not and retain their mercury fillings do improve, but often need six-month therapeutic "tune-ups," he says.

According to Dr. Shelton, mercury toxicity can also result in an underactive thyroid, another contributing factor to chronic fatigue. Specifically, in thyroid cases, the fifth tooth from the mouth's midline (between the two front teeth), upper and lower, in both directions, frequently has a mercury filling or a root canal, or is in a state of degeneration. In other words, potentially four different teeth can have a thyroid connection.

## How Mercury Disrupts the Body

Heavy metals such as mercury act as free radicals—highly reactive, charged particles that can cause damage to body tissues. Since mercury is a cumulative poison, building up in the body with repeated exposure,[6] its effects can be devastating. It can prevent nutrients from entering the cells and prevent wastes from leaving, and it can block enzymes necessary for the body's detoxification processes. Mercury can bind to the DNA (deoxyribonucleic acid) of cells, as well as to the cell membranes, distorting them and interfering with normal cell functions.[7] When this happens, the immune system no longer recognizes the cell as part of the body and will attack it. This is the basis of an autoimmune disease, of which CFS is one.

After elemental mercury from amalgam fillings is inhaled or ingested, it is converted to methylmercury, the organic form of mercury. Methylmercury, because it easily crosses the blood-brain barrier, has been associated with neurodegenerative diseases such as Alzheimer's, multiple sclerosis, and amyotrophic lateral sclerosis. It is important to mention that as toxic as elemental mercury is, methylmercury is 100 times more toxic. Once it has leached from the dental fillings and infiltrated the body, mercury becomes a neurotoxin, according to Dietrich Klinghardt, M.D., Ph.D., a leading specialist in neural therapy (SEE QUICK DEFINITION) based in Seattle, Washington. A neurotoxin is a substance that, strangely, the nerve cells voluntarily absorb, even though it is poisonous. They do this out of a natural function akin to curiosity, Dr. Klinghardt explains.

Nerve endings in the peripheral nervous system constantly scan their environment, engulfing foreign particles and bringing them across the cell membrane for inspection. "These substances may then travel all the way up from the foot to the spinal cord and get presented to the nerve cells there," he says. If the substance is judged to be harmful, the body tries to produce an antitoxin to neutralize it and eliminate it from the body.

But when it comes to mercury there are two problems with this func-

 **QUICK DEFINITION**

**Neural therapy** uses local injections of anesthetics, such as lidocaine or procaine, to remove interferences in the body's electrical network and thus relieve chronic pain, reverse injury, and clear energy blockages. The anesthetics are injected into nerve bundles in the autonomic nervous system, acupuncture points, scars, glands, and other tissues. By clearing the local site of interference, neural therapy helps to regulate energy throughout the body.

tion, Dr. Klinghardt cautions. "First, as it travels up the nerve, mercury destroys the body's mechanism, a substance called tubulin, for transporting along nerves. Burning the bridges behind it, as it were, it effectively destroys the nerve. Second, the body has not yet learned how to make an antineurotoxin against mercury."

Laboratory research using monkeys as subjects has shown that within 24 hours of injecting a minute dose of mercury into a muscle anywhere in the body, it is present in the spinal cord and brain. The mercury is also present in the kidneys, lungs, bloodstream, connective tissue, and adrenal and other endocrine glands. In the brain, it tends to congregate in the hypothalamus, which regulates the sympathetic nervous system, and in the limbic system (associated with the brainstem), believed to be the organic seat of emotions. While mercury levels slowly dissipate in a predictable amount of time from other body tissues and even from the teeth (in six weeks, its levels may be halved), mercury does not have a "half-life" in the nervous system or brain. Instead, it binds firmly to a specific chemical compound which happens to exist there in the body's highest concentrations.

"The main devastating effect of mercury in the nervous system is that it interferes with the energy production inside each cell," says Dr. Klinghardt. "The nerve cell is impaired in its ability to detoxify itself [and excrete the mercury] and in its ability to nurture itself. The cell becomes toxic and dies, or lives in a state of chronic malnutrition. A multitude of illnesses, usually associated with neurological symptoms, result." Among these are chronic viral and fungal illnesses, recurrent episodes of bacterial infections, and chronic fatigue.

Dr. Klinghardt speculates that by a curious self-preservation reflex of the body, the emergence of these conditions can be viewed as a way of accommodating the heavy metal presence. "Most, if not all, chronic infectious diseases are caused not by a failure of the immune system, but by a conscious adaptation of the immune system to an otherwise lethal heavy metal environment," he says. Mercury suffocates the cells and they die, so the immune system cultivates fungi and bacteria that are able to bind large amounts of the toxic metal in their respective cell walls, thereby enabling the patient's cells to breathe again.

The downside, of course, is that the body must now feed these oth-

**Dietrich Klinghardt, M.D., Ph.D.:** American Academy of Neural Therapy, P.O. Box 5023, Bellevue, WA 98004; tel: (425) 462-1777. Website: www.neuraltherapy.com. Dr. Klinghardt regularly instructs physicians in the United States and Europe in neural therapy techniques.

> As soon as anybody has any type of medical illness or symptom, whether medical or emotional, the amalgam fillings should be removed and the mercury residues should be eliminated from the body, especially the brain.
>
> —*Dietrich Klinghardt, M.D., Ph.D.*

Dietrich Klinghardt, M.D., Ph.D.

erwise undesirable microbes and deal with their toxic waste. In addition, a person with mercury contamination often becomes zinc deficient, and the functioning of copper and other minerals in the body will be compromised as well. This perspective leads Dr. Klinghardt to the following strong statement: "As soon as anybody has any type of medical illness or symptom, whether medical or emotional, the amalgam fillings should be removed and the mercury residues should be eliminated from the body, especially the brain."

### Neural Therapy and Herbs for Mercury Detoxification

In Dr. Klinghardt's clinical experience, it is common for heavy metals to migrate to and accumulate in nerve ganglia (nerve bundles that are the nervous system's relay stations). Neural therapy is useful in treating mercury-based problems in the ganglia, he says. As a heavy metal (which means heavier than water), mercury tends to accumulate in the lowest parts of the body, such as the floor of the mouth, the pelvic floor, and the feet. Pelvic symptoms, in both men and women, "are very commonly caused by metal toxicity of Frankenhäuser's ganglion." A mercury accumulation in this nerve plexus can account for premature ejaculation and an enlarged prostate in men, and endometriosis, pelvic pain, and hormonal dysfunction in women, Dr. Klinghardt says.

Neural therapy "cleans up" this area by injecting Frankenhäuser's ganglion (just above the pubic bone) with a local anesthetic. "This opens up most of the ionic channels in the cell wall; the cell is then able to excrete a high number of its toxic components." This painless injection spurs the body to dump a large amount of mercury into the urine, Dr. Klinghardt says.

As an adjunct to neural therapy, Dr. Klinghardt employs botanical substances to assist in removing the mercury. Cilantro and chlorella are particularly effective. The herb cilantro (Chinese parsley) is known to detoxify the brain and central nervous system of heavy metals. Taking it in an alcohol-based tincture guarantees fast delivery of the cilantro to the brain, he says. A typical dose is ten drops of cilantro tincture twice daily. While cilantro mobilizes mercury or tin stored in the brain and spinal cord and moves it out of those tissues, it does not facilitate the removal of these heavy metals from the body. For this, a natural detox-ifying agent such as the algae chlorella is needed to bind up the mercury and carry it out through the feces. Dr. Klinghardt notes that a typical dosage of chlorella for this purpose is 12 330-mg capsules daily.

## Safely Eliminating Mercury from the Body

Although mercury amalgam removal eliminates the source of further contamination, that alone does not put an end to the mercury poison-ing. The mercury that leached from the fillings in the mouth is stored in cells throughout the body and continues to exert its damaging influ-ence. Therefore, amalgam removal should be accompanied by a detox-ification program to rid the body of the mercury accumulation. In this section, Daniel F. Royal, D.O., of Henderson, Nevada, describes his highly successful protocol for mercury detoxification:

In my medical practice, based on urine samples taken during a 24-hour period, I've documented many cases of mercury poisoning. Even if amalgam fillings are no longer present in a patient's mouth, mercury levels can often still be detected. It is not unusual to see patients who had their amalgam fillings removed and replaced 10 to 15 years prior to testing still having elevated lev-els of mercury in the body. Once mer-cury toxicity has been demonstrated—by tests such as high electrogalvanism (SEE QUICK DEFINITION), high mercury vapor emissions, and/or high mercury body burden (tissue deposits)—mercury amalgam removal and replacement with alternate, nontoxic materials is the rec-ommended next step.

The device used to measure **electrogalvanism** is a Gal-vanometer, which in this case was made specifically for Dr. Royal's clinic. The staff use it to determine the amount of positive or negative charges that the vari-ous metals in the patient's teeth are emit-ting. For measuring mercury vapor emis-sions from the teeth, Dr. Royal uses the Jerome Mercury Vapor Analyzer, the same device used by the Environmental Protection Agency to check the mercury levels in den-tal offices.

For more about **chlorella**, see chapter 10, Ending Nu-tritional Deficiencies with Supplements.

While removal of amalgam fillings stops any further source of poisoning from mercury fillings, you still need to detoxify the body to eliminate the residual effect from mercury that remains behind in the body. After all, it has been accumulating for as long as you've had amalgam fillings. First, you "turn off the faucet" by removing the fillings; then you "pull the plug" through oral detoxification; and lastly, you "drain the bathtub" (your body) of all traces of mercury.[9]

Ideally, you should initiate the detoxifying program detailed below at least two weeks before amalgam removal begins and continue it for at least three months after the last amalgams are removed. If you have already had your amalgams removed, then start today. The usual length of time required for elimination of mercury from the body is three to six months.

## A Complete Mercury Detoxification Program

In my practice, I use the following substances that, taken together, successfully remove mercury residues from the body:

*Chlorella.* This medicinal green algae helps move mercury out of connective tissue so that substances such as DMPS can bind with it and eliminate it from the body. Begin with only one chlorella capsule daily for the first few weeks after amalgam removal, then gradually increase to three daily.

*L-glutathione.* This natural detoxifying substance (made from the amino acid cysteine) improves liver function and metabolism, thereby helping the body detoxify. Take 150 mg once daily (for more on glutathione, see chapter 4, Restoring Immune Vitality).

*Kyolic Garlic.* Garlic's high sulfur and cysteine content enable it to bind up (chelate—SEE QUICK DEFINITON) toxic metals and chemicals and to work against harmful microbes. Take one capsule with meals three times daily.

*Silymarin.* Also known as milk thistle seed, silymarin has long been used as a liver-purifying agent. Take one capsule twice daily.

*Vitamin C.* Ascorbic acid has a protective effect against free-radical damage, which can occur as heavy metals are being removed and excreted through the kidneys. On the day before amalgam removal, take your bowel tolerance of vitamin C. This is the amount your system can tolerate before producing diarrhea, usually 8,000 to 16,000 mg daily, divided into hourly doses of about 2,000 mg for a 150-pound

# A Quick Guide to the Nervous System

Standard anatomy describes two components to the nervous system. The **central nervous system (CNS)** comprises the spinal cord, containing millions of nerve fibers, and the brain; the **peripheral nervous system (PNS)** is the network of nerves estimated to extend 93,000 miles inside the body. The PNS is the sensory motor branch that pertains to the five senses and to how sensory information from the outside world gets translated into muscle movements.

The **autonomic nervous system (ANS)**, involving elements of both the CNS and PNS, is controlled by the brain's hypothalamus gland; it pertains to the automatic regulation of all body processes, such as breathing, digestion, and heart rate. It can be likened to the body's automatic pilot, keeping you alive without your being aware of it or participating in its activities. Neural therapy focuses its injections of anesthetics into body structures whose nerve supply is linked with the autonomic nervous system. Within the ANS, there are two branches—the parasympathetic and sympathetic branches—that are believed to counterbalance each other.

The **parasympathetic nervous system** slows heart rate, inhibits activity, conserves energy, and calms the body, but stimulates gastric secretion and intestinal activity. The **sympathetic nervous system** involves the expenditure of energy and is associated with arousal and stress. It prepares us physically when we perceive a threat or challenge by increasing our heart rate, blood pressure, and muscle tension. The sympathetic portion links all the cells of the body together; it regulates the contraction and expansion of blood vessels; the activity of connective tissue necessary for regenerating body systems; and the voltage (membrane potential) across a cell wall. Neural therapy primarily addresses this system.

A **ganglion** is a bundle, knot, or plexus of nerve cell bodies with many interconnections; it acts as a sorting and relay station for nerve impulses. There are several dozen ganglia throughout the body.

**Membrane potential** refers to differing electrical charges, which constantly change around a certain baseline—measured in millivolts (mV)—inside and outside of a cell. This, in turn, influences the ease or difficulty with which substances (nutrients or toxins) can pass into and out of a cell. Sodium ions are pumped out of the cell (to create the normal resting potential of 80 mV) and potassium ions are pumped in. The three means by which substances are transported across the cell membrane are called ion pumping, ionic channel transport, and carrier-protein transport. Transport is voltage dependent; it resembles the ebb and flow of tidal water, with nutrients "washing in" and toxins "washing out" with each pulse of the electrical current every two to five milliseconds.

---

person; decrease the dosage if you get diarrhea. My recommendation is 2,000 to 8,000 mg daily.

*Vitamin B Complex.* Take 25 to 100 mg daily to help replenish nutrients lost when heavy metals are bound up and excreted.

*DHEA.* This is an adrenal hormone precursor. The adrenal glands of patients with mercury toxicity are often weak, contributing to an

> While removal of amalgam fillings stops further poisoning from mercury fillings, you still need to detoxify the body to eliminate the residual effect from mercury that remains behind in the body. After all, it has been accumulating for as long as you've had amalgam fillings. —*Daniel F. Royal, D.O.*

Daniel F. Royal, D.O.

inability to handle stress. My recommended daily dosage is 5 mg for men and 2.5 mg for women, to be taken daily with pregnenolone.

***Pregnenolone.*** This substance (a steroid building block made from cholesterol, usually extracted from soybeans or wild yam) aids in the formation of key brain chemicals associated with memory and thinking. The recommended daily dosage is 10 mg for men and 30 mg for women. This dosage should initially be taken daily and may be decreased as symptoms improve.

***DMSA.*** DMSA (2,3-dimercaptosuccinic acid) is an effective chelating (binding-up) agent for heavy metals because it crosses the blood-brain barrier and thus helps remove the remaining toxic residues from the central nervous system. On the day of amalgam removal, take three 100 mg capsules in the morning prior to removal; take another three on the day after removal. Take them 30 minutes before or after eating. Once the amalgams have been removed and after you have been on this supplement program for three months, on one occasion only, take two capsules (100 mg each) three times daily for three days.

***DMPS*** (2,3-dimercaptopropane-1-sulfonate). This is the chelating (bind-

 On the day of amalgam removal, vitamin C should not be taken until after the procedure; otherwise, it may interfere with the anesthesia.

 **Chelation therapy** refers to a method of binding up ("chelating") toxins (such as heavy metals) and metabolic wastes and removing them from the body, while at the same time increasing blood flow and removing arterial plaque. One type of chelation therapy involves the chelating agent disodium EDTA given as an intravenous infusion over a three-and-a-half-hour period. Usually 20 to 30 treatments are administered at the rate of one to three sessions per week. Chelation therapy is especially beneficial for all forms of atherosclerotic cardiovascular disease, including angina pectoris and coronary artery disease.

ing-up) agent of choice for the removal of elemental mercury from the human body. First developed in China, DMPS was then introduced in Russia, where it was used for workers injured by exposure to heavy metals. DMPS has since been researched for over 40 years in Japan, Germany, and the former Soviet Union, and for the past 25 years it has been used as a treatment for humans in these countries. DMPS can be given orally, intravenously, or intramuscularly, with a maximum dose of 3 mg/2.2 pounds of body weight, with 250 mg being the typical dose. I recommend a single 250 mg capsule taken once a month, or the same amount by injection, also once monthly. On the day of the last amalgam removal, the first DMPS treatment may be given. People who have had exposure to amalgam through their fillings will usually require three to five injections. Those who have never had amalgam fillings, but show evidence or suspicion of heavy metal toxicity through other sources, may require only one or two injections. An injection every four to six months thereafter is recommended for patient maintenance. Usually, the patient will begin to notice improvement within three to four weeks following the DMPS injections.

**CAUTION** As DMPS removes toxins from the cells, it can temporarily aggravate heavy-metal–related symptoms, such as joint pains, depression, burning sensations, digestive problems, and fatigue. This is a transient occurrence. The routine use of intravenous DMPS is not advisable for patients who still have mercury amalgam fillings. This is because DMPS may appear in the saliva and act to dissolve the surface of the existing amalgam fillings. The potential outcome is acute toxicity from heavy metal injury to the lining of the gut.

*Essential Minerals.* DMPS and DMSA unavoidably remove vital nutrients from the body, so to replenish the body's supply, zinc, copper, magnesium, and manganese should be taken in addition to the other vitamin supplements.

*Homeopathic Amalgam Drops.* This is a combination of homeopathically prepared elements found in amalgam fillings, given for the purpose of enhancing the removal of heavy metals from the body. Beginning one week prior to amalgam removal, take ten drops three times daily; continue this dosage for one week after amalgam removal. Once all the amalgams have been removed, begin taking homeopathic mercury (*Mercurius Solubilis* 30C) at the rate of 30 drops two to three times weekly for the duration of the oral detoxification program or until you feel improved.

## Dr. Royal's Additional Supplements and Guidelines

- **Selenium.** Take 50 mcg three times daily between meals and, whenever possible, two hours before or after you have taken vitamin C, to help bind up mercury.

- **Lactobacillus acidophilus.** This helps to restore the microflora of the intestine, which can be adversely affected by the presence of mercury. In my estimation, Torrence Company manufactures the most potent acidophilus, with 250 billion organisms per teaspoon. Take one teaspoon daily, or more if diarrhea or constipation are present.

- **Psyllium Husk.** This acts as a bulk fiber laxative to absorb toxins and facilitate the removal of fecal debris from the intestines. Drink at least six to eight glasses of water daily and slowly build up the amount of psyllium consumed. Begin with one teaspoon in liquid once daily and gradually increase to three teaspoons once daily (three times daily if constipation is present). Take psyllium separately from vitamin and mineral supplements, as the fiber will reduce their effectiveness.

- **Avoid Fish.** This is the largest dietary source of mercury. While some fish have a comparatively lower mercury content (e.g., sardines, herring, pollack, mackerel, cod, redfish, and Greenland halibut), most tuna has a fairly high mercury content.

- **Don't Eat Shellfish.** Individuals who are sensitive to mercury usually have some type of adverse reaction to shellfish.

- **Reduce Consumption of Chicken and Eggs.** Fish meal has become a major feed for chickens. Depending on the mercury content of the fish products used to make the fish meal, chickens and eggs have the potential of having a significant mercury content.

- **Eat a High Fiber Diet.** A high fiber diet, consisting primarily of fruits, vegetables, and legumes, helps decrease fecal transit time and reduces the amount of time that liquids containing heavy metals remain in the colon, thus minimizing the amount reabsorbed from the colon.

- **Decrease Refined Carbohydrates and Saturated Fats.** Refined carbohydrates include simple sugars and white flour; all may reduce the availability of essential enzymes and nutrients required for more beneficial purposes.

### Use a Sauna to Sweat the Mercury out of Your Body

The skin is one of the body's detoxification mechanisms and sweating can help draw mercury from the body. Saunas are a useful adjunct to safe mercury removal because they induce copious sweating. Initiate sweating and increased circulation by exercising 20 to 30 minutes on a stationary bicycle, trampoline, or treadmill. Immediately following the exercise, sit in the sauna for up to 30 minutes, then take a cool (but not cold) shower.

The temperature in a "low heat" sauna should be between 140° F to 180° F, in contrast to the 200° F to 210° F in a nontherapeutic standard sauna. The sauna may be repeated again, followed by a plunge into a bath or under a shower with a water temperature of 65° F. Over a period of three to four days, increase your time in the sauna to a total of up to two hours, divided into 30-minute periods with a short cooling-off period in between. It's important to shower and towel dry, because the removal of sweat prevents reabsorption of toxins.

 **Daniel F. Royal, D.O.**: Royal Center of Advanced Medicine, 2501 North Green Valley Parkway, Suite D-132, Henderson, NV 89014; tel: (800) 326-7692. Website: www.drroyal.com. Dr. Royal's book, *The Royal Treatment*, discusses numerous innovative alternative medicine approaches and is available from the Center. **Homeopathic amalgam drops** are available from the center or by contacting Bio-Energetics, (800) 334-4043.

While doing the sauna program, consume adequate amounts of water to avoid dehydration: this is a minimum of two quarts before and after entering the sauna. Replace your electrolytes lost to perspiration with grape or prune juice and take a cultured milk product to compensate for calcium-magnesium loss through the skin. Take a full range of nutritional supplements to help detoxify and minimize nutrient loss, including the following:

- *Niacin.* 400 mg in divided doses; gradually increase to a daily divided dose of 3,000 to 6,000 mg, depending on your tolerance
- *Vitamin C.* 2,000 to 8,000 mg/day in divided doses
- *Vitamin E.* 400 to 1,200 IU/day
- *Vitamin A.* 25,000 to 50,000 IU (or beta carotene; 15 to 25 mg) daily
- *Magnesium/calcium.* in a 3:1 ratio, with 1,500 mg magnesium and 500 mg calcium daily
- *Multivitamin/mineral.* take daily for trace minerals and B vitamins (minimum 25 mg)

- *Flaxseed oil.* one to two tablespoons daily
- *Lecithin.* two tablespoons daily.

This simple program works quickly. You will derive immediate benefits from sauna detoxification, such as mental alertness, a sense of inner cleanliness, and enhanced well-being.

## The Truth about Quackery in Dentistry

It may surprise you to learn that in 1840, when organized dentistry formed the American Society of Dental Surgeons, members were required to sign "pledges" promising not to use mercury in dental fillings. Several members were suspended from the dental society in New York City in 1848 for "malpractice for using silver mercury fillings."

Mercury was called "quicksilver" in this country and "quacksalver" in some European countries. A "quack" is one who pretends to cure disease and a "salve" is a substance for application to wounds or sores. The derogatory term "quack" was first used in reference to anyone using mercury preparations on the skin to "cure" diseases. When the skin lesions of syphilis were treated with mercury salves, the skin eruptions would disappear, but their disappearance also resulted in the deeper penetration of the dreaded disease to the organs and nervous system, resulting in a painful death. Thus, mercury has been associated with medical quackery from the beginning.

Internal strife over the use of mercury by nineteenth-century dentists led to the formation of a new dental organization, the American Dental Association (ADA) in 1859. Its leaders not only did not oppose the use of mercury but now, 137 years later, the ADA condemns dentists who inform their patients that the mercury they are implanting in their teeth is a poison! Today, dentists in some states believe that the ADA actually sends "undercover agents" into dental offices in which they suspect a dentist is disseminating "negative" (read, truthful) information about mercury. Hence, dentists who attempt to practice "mercury-free" dentistry do so at the peril of losing their licenses.

If mercury is "safe," then why has Sweden banned it and offered to pay for its citizenry to have their fillings replaced? Why is Germany imposing severe restrictions on its use? Why has the world's largest manufacturer of dentistry metals stopped producing amalgam? If we ban mercury in paint and we disallow it in batteries, then why are we still leaving it inside our mouths as a lifetime implant?

To date, the ADA has never scientifically proven its position that mercury in dental fillings is "safe." At best, the ADA's official position is simply a political opinion. Their argument can be summed up in a few words: "We've been using it for over 160 years, so it must be safe." Fortunately for the American public, real scientific evidence refuting the notion that mercury amalgam fillings are safe is mounting every day in opposition to dentistry's politicians.

# eight

# Replenishing Enzyme Deficiencies

Enzyme deficiencies can play a prominent role in chronic fatigue syndrome. This fact was vividly illustrated in several of the cases discussed earlier in the book. The digestive disorders that are common in CFS may stem from an enzyme deficiency. This shouldn't be surprising; because enzymes are proteins necessary for every chemical reaction that takes place in the body, a deficiency in these vital proteins affects every system, organ, and cell. The impact of this deficiency on digestive function alone sets up a reverberation throughout the body. The poor digestion and intestinal dysfunction that result from enzyme deficiencies deplete the immune system by not providing the body with necessary nutrients and by allowing toxins to leak from the intestines into the bloodstream. The immune system then has to expend energy trying to eliminate them.

As more enzymes are needed to help deal with the overload of toxins circulating in the blood, fewer enzymes are available to break down food, so digestive function worsens and more toxins end up in the blood, creating a further burden on the immune system. When immunity is already compromised by the presence of multiple viruses or infections, this deficit adds another load that can tip the balance into creating chronic fatigue syndrome. An enzyme deficiency is yet another factor in what Serafina Corsello, M.D., called the "loading theory" of toxicity and illness.

Again, as with the viruses associated with CFS, it is unclear which

When immunity is already compromised by the presence of multiple viruses or infections, an enzyme deficiency adds another load that can tip the balance into creating chronic fatigue syndrome.

comes first—the weakened immune system or the enzyme deficiencies. In either case, supplementing with plant enzymes can correct the enzyme imbalance and break the cycle of ill health, with dysfunction in one system worsening dysfunction in another. In addition, as explained in chapter 3, enzymes are antiviral agents, capable of digesting the protective protein coating of numerous viruses, leaving the microorganisms open to destruction. Enzymes also help get rid of toxins in the bloodstream. Clearly, enzyme therapy—the precise supplementation with enzymes and other nutrients—can be an important component in a CFS treatment plan.

Being precise means developing a personalized program of recovery for the individual patient. Maile Pouls, Ph.D., a clinical nutritionist, health educator, and cofounder of the Health Enhancement Center in Santa Cruz, California, explains the importance of gathering information on digestive function as a basis for designing a precise treatment program. Dr. Pouls demonstrates the success of this approach in three cases of patients who had typical CFS symptoms.

## Digestion Is the Key

We're born with a "bank account" of pancreatic enzymes necessary for digestion, but if over a lifetime we eat too many cooked and processed foods (known to be enzyme deficient), this pancreatic enzyme reserve gets depleted. Then the pancreas has to make more enzymes, but it does this at the expense of the enzymes in your white blood cells. Some people report feeling very tired, run down, and even a little shaky after eating; this is because their system is pulling enzymes from the immune system. With the immune system taxed in this way, you can become more susceptible to illness.

In an illness as complex as chronic fatigue syndrome, it is crucial to look at as many factors that may be involved in the health problem as possible. For this, a 24-hour urine analysis is indispensable. A standard blood test can often read "normal," even if a patient is becoming sick or is already ill; it doesn't always reveal the true biochemical status. A 24-hour urinalysis can indicate predispositions to diseases long before they manifest and show why a person has multiple, even confusing, symptoms, many of them founded on digestive problems.

With my patients, the first thing I check is digestive competence, because over 90% of the patients I treat either have digestive problems or digest less than optimally. If your digestion is not functioning well, it doesn't matter how healthy the food you eat is, or how high the quality of supplements you take. If you can't assimilate nutrients from food and/or supplements, the body becomes deficient—not to mention toxic—as a result of this poor digestion.

The body needs three factors for optimal digestion: enzymes, *Lactobacillus acidophilus*, and the correct pH (SEE QUICK DEFINITION). If you lack any of these, the foods you eat are prone to ferment, putrefy, and create acid indigestion, gas, bloating, diarrhea, or constipation. Even worse, the toxins from poorly digested food can migrate into your bloodstream, creating a bodywide state of toxicity. To address digestive problems, it is important not to treat symptoms, but rather to focus on what is setting the person up for poor digestion and bowel toxicity.

Once you know how a person is digesting food, then precise supplementation with enzymes and nutrients can bring about rapid and permanent beneficial changes in a wide range of symptoms seemingly unrelated to digestion, as is true of many CFS symptoms such as headaches, depression, and yeast infections. It may seem paradoxi-

## Conditions Associated with an Enzyme Deficiency

allergies
anxiety, irritability, mood swings
bacterial and viral infections
bronchial and respiratory conditions
candidiasis
chronic fatigue syndrome
depressed immunity
depression
environmental illness
frequent sore throats
gastrointestinal problems, indigestion
hypothyroidism
insomnia
lack of concentration, memory loss, or mental sluggishness
lymphatic congestion with swollen glands
sinusitis and sinus infections

 The term **pH**, which means "potential hydrogen," represents a scale for the relative acidity or alkalinity of a solution. Acidity is measured as a pH of 0.1 to 6.9, and alkalinity is 7.1 to 14; a pH of 7.0 is considered neutral. The numbers refer to how many hydrogen atoms are present compared to an ideal or standard solution. Normally, blood is slightly alkaline, at 7.35 to 7.45; urine pH can range from 4.8 to 7.5, although normal is closer to 7.0.

> If your digestion is not functioning well, it doesn't matter how healthy the food you eat is, or how high the quality of supplements you take. If you can't assimilate the nutrients, the body becomes deficient—not to mention toxic—as a result of this poor digestion. —*Maile Pouls, Ph.D.*

cal, but the more extreme the patient's condition, the faster their response to treatment. They may have such a serious imbalance that as soon as you start providing the missing essential nutrients, combined with enzymes, they feel the changes almost immediately. This was the case for Holden, as described below.

### Success Story: Ten Years of Fatigue and Indigestion Reversed with Enzymes

Holden, 41, came to me with long-standing symptoms of fatigue and very low energy, a lingering viral infection, chronic indigestion, stomach and kidney pain, and headaches. His indigestion was so severe that he had been taking six to ten Rolaids® every day for ten years in an attempt to relieve it. A 24-hour urine test provided the following information about Holden's problem: (1) both his liver and kidneys were distressed, as indicated by his urine's high specific gravity and its protein and ketone acid content; (2) his organs were malfunctioning without the proper amount of water, which led to severe bowel toxicity; (3) at 5.9, his pH was highly acidic; and (4) his protein, carbohydrate, and fat digestion were poor.

Before laying out his treatment plan, I had Holden checked for ulcers and gastritis because certain enzyme formulas can aggravate an irritated stomach; he had neither condition.

Holden began taking four different enzyme formulations from the Ness line of enzymes: #18 would optimize fat digestion and address his acidic pH and the high levels of calcium oxalates (indication of how fats are being digested; in this case, poorly); #6 was to increase protein utilization and reduce the amount of uric acid crystals in his urine (signifying the status of protein digestion); #301 would support his kidneys and lymphatic system; and #416 would help detoxify his system and bolster his immune response. The effect of taking the #416 formula is like getting a second set of white blood cells. After so many years on Rolaids,

## A Glossary of Urine Analysis Terms

The following are specific values measured in a 24-hour urine analysis:

**Volume.** The total urine output, either excessive (polyuria) or minimal (oliguria), in relationship to the specific gravity indicates how well the kidneys are functioning.

**Indican.** This indicates the degree of toxicity, putrefaction, gas, and fermentation in the intestines. Indican comes from putrefying proteins in the large intestine that are kicked back into the blood and excreted through the kidneys. Indican is extremely toxic and causes many symptoms; the higher the level, the greater the intestinal toxemia or inflammation in the digestive tract. Readings as close to zero as possible are desirable.

**pH.** Based on hydrogen ion concentration, this value indicates the degree of urine acidity versus alkalinity on a scale of zero to 14, with urine pH usually ranging from 4.5 to 8.0 and 7.0 being neutral.

**Chlorides.** These are salt residues in the urine; these values give information on salt intake and assimilation.

**Specific gravity.** This value measures the weight of total dissolved substances (solutes) in the urine against an equal amount of water, such that a normal reading of 1.020 means the urine is 20% heavier than water. Specific gravity shows the general water content (hydration) of the body. Values can typically range from 1.005 to 1.030; a high reading indicates solute concentration and kidney stress.

**Total sediment analysis.** This indicates the amount of dissolved organic and mineral substances remaining in the urine after digestion; an optimal total reading for the three sediment categories is 0.5.

**Calcium phosphate.** This reading indicates the status of carbohydrate digestion; a level of 0.5 signifies normal carbohydrate digestion.

**Uric acid.** Levels of uric acid signify the status of protein digestion; optimal digestion yields a reading of zero.

**Calcium oxalate.** This value indicates the status of fat digestion; a reading of zero signifies optimal fat digestion.

**Vitamin C.** Levels of vitamin C indicate body reserves of this key nutrient; a reading of 1 is high, 2 to 5 normal, and 6 to 10 deficient.

---

antibiotics, and other drugs, Holden's natural resistance was low; as a result, he tended to go from one infection to the next.

Enzymes are an energy source, a kind of "workhorse" for the body. If you take them with food, the first thing that any enzyme supplement will do is to begin predigesting this food in the upper stomach. However, when enzymes are taken on an empty stomach, they enter the bloodstream and the targeted tissues often in as little as 15 minutes.

You might think of enzymes as little "Pac-Men"—they can eat up undigested protein, cellular debris, chemicals, toxins, free radicals, and antigen-antibody complexes resulting from allergic reactions. This

We will balance your chemistry, build up your enzyme and nutrient reserve, improve your digestion, and then watch many of the symptoms disappear as the body's innate wisdom takes charge.
—*Maile Pouls, Ph.D.*

Maile Pouls, Ph.D.

spares the immune system these tasks; it is then free to concentrate its full action on the bacterial or viral problems.

Holden took these enzymes daily for a month, reduced his dietary salt intake, ate more alkaline foods (some examples are salad greens, raw vegetables, potatoes, and fresh fruits), and drank more water. His system's response was quick and decisive. Within a week, he no longer needed Rolaids; after a month, his energy level was much improved; he no longer had indigestion or stomach and kidney pains; and instead of daily headaches, he had only one in 30 days. His pH measured 6.7, which is acceptably close to a healthy alkaline level. His levels of chloride and sediment ratios (indicating how well he was handling fats, proteins, and carbohydrates) dropped to normal and his digestion was greatly improved. Now it was time to shift his enzyme formulas.

I started Holden on two products, UltraFiber and Ness #401 with *acidophilus*, to detoxify his intestines. He took two scoops of UltraFiber in water, two times daily, on an empty stomach. Within two months of taking these, Holden's intestinal toxicity (measured by the level of indican) dropped from 3 to 1—an excellent improvement, though not yet optimal, which would be a value of zero. To accomplish this, three months after beginning the enzyme program, Holden started a more extensive colon cleanse program called Cleanse Thyself™ by Arise and Shine, which included a specific *acidophilus* formula (Flora Grow), a psyllium product, bentonite clay, and two herbal mixtures for clearing the deposits from the colon wall and for healing the intestinal lining. I also shifted a few of his enzyme mixtures to combinations more suitable for maintenance.

Holden continued to improve, his symptoms gradually disappearing.

After three months, his urine analysis values had shifted to normal readings.

I never tell my patients that enzymes are a magic bullet or that we're going to "cure" anything. Rather, I say we will balance your chemistry, build up your enzyme and nutrient reserve, improve your digestion, and then watch many of the symptoms disappear as the body's innate wisdom takes charge. The urine analysis enables me to continually monitor progress and play detective with the patient's biochemistry. I do expect many positive improvements, but I never know how long it will take to achieve these changes; it might take another person with similar conditions four months to get the results Holden started having in the first month.

## A Guide to Ness Enzyme Formulas

| | |
|---|---|
| #6: | Marshmallow root, rosehips, amylase, protease |
| #11: | Citrus bioflavonoids, rosehips, acerola cherries, amylase |
| #14: | Kelp, Irish moss, protease |
| #17: | Pau d'arco, yellowdock, echinacea, mullein leaf, amylase, organic germanium |
| #18: | Lipase, amylase, protease, cellulase |
| #301: | Rosehips, alfalfa juice concentrate, echinacea, lipase, protease, mullein |
| #401: | Horsetail, *L. acidophilus*, lipase |
| #416: | Protease, calcium lactate, amylase, lipase |
| #801: | Cellulase, *L. acidophilus*, *L. bifidus* (nondairy source) |

## Success Story:
### Getting to the Root of Fatigue

Muriel, 47, came to me with a lengthy list of problems, including severe fatigue, low stamina, low blood sugar (hypoglycemia), nervousness, irritability, premenstrual syndrome (PMS—SEE QUICK DEFINITION), muscle cramping, heart palpitations, insomnia, stress, constipation, a vaginal yeast infection, an inability to gain weight, bleeding gums, and a tendency to bruise easily. Whenever she exercised, Muriel felt exhausted and sick afterward; she had virtually no muscle strength. (You may recall that post-exercise exhaustion is one of the symptoms of chronic fatigue syndrome.)

Muriel's urine analysis indicated she had severe bowel toxicity and poor nutrient assimilation. A serious calcium and magnesium deficiency accounted for her inability to relax her muscles or feel calm. Her overly alkaline pH con-

 **Premenstrual syndrome (PMS)** symptoms include bloating, cramping, achiness, irregular bleeding, headaches, short temper, irritability, sudden mood swings, depression, frustration, breast tenderness, weepiness, and abdominal discomfort. An estimated 5% of American women have such severe PMS symptoms that they are incapacitated for a few days every month.

tributed to her poor digestion of proteins, causing an amino-acid (SEE QUICK DEFINITION) shortage that, in turn, affected the amino acid levels needed to transport calcium and magnesium into the tissues.

Muriel was radically deficient in vitamin C, showing the lowest possible reading on the scale (a reading of 6 to 10 is deficient); this accounted for her bleeding gums and the tendency to bruise easily. Her total urine sediment was very low, which means she was starving for nutrients and severely deficient in enzymes. Muriel's low levels of calcium phosphate (indicating problems with carbohydrate digestion) contributed to her low blood-sugar level.

At the top of Muriel's supplement program, I used Ness #21 to address her chronic low blood sugar and intolerance for dairy products and sugar. To rebuild her amino acid reserves, speed up muscle repair (addressing the exhaustion after exercise), and improve her stamina, I put her on an amino acid formula called Aminoplex. This would also help correct Muriel's hypoglycemia. Approximately 70% of the amino acids in this mixture are digested in about 15 minutes after consumption and start forming glucose, which, in turn, restores normal blood-sugar levels and reduces sugar cravings.

Muriel also started taking Calcium+ (containing "nutrient partners" such as magnesium, manganese, iron, and vitamins) to ease her nervous system, reduce constipation, and enhance her ability to sleep restfully at night. In addition, she took a product called Trace Minerals (20 drops in a quart of water), which contains plant-based minerals derived from ancient seabeds in Utah. This supplement would replenish electrolytes (SEE QUICK DEFINITION), as Muriel's urine test showed her electrolyte levels were deficient.

To improve her vitamin C levels, Muriel took Ness #11; in two

 **Amino acids** are the basic building blocks of the 40,000 different proteins in the body, including enzymes, hormones, and the key brain chemical messenger molecules called neurotransmitters. Eight amino acids cannot be made by the body and must be obtained through the diet; others are produced in the body but not always in sufficient amounts. The body's main "amino acid pool" consists of alanine, arginine, aspargine, aspartic acid, carnitine, citrulline, cysteine, cystine, GABA, glutamic acid, glutamine, glycine, histidine, isoleucine, leucine, lysine, methionine, ornithine, phenylalanine, proline, serine, taurine, threonine, tryptophan, tyrosine, and valine.

**Electrolytes** are substances in the blood, tissue fluids, intracellular fluids, or urine that conduct an electrical charge, either plus or minus. Examples include acids, bases, and salts, such as potassium, magnesium, phosphate, sulfate, bicarbonate, sodium, chloride, and calcium. Electrolytes provide inorganic chemicals for cellular reactions and control mechanisms, such as the conduction of electrochemical impulses to nerves and muscles. Electrolytes are also needed for key enzymatic reactions involved in metabolism, or the release of energy from food.

> After two months on these supplements, Muriel's urine sediment level was almost normal, her bowel toxicity was much reduced, and many of her other symptoms had abated as her urine test measures improved. — *Maile Pouls, Ph.D.*

months, this brought them back up to a 3, within the normal range. Ness #801 uses acidophilus and cellulase enzymes to kill yeast and eliminate vaginal yeast infections. I had her take this supplement orally (½ teaspoon with each meal) and internally, in the form of a douche or a vaginal suppository at night. She made a paste from the powder and inserted it into her vagina. In three days, her yeast infection cleared up.

After two months on these supplements, Muriel's pH shifted to a more appropriate 6.8. Her urine sediment level was almost normal, her bowel toxicity was much reduced, and many of her other symptoms had abated as her urine test measures improved. As her problem with low blood sugar started to ease off and Muriel began a more intensive weight-lifting and exercise program, I switched her amino acid formula to AminoStasis, which contains a different balance of specific amino acids more suited to muscle repair.

To complement her vitamin C intake at this point, I put Muriel on Pycnogenol C, a supplement made from grape seed and pine bark that is many times more potent as an antioxidant than vitamin C alone. As her calcium levels were approaching normal, I switched her from Calcium+ to Osteoprime Forte; this would work as a longtime preventive strategy against osteoporosis, a condition toward which her extreme calcium deficiency had been leading her. After another two months, most of Muriel's key biochemical factors (including her electrolyte levels) became normal and nearly all of her multiple symptoms disappeared.

### Success Story: Ending Maryann's Fatigue and Depression

Like Holden and Muriel, Maryann, 31, complained of many symptoms typical of CFS, beginning with great fatigue. She also had constant headaches, anemia, constipation, PMS, kidney and intestinal pain, dry skin, and low body temperature along with cold hands and feet, which can be a sign of hypothyroidism. She was unable to lose weight and was taking the antidepressant Prozac® for serious depression. More seriously, she had all the signs of irritable bowel syndrome, which in her case exhib-

> Maryann's low level of water intake created considerable prob-
> lems for her. She was becoming toxic from lack of water, as
> water is needed to flush waste products out of the tissues and
> to absorb nutrients. — *Maile Pouls, Ph.D.*

ited as bleeding and inflammation of the intestines; she also had symptoms suggesting an ulcer in the small intestine. She was on Tagamet®
for stomach ulcers and an iron supplement for her anemia.

This case demonstrates another aspect of biochemical functioning
revealed by a urine analysis. In Maryann's case, she had high values for
specific gravity and total sediment, indicating a heavy concentration of
substances in her urine. It turns out Maryann drank very little water and,
as a result, passed very little urine, a condition clinically called oliguria,
or underproduction of urine. Her low level of water intake created considerable problems for her. She was becoming toxic from lack of water,
as water is needed to flush waste products out of the tissues and to absorb
nutrients. Water also acts as an intestinal lubricant; Maryann's constipation and high level of bowel toxicity were partly due to this deficiency.

In treating Maryann, I had to keep in mind the fact that a strong
enzyme formula, especially one containing higher amounts of protease
(which digests proteins), could irritate her inflamed stomach wall. I
started her on Gastritis Complex, a plant enzyme formula containing
gamma oryzanol, marshmallow root, and slippery elm. I also prescribed
Chlorophyll Perles for her intestinal ulcer. In this form, the chlorophyll
is fat soluble, which means it does not get digested in the stomach but
moves on to the intestines, where it literally adheres to the gut wall, forming a kind of lubricating film and healing ointment.

To address Maryann's depression and to provide an alternative to
Prozac, Maryann started taking Stabilium, a form of essential fatty acids
(EFAs). With this product, I have been able to assist over 40 patients in
getting off of Prozac, with their physician's supervision. Stabilium helps
boost physical energy and stamina, decrease mood swings, lessen anxiety, agitation, and melancholia, and improve the quality of sleep. For
the continuing fatigue, I put her on Adaptogen, which contains a variety of energy-balancing Chinese herbs. To eliminate the PMS, Maryann
took natural progesterone (SEE QUICK DEFINITION) in the form of a
cream called ProGest™.

Maryann took Ness #17 to address her headaches and anemia, as she was not absorbing the iron from the conventional supplement she had been taking. Ness #17 contains the herb yellowdock as an easily assimilated form of plant-based iron. It also contains germanium, which gets oxygen into the cells including those in the brain, thereby helping to relieve tension-type headaches that result from too little oxygen being available in the brain.

Maryann had low body temperature, especially in her hands and feet. To rebalance this, I put her on Omega EFA (containing both omega-3 and omega-6 essential fatty acids [SEE QUICK DEFINITION], plus borage oil and vitamin E), two capsules twice daily with meals. Since EFAs bind oxygen to hemoglobin (made of iron and amino acids, hemoglobin's job is to transport oxygen in the blood), getting more EFAs into the body will improve circulation and thus bring warmth to the hands and feet. To address Maryann's underactive thyroid and still-deficient electrolyte levels, I gave her Ness #14.

Within two months on this program, Maryann was no longer tired and depressed, nor was she taking Prozac or Tagamet. She passed a normal volume of urine after increasing her water intake; in fact, her urine output more than doubled. Marked changes also occurred in her readings for specific gravity, which dropped from 1.033 to 1.018 (normal is 1.020), and in her total sediment, which went down from 1.1 to 0.60 (normal is 0.5). Even the color of

 **Progesterone** is a female "sex" hormone produced in the ovaries that prepares the uterus for a fertilized egg and, when a pregnancy does not occur, stops the cell proliferation in the uterus begun under estrogen. When estrogen is high during days 7 to 14 of a woman's menstrual cycle, progesterone levels are at their lowest. Progesterone then climbs to a peak from about day 14 to 24, before dramatically dropping off again just before the start of menstruation. When the cells stop producing progesterone, it's a signal to the uterus to start the menstrual cycle anew. By age 35, the amount of progesterone that a woman's body produces usually starts to decline.

**Omega-3** and **omega-6 oils** are the two principal types of essential fatty acids, which are unsaturated fats required in the diet. The digits "3" and "6" refer to differences in the oil's chemical structure with respect to its chain of carbon atoms and where they are bonded. A balance of these oils in the diet is required for good health. The primary omega-3 oil is called alpha-linolenic acid (ALA) and is found in flaxseed (58%), canola, pumpkin and walnut, and soybeans. Fish oils, such as salmon, cod, and mackerel, contain the other important omega-3 oils, DHA (docosahexaenoic acid) and EPA (eicosapentaenoic acid). Omega-3 oils help reduce the risk of heart disease. Linoleic acid or cis-linoleic acid is the main omega-6 oil and is found in most plant and vegetable oils, including safflower (73%), corn, peanut, and sesame. The most therapeutic form of omega-6 oil is gamma-linolenic acid (GLA), found in evening primrose, black currant, and borage oils. Once in the body, omega-3 and omega-6 are converted to prostaglandins, hormone-like substances that regulate many metabolic functions, particularly inflammatory processes.

> By getting a complete picture of exactly what is happening in the body, as can be obtained through a 24-hour urine analysis, the specific components of even a complex, multilayered disorder such as chronic fatigue syndrome can systematically be addressed and the body restored to health.
>
> — *Maile Pouls, Ph.D.*

Maryann's urine showed the change: before it had been a hazy yellow brown; now it was a more normal yellow. Her constipation disappeared, her skin was less dry, her extremities were not cold all the time, and she lost five pounds.

As a result of taking Prozac, Tagamet, and other drugs, which can tax the liver, Maryann needed nutritional support, so I put her on a product called Liverguard. After four months on the program (the components of which I shifted as she progressed), most of Maryann's urine readings fell within the normal range and nearly all of her symptoms disappeared.

These three cases give a clear idea of what nutrients and enzymes can do in shifting body chemistry to relieve health problems. By getting a complete picture of exactly what is happening in the body, as can be obtained through a 24-hour urine analysis, the specific components of even a complex, multilayered disorder such as chronic fatigue syndrome can systematically be addressed and the body restored to health.

For a personalized nutritional program, a urine analysis to evaluate your individual nutritional needs, and specific nutrients and plant enzymes to optimize your body chemistry (via phone consultation), contact **Maile Pouls, Ph.D.**: Health Enhancement Center, 2315A Mattison Lane, Santa Cruz, CA 95060; tel: (866) 424-4325. Website: www.yournutrition.com.

## Signs and Symptoms of Enzyme Deficiency

"Depletions of plant enzymes lead to a host of chronic diseases that could in part be avoided if we provided the body with the enzymes it needs," says Lita Lee, Ph.D., an enzyme therapist based in Lowell, Oregon. "As it is, we are not aware of enzyme deficiencies because they take so long to manifest. When there are signs, the body is already in a state of exhaustion." If you are wondering whether a shortage of enzymes may be contributing to your CFS, Dr. Lee states, "If you have fatigue, allergies, bloating, gas, constipation, indigestion, or any symptom of undigested food, then you most likely have an enzyme deficiency."

As mentioned above, a simple urine analysis can precisely pinpoint your deficiencies, but here, in the following section, Dr. Lee explains the signs and symptoms associated with deficiencies of the main digestive enzymes: protease, amylase, lipase, cellulase, and disaccharidase:

## Protease

Protease digests protein; not only protein from food, but also other organisms that are composed of protein, such as the protein coating on certain viruses, toxins from dead bacteria and other organisms, and certain harmful substances produced at sites of injury or inflammation. Protease is especially effective during inflammatory processes to control swelling, redness, heat, fever, and pain. Due its ability to bolster immunity, protease is an important line of defense in the immune system. Consequently, immune system disorders are among the most common symptoms of protease deficiency. Additionally, since about half the protein you eat is converted to sugar, protease deficiency and inadequate protein digestion lead to hypoglycemia (low blood sugar), with such symptoms as moodiness, depression, anxiety, irritability, and attention deficit disorder (ADD).

Toxic colon syndrome, also called indicanuria or intestinal toxemia, is another result of protease deficiency and the inability to digest protein. Undigested protein decomposes at the intestinal level. The products of this putrefaction (called indican) leak into the blood from the intestines. From there, they reach the liver. The liver can detoxify only some of these products, and in doing so becomes stressed. Those substances that cannot be processed are excreted through the urine.

Indicanuria is identified by elevated levels of indican in the urine, as determined by a 24-hour urine analysis. Research has found that numerous inflammatory or pathological conditions can result from elevated indican. In fact, indicanuria can cause more than 100 symptoms or conditions. The following (all are associated with CFS)

> ### Conditions Associated with Protease Deficiency
>
> anxiety
> cold hands and feet
> water retention (edema)
> frequent bacterial/viral infections
> colon problems
> kidney disease
> bone problems (osteoporosis, spurs)
> blood clots
> low blood sugar (hypoglycemia)

> We are not aware of enzyme deficiencies because they take so long to manifest. When there are signs, the body is already in a state of exhaustion.　　　　— Lita Lee, Ph.D.

are among those that have been linked to high indican levels: fatigue, allergies, gastrointestinal problems, hypothyroidism, lack of concentration, memory loss, and sinusitis and sinus infections.

### Amylase

Amylase digests carbohydrates, breaking them down into smaller units, which are later converted into monosaccharides (simple sugars) such as glucose and fructose. People who can't digest fats often eat large amounts of sugar and carbohydrates to make up for the lack of fat in their diet. If their diet is excessive in carbohydrates, they can develop an amylase deficiency. Amylase is important in preventing the proliferation of dead leukocytes (white blood cells), which manifests as pus. Amylase is used in combination with lipase, fatty acids, and herbs to reduce certain viral problems, including all types of herpes, and to remove the pus from inflamed areas. Additionally, amylase aids in clearing the lungs.

**Conditions Associated with Amylase Deficiency**

skin problems (hives, rashes)
eczema
psoriasis
herpes
allergies to bee stings and insect bites
muscle soreness and pain
joint stiffness
thick blood

**Conditions Associated with Lipase Deficiency**

cardiovascular problems
diabetes
dizziness
high blood pressure
high cholesterol
obesity
difficulty losing weight

### Lipase

Lipase is the enzyme responsible for digesting fats. This includes fat in foods and the fat-based coatings of certain viruses—lipase can effectively destroy some viruses by digesting their outer coating. Certain viral infections may accompany a lipase deficiency; they are characterized by symptoms including fatigue, sore throat, and swollen glands. People who are diagnosed with chronic fatigue syndrome fall into this category. A prominent

A prominent indicator of lipase deficiency is chronic fatigue syndrome or "hidden" viruses.

indicator of lipase deficiency is chronic fatigue syndrome or "hidden" viruses. A lipase-deficient person is also likely to have irritable bowel symptoms.

Here is a classic case of chronic fatigue and lipase deficiency: A frail, 47-year-old woman came to me with chronic fatigue, allergies, and abdominal pain of 20 years' duration. She had been to countless doctors and health clinics, all to no avail. She had been trying to gain weight for years, and she was so painfully thin and listless, I wondered how she mustered up enough energy to come to my office. Her diet was mainly liquefied greens, sprouted seeds, salad, potatoes, yams, corn, fresh vegetables, and raw juices. Her tests indicated a toxic colon, poor digestion, and extreme lipase deficiency. I recommended a high lipase formula required in cases of fiber-intolerant, lipase-deficient clients. When she started taking the high-lipase multiple-digestive formula, she began to gain weight and her abdominal pains diminished.

## Cellulase

Cellulase digests fiber. It also "eats" pathogenic yeast, so candidiasis from a *Candida* overgrowth is often the result of inadequate "friendly" bowel bacteria coupled with a cellulase deficiency. Sudden, acute allergies can also be an outcome of cellulase deficiency. Candidiasis sets the stage for leaky gut syndrome, which in turn can lead to the development of food allergies, as undigested food particles make their way into the bloodstream and trigger an immune response. Once these food particles have passed from the digestive system to the circulatory system, the brain no longer interprets them as "food"; instead, they are considered foreign substances that must be eliminated from the body.

### Conditions Associated with Cellulase Deficiency

acute food allergies
candidiasis
facial pain or paralysis
gas and bloating

 For more on **candidiasis and allergies**, see chapter 9, Addressing the Allergy Connection.

## Conditions Associated with Disaccharidase Deficiency

asthma

bronchitis and other lung problems

chronic diarrhea

dizziness

environmental illness

hyperactivity

insomnia

mood swings

seizures

### Disaccharidase

Disaccharidase digests sugars. The sugar intolerance that results from a deficiency in these enzymes can lead to various health conditions. The inability to digest complex sugars (sucrose, lactose, and maltose) and convert them into the simple sugars (glucose and fructose) lowers the blood-sugar level and starts starving the brain of nourishment. The end result can be a range of problems, including depression, attention deficit disorder (ADD), and even seizures. Disaccharidase deficiency is also associated with environmental illness, asthma, and diarrhea.

## The Essentials of Enzyme Therapy

The human body makes approximately 22 different digestive enzymes, capable of digesting protein, carbohydrates, sugars, and fats. The body digests food in stages: beginning in the mouth, moving to the stomach, and finally through the small intestine. At each step, specific enzymes break down different types of food. An enzyme designed to digest protein, for example, has no effect on starch, and an enzyme active in the mouth will not be active in the stomach. This process is balanced through acidity; each site along the digestive track has a different degree of acidity that allows certain enzymes to function while inhibiting others.

As enzymes begin digesting food in the mouth and continue their work in the stomach, plant enzymes (derived from food itself or taken as a supplement) become active. The food then enters the upper portion of the small intestine, where the pancreatic enzymes supplied by the pancreas (a digestive organ that feeds enzymes into the gut) further break down the food. Final breakdown of remaining small molecules of food occurs in the lower small intestine.

Ideally, plant and pancreatic enzymes work together, digesting food and delivering nutrients to cells to maintain their health. Protocols for enzyme therapy are based on this sequence of events. "One of the most important processes in the metabolism of food is the chain of reactions

## Metabolism and the Life of Enzymes

**Metabolism** is the biological process by which energy is extracted from the foods consumed, producing carbon dioxide and water as by-products for elimination. Biochemically, metabolism involves hundreds of different chemical reactions, necessitating the involvement of hundreds of different enzymes, each of which handles a specific reaction. There are two kinds of metabolism constantly under way in the cells: anabolic and catabolic. In anabolic metabolism, the upbuilding phase, larger molecules are constructed by joining smaller ones together; in catabolic metabolism, the deconstructing phase, larger molecules are broken down into smaller ones. The anabolic function produces substances for cell growth and repair, while the catabolic function controls digestion (called hydrolysis), disassembling food into forms the body can use for energy.

**Circulating immune complexes (CICs)** form in the body when poor digestion results in undigested food proteins "leaking" through the intestinal wall and into the bloodstream. The immune system treats these foreign substances or antigens as invaders, causing antibodies to form and couple with them. This antigen and antibody combination is known as a CIC. In a healthy person, CICs are neutralized, but in someone with a compromised immune system, they tend to accumulate in the blood, where they burden the detoxification pathways or initiate an allergic reaction. If too many CICs accumulate, the kidneys cannot excrete enough of them via the urine. The CICs are then stored in soft tissues, causing inflammation and bringing stress to the immune system. The overload can lead to a variety of chronic health conditions.

that convert glucose to energy," states Dr. Lee. "Several vitamin and mineral coenzymes are necessary for these reactions. Coenzymes are consumed in the process. Our bodies need a continuing supply. All the food we eat, which eventually becomes energy, passes through this same set of reactions, whether the food is a fast-food hamburger or a raw carrot. Coenzymes are always needed, and when the food doesn't provide these, we use the vitamins and minerals stored in our body until these reserves are used up. Only when we eat whole and raw foods can we maintain a good supply of the parts that keep the metabolic machinery going."

 **Lita Lee, Ph.D.:** Enzyme Therapy, P.O. Box 516, Lowell, OR 97452; tel: (541) 937-1123. Website: www.litalee.com.

When the body receives plentiful supplies of enzymes, says Edward Howell, M.D., an accomplished author and pioneer in the field of enzyme therapy in the United States, "its internal enzyme supplies are preserved for the important work of maintaining metabolic harmony." As a result, many body systems are strengthened.[1]

The importance of raw foods becomes clear once you understand that plant enzymes—which are more heat-sensitive than vitamins—

are destroyed in the process of cooking food at temperatures above 118° F and, as Dr. Lee points out, "are deactivated or destroyed by pasteurizing, canning, and microwaving." Given the predominance in our diet of these methods of food preserving and preparation, you can see how enzyme deficiency can easily develop. However, while raw foods are recommended, a 100% raw foods diet is not necessary. Some people may have problems digesting uncooked food because of a lack of cellulase in their bodies.

According to Dr. Lee, when a patient's plant enzyme deficiencies are addressed, many other conditions can be resolved, from digestive ailments and common sore throats to candidiasis, a common complaint of chronic fatigue syndrome sufferers. Howard F. Loomis, Jr., D.C., founder and president of 21st Century Nutrition in Madison, Wisconsin, agrees. "It cannot be said that a *particular* enzyme can help a *particular* illness, but by clearing up digestive problems, we've found that many other problems seem to go away and new ailments may be prevented," he says.

Dr. Loomis developed a line of plant enzyme formulas after a personal experience with the healing abilities of enzymes. He had been searching for years for a solution to his chronic ear problems—hearing loss and continual ear infections that had plagued him since infancy, when he had severe whooping cough. Medications had proven ineffective against the infection and he was unable to wear hearing aids because his ears were constantly draining. He finally treated himself with massive doses of protease enzymes and his 43-year-old ear infection cleared up within 36 hours.

As discussed previously, in addition to their crucial role in digestion, enzymes directly assist the defense mechanisms of the immune system.[2] When taken between meals, enzymes—whether produced by the pancreas or from supplements of plant or pancreatic (animal-derived) enzymes— act, as Dr. Pouls says, like "little Pac-Men" in the bloodstream, getting rid of unwanted material. With their ability to digest foreign proteins, enzymes are useful in clearing out infecting organisms, scar tissue, and the products of inflammation.

For example, CFS sufferers characteristically have high Epstein-Barr virus (EBV) antibody levels. Enzymes can digest the protective protein coat of EBV so the virus can be destroyed. Enzymes are also helpful in the removal of the CICs that are abundant in viral disease and, in particular, in patients with immune deficiencies.[3] Supplemental enzymes share the workload of the body's own pancreatic enzymes and therefore ease the burden of that organ's production of the enzymes needed for digestion, immune function, and all other chemical reactions in the body.

**Howard F. Loomis, Jr., D.C.:** 21st Century Nutrition®, 6421 Enterprise Lane, Madison, WI 53719; tel: (800) 662-2630. Website: www.loomisenzymes.com. Dr. Loomis's first line of enzymes was marketed under the brand name of Ness. His second-generation line of 29 enzyme formulas, called Natural Enzymes™, is available from 21st Century Nutrition.

For more on **enzymes and allergies**, see chapter 9, Addressing the Allergy Connection.

Further research into the benefits of enzyme therapy is needed, as it has been clinically proven to alleviate a wide range of conditions, including chronic fatigue syndrome.

# nine

# Addressing the Allergy Connection

Allergies are a common complaint of people who suffer from chronic fatigue syndrome and fibromyalgia, and they are the defining feature of environmental illness. Characterized by multiple and extensive allergies, environmental illness could be called the "ultimate allergy." Allergies in all three syndromes contribute to an already taxed immune system. Allergies and the immune response they generate can be a factor in up to 80% of patients with chronic fatigue.[1] As a contributor to immune overload, ongoing allergic reaction is an essential condition to address in the treatment of CFS.

Previous chapters have shown how immune dysfunction and enzyme deficiencies are related to intestinal problems. Allergies are closely linked to intestinal disorders as well. For example, candidiasis (overgrowth of the intestinal fungus *Candida albicans*) and allergies are often paired. As in the domino effect of mercury toxicity (see chapter 7, Eliminating Heavy Metal Toxicity), the intestinal dysfunction created by candidiasis can lead to "leaky gut" syndrome.

With leaky gut, undigested food particles pass through the intestinal walls into the bloodstream, and the body launches an allergic reaction against these foreign substances. When the condition is chronic, the patient may develop an allergy to that food. A delayed allergic reaction (hours to days after eating a food) is common; thus, you can have food allergies and not know it. Continued dysbiosis (imbalance of intestinal flora) leads to more allergies and serious health disorders such as chronic

> Dysbiosis [imbalance in intestinal flora] and delayed food allergies are almost universally present in people with autoimmune disorders.
> — *Serafina Corsello, M.D.*

fatigue syndrome. "Dysbiosis and delayed food allergies are almost universally present in people with autoimmune disorders," observes Serafina Corsello, M.D., director of the Corsello Centers for Nutritional Complementary Medicine in New York City and Huntington, New York.

In this chapter, you will learn about Nambudripad Allergy Elimination Technique (NAET) (SEE QUICK DEFINITION), a highly effective technique for permanently getting rid of your allergies, developed by Devi Nambudripad, D.C., L.Ac., R.N., Ph.D. You will also learn how other alternative medicine physicians treat the underlying causes of allergies and the attendant CFS. One of these physicians, Susan Lange, O.M.D., L.Ac., explains how "sick building syndrome" can be a contributing factor in environmental illness and describes how she healed herself of this debilitating condition.

We begin with Elinor, whose story vividly illustrates how unidentified allergies and untreated candidiasis can prevent recovery from chronic fatigue syndrome.

 The **Nambudripad Allergy Elimination Technique (NAET)** is used for the detection and elimination of allergies. Developed by Devi Nambudripad, D.C., L.Ac., Ph.D., R.N., this noninvasive method combines kinesiology's muscle response testing, acupuncture, and chiropractic. After identifying allergenic substances through muscle-response testing, the NAET practitioner uses acupuncture (or acupressure if the patient dislikes needles) to retrain the brain and nervous system to no longer respond allergically to those substances. For the treatment to become permanent, the patient must stay away from the offending substance for at least 24 hours, and sometimes more than one treatment is necessary.

## Success Story: Uncovering Hidden Allergies to Reverse Chronic Fatigue

When Elinor, 45, came to see Milton Hammerly, M.D., medical director of Integrative Global Medicine in Englewood, Colorado, she had been suffering from a long list of symptoms for 18 years. They included severe fatigue, depression, brain fog, concentration troubles, muscle spasms and aches, night sweats, premenstrual syndrome (SEE QUICK DEFINITION), frequent infections including bronchitis and sore throats, "migratory" rashes that sprang up on different areas of her body, and

# A Primer on Allergies

**Allergy**—This is an adverse immune system reaction—sometimes mild, sometimes severe—to a substance that other people may find harmless. Quite often, an allergen (a substance provoking an allergy symptom) is a protein that the body judges to be foreign and dangerous. The adverse reaction that follows is called an allergic response.

Common manifestations of this allergic response include fatigue, headaches, sneezing, watery eyes, and stuffy sinuses following exposure to an allergen. Allergies fall into two categories: those caused by environmental factors and those caused by food. The most common source of environmental allergies is the pollen of plants, particularly trees, weeds, and grass. The most common culprits in food allergies are wheat, corn, milk and other dairy products, egg whites, tomatoes, soy, shellfish, peanuts, chocolate, and food dyes and additives.

**Common Symptoms of an Allergic Reaction**—Breathing congestion; inflamed, bloodshot, scratchy, or watery eyes; runny nose; sneezing; nosebleeds; coughing; itching; puffy face; flushing of the cheeks; dark circles under the eyes; swelling; hives; vomiting; stomachache; intestinal irritation or bloating.

**Common Health Problems Partly Caused by Allergens**—Acne, allergic rhinitis (inflammation of mucous lining of nose), chronic runny nose, hay fever, ear infections, bedwetting, diarrhea, asthma, eczema, fatigue, headache, irritability, hyperactivity, concentration problems, attention deficit disorder.

**The Cycle of Food Allergies**—Food allergies present a paradox: often a person becomes addicted to a food that produces an allergic response. When a person stops eating an allergy-producing food to which their body is "addicted," such as coffee or chocolate, there is a three-day period in which they experience unpleasant withdrawal symptoms, such as fatigue; eating more of this addictive substance can actually improve the situation by suppressing these withdrawal symptoms. This of course becomes an unhealthy cycle of addiction, craving, and fulfillment that eventually leads to more serious health problems. Allergy experts call this suppression of symptoms by an allergy-producing (allergenic) food "masking," because it masks or disguises the true allergic symptoms.

**What Happens in an Allergic Response**—The typical allergic responses many people have to foods, dust, pollen, and other substances are the body's way of fending off the intrusion of toxins that disrupt its equilibrium. Allergens enter the body through the skin, through breathing, eating, or drinking, or by injection, such as insect bites or vaccinations. Because the body judges the allergens to be dangerous to its health, the immune system identifies them as antigens. Antigens trigger an allergic inflammatory response. The immune system then releases specific forms of protein called antibodies to deactivate the allergenic antigens, setting in motion a complex series of events involving up to 12 different biochemicals. These chemicals then produce the inflammation or other typical symptoms of an allergy response.

An antibody known as IgE is most commonly involved in the allergic response to pollens and foods. IgE is one of five immunoglobulins, or antibodies, involved with allergic responses. An immunoglobulin is one of a class of five specially designed antibody proteins produced in the spleen, bone marrow, or lymph tissue and involved in the immune system's defense response to foreign substances (technically, all antibodies are immunoglobulins). The main types of immunoglobulins, in the order of their concentration in the blood, are IgG (80%), IgA (10% to 15%), IgM (5% to 10%),

IgD (less than 0.1%), and IgE (less than 0.01%).

Mast cells, which produce the allergic response and are found throughout the body's tissues, next come into play; they tend to be concentrated in the skin, nose and lung linings, gastrointestinal tract, and reproductive organs. To respond to the IgE antibody, for example, a single mast cell has between 100,000 and 1 million receptor sites on its surface; it also has about 1,000 granules containing a substance called histamine. When the IgE antibody senses an allergen, it triggers the mast cells to release histamine and 28 other chemicals, and the allergic response flares into action. The IgE molecules also attach themselves, like a key fitting a lock, to the allergens.

**Histamine**—This is the substance that causes the blood vessels to widen, enabling more fluid to pass into body tissues, resulting in swelling; it also triggers the smooth involuntary muscles in the lungs, blood vessels, heart, stomach, intestines, and bladder to contract. Histamine gives us runny noses; red itchy eyes; hot, tender, or swollen body parts; flushed skin; and the other symptoms associated with allergic reactions.

In general, the allergic response—in the form of an inflammation, swelling, heat, redness, or tenderness—is the body's attempt to heal itself from the effect of the allergen. In other words, these responses are normal ways the body takes care of itself, albeit that in the process they can make us feel miserable. They may be the body's protective mechanism, but if they continue unchecked for too long your health will suffer.

The allergic response can happen as quickly as 15 minutes after your initial exposure to an allergenic substance. If the histamine and related biochemicals are released in the chest, you may experience coughing or asthma-like symptoms; if they come out through the skin, the symptoms may be hives or eczema; if in the intestines, the allergic response may show up as diarrhea; and if in the brain, it may result in a migraine headache.

**Other Chemicals Released During an Allergic Response:**

- **Heparin:** Increases blood flow to the site of inflammation or swelling.

- **Platelet Activating Factor:** Causes blood platelets to group together so that they release chemicals to change the diameter of blood vessels, thereby affecting blood pressure.

- **Serotonin:** A brain chemical known as a neurotransmitter, found mostly in the mucous membrane cells of the gastrointestinal tract, and involved in the allergic response to foods.

- **Lymphokines:** Produced by white blood cells (lymphocytes) and involved in communications among cells.

- **Leukotrienes:** Found in cell membranes and involved in making the lung muscles contract and the lungs retain more air, as in the bronchial spasm of asthma.

- **Prostaglandins:** Hormone-like substances that help dilate blood vessels, affect smooth muscle contraction, increase pain in affected areas, and heat up inflamed tissues.

- **Thrombaxanes:** Chemicals that cause the blood vessels and bronchial tubes to contract.

- **Bradykinin:** Supports the cascade of inflammatory symptoms set in motion by the mast cells.

- **Interleukins:** Antigens involved in the activity of lymphocytes, including the irritation of tissues.

- **Interferons:** Produced by lymphocytes to regulate the speed of immune responses.

not feeling refreshed after sleeping. Elinor also had digestive problems, including frequent constipation and bloating, indicating a probable imbalance in the microfloral population of her intestines (called dysbiosis).

**Premenstrual syndrome (PMS)** symptoms include bloating, cramping, achiness, irregular bleeding, headaches, short temper, irritability, sudden mood swings, depression, frustration, breast tenderness, weepiness, and abdominal discomfort. An estimated 5% of American women have such severe PMS symptoms that they are incapacitated for a few days every month.

She had been taking Synthroid, a synthetic thyroid drug for an underactive thyroid (a condition called hypothyroidism), for 12 years. Elinor was also taking a battery of standard drugs to address her other symptoms, including prescription synthetic progesterone for her PMS, and had become dependent on many of them. Elinor was generally unable to function; she couldn't hold a job or engage in normal social interactions. Elinor's husband had to drive her around and handle most of the domestic chores. Over the years, Elinor had seen many specialists and experimented with many drugs, but nothing had really helped. "Her symptoms were typical of CFS and fibromyalgia, both of which have come to be umbrella-like terms for this type of condition," observes Dr. Hammerly.

A blood test revealed that Elinor was deficient in DHEA, a hormone produced by the adrenal glands. While the range for DHEA is 130 to 980, Elinor's 136 was characteristic of a woman of 80, not 45, notes Dr. Hammerly. To start off her treatment, he put her on 25 mg of DHEA once daily. After a month of supplementation, a follow-up blood test showed her levels had climbed to a more acceptable 522.

With the raising of her DHEA levels, Elinor observed that her sleeping was improved and she had fewer aches and pains, but she was still very tired. At the same time that Dr. Hammerly had Elinor taking DHEA, he started her on digestive enzymes, taken with meals, to address her gastrointestinal disorders. He also gave her a product called Bioflora (containing beneficial bacteria needed by her intestines for better digestion and absorption); and 500 mg twice daily of chelated magnesium citrate (to help reduce muscle spasms). To complete his nutritional recommendations, Dr. Hammerly suggested a variety of key antioxidants, such as vitamin A (15,000 to 25,000 IU daily), vitamin C (2,000 mg daily), vitamin E (400 to 800 IU daily), and grape seed extract (100 mg daily).

Dr. Hammerly taught Elinor a pain-relief healing technique called electrostatic massage (SEE QUICK DEFINITION). He also suggested an energy therapy in the form of magnets (SEE QUICK DEFINITION), which he had Elinor apply to the pained muscles. A negative magnetic field has been found to be therapeutic for a range of conditions, including chronic pain and sleep disorders. Dr. Hammerly also recommended that Elinor get a magnetic mattress pad so that the energy of the magnets could gently work on her physiology (organs, tissues, and cells) during sleep. After using this mattress for only a week, she reported sleeping better, and she decided to continue using the pad regularly.

Yet, Elinor was still very tired. At this point, two months into Dr. Hammerly's program, a registered nurse at the center treated Elinor with Therapeutic Touch, which is a way of delivering subtle healing energy through the hands. "Due to her degree of soreness, Elinor would not have responded well to massage, but needed a gentler 'hands off' approach, such as therapeutic touch, which works with the body's energy fields rather than muscles." Dr. Hammerly notes that after the healing touch session, Elinor reported having a lot more energy, and for the first time in 18 years she felt ready and able to start an exercise program.

The healing benefits of Therapeutic Touch were working synergistically with the other components of the program. Elinor continued with this program, but three months later, her fatigue returned, accompanied by pressure in her head, sores in her nose and mouth, upper respiratory problems, and hair loss. When he examined her, Dr. Hammerly found swollen lymph nodes and muscle tenderness. A food allergy test, called the IgG-Antibody, which shows a patient's delayed reaction (hours to days after exposure) to allergenic substances and screens for reactions

**Electrostatic massage (EM)** is a therapeutic technique that uses static electricity to relieve pain by normalizing the malfunctioning nervous system, organs, and cells. A negatively charged PVC pipe is moved over the painful area of the body; this pushes electrons to the symptomatic area, where they facilitate the normal healing process, stimulating the metabolism and increasing the amount of oxygen to the cells. EM can reduce swelling due to water retention or edema by moving the water that accumulates in an area of inflammation. EM is used on patients suffering from general muscular pain, arthritis, fibromyalgia, headaches (tension and sinus), and tendinitis.

**Magnet therapy** works with the body's own electromagnetic fields to effect important metabolic changes in the body. Commonly, small, simple magnets are employed, providing a "calming" negative charge that helps normalize pH, oxygenate the blood, reduce swelling, and negate free radical damage, among other benefits.

For more on **hormone testing**, see chapter 2, Testing. For more on **the role of the thyroid and CFS**, see chapter 6, Reversing Hidden Thyroid Problems.

to 96 foods and 24 spices, indicated she was allergic to dairy products, eggs, gluten, and wheat.

Another test—the Candida Antibodies Panel, which measures *Candida albicans* levels—showed that there was a yeast overgrowth in Elinor's mucosal cells lining the intestines, lungs, and mouth. As discussed previously, candidiasis can create leaky gut syndrome, which can, in turn, lead to the development of allergies, as undigested food particles find their way from the intestines into the bloodstream where the immune system launches an allergic reaction against them. *Candida* infestation was also robbing Elinor's system of needed energy.

To treat Elinor for candidiasis, Dr. Hammerly employed an integrative approach, prescribing Nystatin—a conventional antifungal drug commonly given for candidiasis—and instructing Elinor to stop eating sugar, as well as the foods to which she was allergic. In addition, Dr. Hammerly wanted to build her nutrient status, as it is the foundation for energy and was depleted by the candidiasis and continual allergic reaction. He started Elinor on a series of Meyers' Cocktails (SEE QUICK DEFINITION), which involve a slow injection (lasting ten minutes) of mainly B-complex and C vitamins and magnesium. After four "cocktails" given over a four-week period, "her energy was significantly better." Elinor's *Candida* symptoms had also cleared up.

The **Meyers' Cocktail** is an intravenous vitamin and mineral protocol developed in the 1970s by John Meyers, M.D., a physician at Johns Hopkins University in Baltimore, Maryland. It contains magnesium chloride hexahydrate (5 cc given), calcium gluconate (2.5 cc), vitamin B2 (1,000 mcg/cc; 1 cc given), vitamin B5 (100 mg/cc; 1 cc given), vitamin B6 (250 mg/cc; 1 cc given), the entire vitamin B complex (100 mg/cc; 1 cc given), and vitamin C (222 mg/cc; 6 cc given). The solution is slowly injected over a 5- to 15-minute period. The "Cocktail" is indicated for patients with chronic fatigue, depression, muscle spasm, asthma, hives, allergic rhinitis, congestive heart failure, angina, ischemic vascular disease, acute infections, and senile dementia.

At this point, Elinor's psychiatrist started to reduce her antidepressants, telling Dr. Hammerly this was the first time in many years that Elinor had not seemed depressed to him. Her husband called Dr. Hammerly to exclaim, "I have my wife back for the first time in 18 years!" Two months later, Elinor had a slight relapse, feeling tired again, so Dr. Hammerly put her through a series of six Meyers' Cocktails, one per week; after this, she was fine. "She is out in the world, doing things. She's exercising. Her aches and pains are gone and her energy is good. Her husband is having a hard time keeping up with her," says Dr. Hammerly.

Elinor is one of many chronically ill

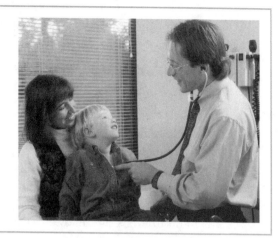

With alternative medicine, I actually have something to offer my patients.
—*Milton Hammerly, M.D.*

patients Dr. Hammerly has successfully helped. However, his results weren't always so promising. Before he joined the world of alternative medicine, Dr. Hammerly endured great frustration in his conventional medical practice at not being able to offer many of his patients lasting relief. Typically, Dr. Hammerly would see 25 patients a day and routinely prescribe at least 30 drugs. Many patients had chronic problems and didn't respond to conventional treatments.

"These were people who had already been through the mill of specialists, had tried everything. They were frustrated. I was frustrated. I would roll my eyes and ask myself, 'What am I going to do for this person?'" But now, after becoming versed in alternative medicine, Dr. Hammerly says with pleasure, "I actually have something to offer them." Most of his chronic illness patients— 70% to 80%, he estimates—get a good response and heal.

For more on **candidiasis testing**, see chapter 2, Testing. For more on **treating candidiasis**, see chapter 3, Eliminating Viruses, Infections, Candidiasis, and Parasites.

**Milton Hammerly, M.D.**: Integrated Global Medicine, 3464 South Downing, Englewood, CO 80110. For the **Candida Antibodies Panel**, contact: National BioTech Laboratory, 13758 Lake City Way N.E., Seattle, WA 98125; tel: (800) 846-6285.

## What Causes Allergies?

One of the primary causes of allergies is an impaired immune system, which substantially increases the risk of allergic reactions. "This occurs when the immune system becomes stressed due to an overload of toxins," says Charles Gableman, M.D., a former practitioner of environ-

> As with other body systems, allergic response and immune impairment are interlocking and form a vicious cycle of each worsening the other. As the immune system falters further, more allergies develop.

mental medicine, now living in Lake Forest, California. Many alternative practitioners agree.

In researching allergies, Leon Chaitow, M.D., D.O., based in London, England, has found that a number of factors have a negative impact on the immune system, including pollution in all its forms, vaccinations and immunizations, and an over-reliance on steroids, birth-control pills, and antibiotics. "Antibiotics further add to the confusion the immune system is facing," states Fuller Royal, M.D., of Las Vegas, Nevada, "until the immune system is no longer able to tell friend from foe. When that happens, it starts reacting to all sorts of things that are not foes, which then become treated as allergens. This leads to fatigue and allows viruses, bacteria, and so forth to come in and wreak havoc."

Dr. Royal also believes that the immune system may be weakened by hereditary problems. "Usually this will be reflected in the gastrointestinal tract. The nutrients are not able to be absorbed and utilized properly and this sets you up for food allergies." As with other body systems, allergic response and immune impairment are interlocking and form a vicious cycle of each worsening the other. Histamine, which is released during an allergic reaction, is an immune suppressant. As the immune system falters further, more allergies develop.

"A repetitive diet can contribute greatly to the development of allergies," says Marshall Mandell, M.D., medical director of the New England Foundation for Allergies and Environmental Diseases. The late Theron Randolph, M.D.—the founder of environmental medicine (SEE QUICK DEFINITION)—

 **QUICK DEFINITION** **Environmental medicine** (formerly called clinical ecology) explores the role of dietary and environmental allergens in health and illness. Dust, molds, chemicals, certain foods, and many other substances can cause allergic responses that can be linked to disorders such as chronic fatigue, asthma, arthritis, headaches, depression, gastrointestinal problems, and environmental illness. Environmental medicine physicians identify and treat patients' allergies as a means to resolve their health condition. Environmental medicine also addresses "sick building syndrome," a term applied to situations in which the physical environment of a building—its construction materials, furnishings, paints, lighting, ventilation—directly contributes to the ill health of those living or working in it.

discovered that the diets of allergy patients normally consist of 30 foods or less, which they eat repeatedly. "These 30 foods then become the basis for the most common food intolerances," says Dr. Mandell. "If someone eats bread every day, for instance, he could easily develop a wheat allergy due to the immune system's continuous exposure to it."

As mentioned earlier, leaky gut syndrome, or excessive permeability in the digestive tract, is another major factor that can lead to allergies. Among the causes of leaky gut syndrome, James Braly, M.D., of Fort Lauderdale, Florida, cites poor digestion, viral and bacterial infections, parasitic infestation, deficiencies in vitamins, minerals, amino acids and/or essential fatty acids, excessive stress, antibiotics, and candidiasis, all of which can be factors in CFS.

## Treating Allergies in Chronic Fatigue and Related Disorders

Alternative medicine offers a range of techniques for treating allergies and thus reducing the immune load of a person with CFS or similar illness. Among the most effective are NAET, nutritional supplements to address the deficiencies that help to create allergies, and Ayurvedic medicine treating digestive dysfunction as the source of allergies.

### The Nambudripad Allergy Elimination Technique (NAET)

To immediately alleviate the burden on the immune system created by allergies, it is necessary to eliminate the allergic reaction. Many practitioners accomplish this first through an often laborious process of identifying the offending substances and then by advising the patient to avoid these allergens. NAET, developed by Dr. Nambudripad in her journey back from healing her own severe allergies, eliminates both the laborious first step and the second step by permanently clearing the body of its allergic reaction to a substance.

NAET was discovered by chance when Dr. Nambudripad, who at one point in her life was found to be allergic to all foods but white rice and water, accidentally kept a trigger substance in her hand as she gave herself acupuncture in the middle of an intense reaction. To her astonishment, she recovered so fully that the next time she came into contact with the food it no longer bothered her. Through subsequent trial and error, she determined that the treatment worked because she was holding the substance within her own electromagnetic field. She went on to develop NAET, which uses applied kinesiology's (see QUICK DEFINI-

> Allergic response to foods, chemicals, or environmental sub-
> stances is often the cause of chronic fatigue syndrome.
>
> —-*Devi Nambudripad, D.C., L.Ac., R.N., Ph.D., developer of NAET*

TION) muscle response testing, acupuncture, and chiropractic to retrain the brain and nervous system not to launch an allergic response to a previously problematic substance.

What is unique to NAET is that through a simple, noninvasive procedure allergies can be permanently eliminated. Here's how it works. The practitioner using NAET has the patient lie down on the table, then tests the muscle strength in the patient's arm or leg as they hold a substance in a vial in one hand. Once an allergy-causing substance has been identified, the patient again holds it in one hand while the practitioner uses acupuncture, or acupressure if the patient prefers, on specific acupoints to "clear" the charge on that substance. For the treatment to become permanent, the patient must stay away from the offending item for at least 24 hours. Usually, a single treatment is enough to eliminate the allergy, but occasionally it takes more than one.

For the last 15 years, Dr. Nambudripad has used her technique to permanently eliminate the allergies of between 80% and 90% of her patients. Today, over 600 practitioners—including M.D.s, acupuncturists, and chiropractors—have joined her and are using NAET with equal success. They have seen numerous cases of CFS reversed by getting rid of the person's allergies; many of these patients had been going to CFS clinics for years with little result.

Dr. Nambudripad points to genetic susceptibility and the toxic environment

**Applied kinesiology**, first developed by George Goodheart, D.C., of Detroit, Michigan, is the study of the relationship between muscle dysfunction (weak muscles) and related organ or gland dysfunction. Applied kinesiology employs a simple strength-resistance test on a specific indicator muscle that is related to the organ or part of the body that is being tested. If the muscle tests strong, maintaining its resistance, it indicates health. If it tests weak, it can mean infection or dysfunction. For example, the deltoid muscle in the shoulder is related to the lungs and therefore is a good indicator of any problems there.

For more information about **NAET testing**, see chapter 2, Testing.

**Devi Nambudripad, D.C., L.Ac., R.N., Ph.D.** (for appointments or referrals for other doctors using NAET): Pain Clinic, 6714 Beach Boulevard, Buena Park, CA 90621; tel: (714) 523-0800. Website: www.naet.com. Dr. Nambudripad's book about NAET, *Say Goodbye to Illness*, is available from her clinic.

in which we live as the sources behind the current epidemic of allergies in the United States. "We are living today in an environment of electromagnetic pollution," she states. "All types of energies are bombarding our bodies from all directions and causing a wide range of psychological and physiological disorders, resulting in a weakening of the immune system that leaves people prey to debilitating illnesses," she says.

Allergic reaction to foods, chemicals, or environmental substances is often the cause of one such illness, chronic fatigue syndrome, says Dr. Nambudripad. Although the role of allergies in CFS has long been overlooked in the medical profession, she observes that "the connection between allergies and chronic fatigue syndrome is beginning to get the attention it deserves."

Frequently, offending substances are seemingly innocuous ones used in everyday life. For example, allergies to acetic acid and formic acid—present in most rubber goods, including the erasers on pencils, as well as in office correction fluid—can trigger extreme fatigue and chronic fatigue syndrome. Some people with CFS are allergic to their own body secretions (saliva, blood, urine, mucus), Dr. Nambudripad reports. Clearly, the allergies involved in cases of chronic fatigue can be to nearly anything and, as CFS is a serious disorder that has progressed over a long period, are often to many substances. The following brief case histories demonstrate the effectiveness of NAET in reversing CFS and related illnesses, despite the severity of the allergies:

A 35-year-old woman had been treated for CFS for three years. In spite of her treatment and a healthy diet, she was getting progressively worse and had already been on disability for three years when she came to Dr. Nambudripad. A thorough evaluation determined that she was allergic to almost all foods and fabrics. However, she was relieved to learn that she was suffering from allergies rather than some incurable illness. Within a couple of months of beginning NAET treatment, she started showing marked improvement. In all, it took six months (three to four visits per week) to clear all of her allergies. At the end of that period, she felt almost normal and began to work at a regular job.

Another woman, a 28-year-old teacher, had been disabled by Epstein-Barr for seven years. She was also found to be allergic to a great many substances—foods, physical agents, fabrics, and especially tap water. It took almost a year of continuous treatment to eliminate her allergies. She was then able to return to teaching full-time.

A 48-year-old computer programmer complained of extreme fatigue, frequent headaches, insomnia, and irritable bowel syndrome—condi-

> We are living today in an environment of electromagnetic pol-
> lution. All types of energies are bombarding our bodies from
> all directions and causing a wide range of psychological and
> physiological disorders, resulting in a weakening of the immune
> system that leaves people prey to debilitating illnesses.
> — *Devi Nambudripad, D.C., L.Ac., R.N., Ph.D.*

tions he had had since the age of eight. In addition to uncovering various environmental allergies, NAET found this patient to be allergic to
the electromagnetic emissions of the computer. All 12 acupuncture
meridians were implicated in his disability, meaning that his allergies
were so extensive that all the energy channels in his body showed an
imbalance. When he was treated with NAET for allergies to radiation
and the other substances, he was able to lead a normal life again.

**Success Story: Enzymes and NAET Cleared Up Chronic Fatigue and
Candidiasis.** Elizabeth, 35, had been struggling with chronic fatigue,
recurrent candidiasis, and a weight problem for a period of years when
she finally went to see Ellen Cutler, D.C., a chiropractor, enzyme therapist, and NAET practitioner at the Tamalpais Pain Clinic in Corte
Madera, California. In recent months, Elizabeth had also developed a
bladder infection for which she had been taking antibiotics. Soon after
beginning the medication, her symptoms disappeared, but the infection returned a few weeks later. This time, she wanted a permanent
solution to her chronic problems.

Dr. Cutler was not surprised to hear of Elizabeth's bladder infections.
"Women who suffer from chronic candidiasis eventually develop infections of the bladder," says Dr. Cutler. "The one causes the other. If you
cure the bladder symptoms without addressing the candidiasis, the bladder infection will simply come back." Similarly, treating Elizabeth's
chronic fatigue and candidiasis without addressing the underlying causes
of these ailments would relieve them only temporarily as well. To pinpoint these causes, Dr. Cutler performed an enzyme evaluation and a
urine analysis. The tests revealed that Elizabeth's diet might be a key
factor in her medical problems; specifically, she was not digesting fats,
proteins, and sugars well and she was eating a lot of sugar-rich carbo-

hydrates. Poor absorption of sugars is common in women suffering from candidiasis.

To address Elizabeth's digestive problems, Dr. Cutler put her on a special "sugar-intolerant diet." Elizabeth began eating less sugar and fewer starchy sugar-containing vegetables, such as potatoes, corn, and peas; emphasized protein over carbohydrates; and limited her intake of complex carbohydrates (such as breads and grains) and fruit to two daily servings each. To help break down food, Dr. Cutler recommended an enzyme formula containing amylase (digests carbohydrates), protease (digests proteins), and lipase (digests fats). After a few weeks, the dietary changes and enzyme supplementation noticeably improved Elizabeth's condition. Now her system was strong enough to begin addressing the fatigue and candidiasis.

Dr. Cutler treated Elizabeth's candidiasis by prescribing two enzyme formulas: *L. acidophilus* cellulase magnesium enzyme and an antifungal called Combat Fung. Elizabeth continued to improve, but Dr. Cutler suspected her problem might have causes other than the *Candida* yeast. "A lot of times the reason people don't succeed in treating *Candida* is that they're just looking at one type of fungus," Dr. Cutler notes. "There are ways of testing that can identify all the different fungi that might be causing an infection." For this, Dr. Cutler relies on NAET. Using NAET, Dr. Cutler identified and desensitized Elizabeth to over 50 different kinds of fungus and mold. "I've been in practice 20 years," says Dr. Cutler, "and I've never found any other way to get rid of fungus permanently." After the NAET treatment, Elizabeth never had another yeast infection. During the course of the NAET, Dr. Cutler also discovered that Elizabeth was allergic to B vitamins. NAET cleared her of this allergy as well.

Elizabeth now reported feeling less tired all the time. To supplement the probable nutritional deficiencies Elizabeth had developed as a result of her faulty digestion and allergy to B vitamins, Dr. Cutler prescribed a multivitamin (two capsules daily). To give her energy a boost by supporting her adrenal glands, Dr. Cutler recommended an enzyme for-

> **A Patient Speaks: No More Allergies**
>
> Jill Thompson, of Anaheim, California, says, "I was diagnosed as having Epstein-Barr virus/chronic fatigue syndrome and told there was no cure. Medical doctors were unable to offer me any hope. Some specialists believe that the root of CFS has something to do with allergies, and my experience with NAET confirms that. Since being treated, my CFS symptoms have ceased."

> **Ellen Cutler, D.C.:** P.O. Box 5356, Larkspur, CA 94977; tel 877-927-0741.

> What is unique about NAET is that through its simple, noninvasive procedure, allergies can be permanently eliminated.

mula called Chirozyme Adrenal (two capsules per dose, to be taken as needed). Soon, Elizabeth's symptoms of chronic fatigue disappeared entirely. "I've run into her a couple of times since we finished the treatment," says Dr. Cutler. "Elizabeth tells me that her fatigue is no longer a problem, and that she's 'religious' about staying on her enzymes."

*Success Story: Environmental Illness Reversed with NAET.* When Marilyn, 42, consulted Helen Thomas, D.C., a chiropractor and NAET specialist practicing in Santa Rosa, California, she had been enduring the serious symptoms of environmental illness for five years. After the birth of her child five years previously, she had became nauseous and developed chronic fatigue syndrome; her hands and feet swelled, and she experienced severe dizziness and headaches. Marilyn had also suffered toxemia during her pregnancy and two days before delivery had slipped into a coma and almost died. Her conventional physicians kept her on numerous medications in an attempt to reduce her symptoms, but her condition had worsened to the point where she was considered to be suffering from environmental illness.

Using NAET testing, Dr. Thomas determined that Marilyn was allergic to 40 different items. The list of substances producing an allergic reaction in her was formidable, including all egg and chicken products, calcium, milk protein, all fruits and vegetables containing vitamin C and B complex, all sugars, iron, vitamin A, fish, most minerals, salt, wheat gluten, and corn. In addition, Marilyn was allergic to most of the key brain chemicals known as neurotransmitters (SEE QUICK DEFINITION).

According to Dr. Thomas, Marilyn had major imbalances in her nervous, endocrine, and immune systems, such that her stress mechanism (her system's ability to tolerate the stress of allergic

> **QUICK DEFINITION**
> A **neurotransmitter** is a brain chemical with the specific function of enabling communications to happen between brain cells. Chief among the 100 identified to date are acetylcholine, gamma-aminobutyric acid (GABA), serotonin, dopamine, and norepinephrine. Acetylcholine is required for short-term memory and all muscle contractions. GABA works to stop excess nerve signals and thus keeps brain firings from getting out of control; serotonin does the same and helps produce sleep, regulate pain, and influence mood, although too much serotonin can produce depression. Norepinephrine is an excitatory neurotransmitter.

reactions) was incapacitated. Dr. Thomas systematically cleared each of Marilyn's allergies with NAET. Progress was unmistakable and steady during this process.

In about three weeks, her nausea began to recede; then within two months, her headaches lessened and her energy level started to pick up considerably. Five months after beginning the NAET treatments, Marilyn was able to wash every window in her house, clean all the rooms, and host a dinner party. In a subsequent letter to Dr. Thomas, Marilyn wrote: "I feel well and truly cared for, eased and comforted. Your treatments allowed my body to remember how well it could be."[2]

## Nutritional Supplements

According to James Braly, M.D., if digestive disorders are compounding the allergies, which is usually the case, they will also need to be corrected before any significant improvement can occur. "I find that many people with such complaints suffer from deficiencies in vitamin A, certain B vitamins, zinc, magnesium, and/or essential oils," Dr. Braly says. "Some people, especially as they get older or if their allergies are severe, also require digestive assistance in the form of pancreatic enzymes and/or hydrochloric acid (HCl), so supplementing each meal with them can be helpful as well."

Both zinc and vitamin A play an important role in the production of secretory IgA (immunoglobulin A) (SEE QUICK DEFINITION), a gastrointestinal antibody secreted from the salivary glands in the mouth and from cells that line the digestive tract. "The IgA antibody latches on to what is perceived in the body as allergens or potential allergens in the foods that we eat," Dr. Braly explains. "This action results in a protective coat of mucus being formed around these allergens, which prevents them from being absorbed into the bloodstream. If you're zinc and vitamin-A deficient, you produce less secretory IgA, and therefore your sus-

 An **immunoglobulin** is one of a class of five specially designed antibody proteins produced in the spleen, bone marrow, or lymph tissue and involved in the immune system's defense response to foreign substances. (Technically, all antibodies are immunoglobulins.) The main types of immunoglobulins, in the order of their concentration in the blood, are IgG (80%), IgA (10% to 15%), IgM (5% to 10%), IgD (less than 0.1%), and IgE (less than 0.01%).

ceptibility to food allergies increases." Zinc also plays a role in the production of the body's hydrochloric acid, which the body also needs for proper digestion to occur, says Dr. Braly.

Other nutrients that Dr. Braly employs to treat allergies are bioflavonoids (SEE QUICK DEFINITION). "Certain bioflavonoids are some of the most effective anti-allergy nutrients that I've come across," he says. "Many of my patients who are allergy prone, both to their diet and their environment, over a period of time stop having allergic reactions once these bioflavonoids start taking effect. Quercetin, my favorite bioflavonoid, taken orally along with bromelain, vitamin C, and glutamine, has produced wonderful results." Quercetin is a natural bioflavonoid and nontoxic alternative to allergy and anti-inflammatory drugs. It works by stabilizing the mast cells, effectively preventing them from releasing histamine. Histamine produces the common symptoms of an allergic reaction.[3]

Finally, vitamin C in high doses can have a dramatic effect in improving allergy symptoms, due to its ability to counteract the inflammation responses that are part of the allergic condition.

 A **bioflavonoid** is a pigment within plants and fruits that acts as an antioxidant to protect against damage from free radicals and excess oxygen. In the body, bioflavonoids enhance the beneficial activities of vitamin C; they are often formulated with this vitamin in supplement form. Originally called vitamin P up until 1950, these vitamin C "helper" substances include citrin, hesperidin, rutin, quercetin, epicatechin, flavones, and flavonols. When taken with vitamin C, bioflavonoids increase the absorption of vitamin C into the liver, kidneys, and adrenal glands. Acting as antioxidants, they also protect vitamin C from destruction by free radicals.

 For more on **supplements**, see chapter 10, Ending Nutritional Deficiencies with Supplements. For more on **probiotics**, see chapter 5, Detoxifying the Body.

*Probiotics.* Since imbalances of intestinal flora are common among allergy sufferers, Dr. Leon Chaitow stresses the need to restore bowel flora balance with a daily program of probiotics—the friendly or beneficial bacteria that inhabit the intestines under healthy conditions. "*Lactobacillus acidophilus, Lactobacillus bulgaricus,* and the *bifidobacteria* are the key players in this process," Dr. Chaitow says. "But care must be taken to select the proper strains," he cautions. "To be effective, probiotic supplements should be freeze-dried, contain only the declared and desirable strains of the species, and have concentrations of the friendly bacteria of about one billion parts per gram. They should also be kept refrigerated."

### Ayurvedic Medicine

In Ayurvedic medicine (SEE QUICK DEFINITION), allergies are viewed as a result of impaired digestion. "This is known as an *ama* condition," explains Virender Sodhi, M.D. (Ayurveda), N.D., of Bellevue, Washington. "In other words, the person with allergies is having trouble digesting proteins, carbohydrates, or fats, and this leads to a breakdown in the system that eventually creates the allergy." Dr. Sodhi points out that the digestive system has a link to all allergies, not just those caused by food. "Proper digestion aids the body in clearing out toxins," he says. "When digestion becomes impaired, a greater threshold of toxins have to be dealt with and eventually the body becomes overwhelmed. This is what leads to the allergies. So, in Ayurvedic medicine we always start with the digestive system in order to treat allergies."

 **Ayurveda** is the traditional medicine of India, based on many centuries of empirical use. Ayurveda describes three metabolic, constitutional, and body types (doshas), in association with the basic elements of Nature—*vata*, *pitta*, and *kapha*—and uses them as the basis for prescribing individualized formulas of herbs, diet, massage, and detoxification techniques.

In the case of CFS, Dr. Sodhi's treatment focuses on eliminating toxins and allergies and improving digestion. He puts patients on diet modification and cleansing programs to get rid of the toxins and also works on psychosomatic elements to improve sleep patterns. Dr. Sodhi states, "If patients don't sleep well, growth hormones don't get triggered and the body cannot be repaired."

Some of the herbs used in Dr. Sodhi's treatment include *ashwaganda*, *amla*, *bala*, *triphala*, and *lomatium*, which are combined according to each patient's particular needs. *Acidophilus* is also part of the program. According to Dr. Sodhi, *vata* metabolic body types are more susceptible to CFS. Physically, *vata* people tend to be slender, with prominent features, joints, and veins. Temperamentally, they are vivacious, energetic, and moody. Their energy characteristically fluctuates, with jagged peaks and valleys.

Maria, 45, had been experiencing progressively worsening fatigue for five years, to the point where she could not work at all. After being tested by hospitals and doctors, she was told nothing could be done for her and was given a prescription for antidepressants. Maria refused the medication and came to Dr. Sodhi. He placed her on his program, including a diet tailored to her specific medical history and body type. The diet consisted of vegetables, fruits, and fish, with no meat or dairy products. "Within three months of treatment, we were able to bring her test results down to normal. Now, she is working and functioning fine," reports Dr. Sodhi.

## Environmental Illness
## and the Sick Building Syndrome

Left untreated, chronic fatigue syndrome can progress to environmental illness, in which the person becomes allergic to almost everything around them. Many sufferers of environmental illness are so reactive that they are forced to barricade themselves in a home cleared of all chemical products. Until fairly recently, no medical solutions were to be found for this perplexing disorder. Now, however, there are alternative medicine physicians who, in the course of treating the rising number of patients seeking their help after conventional medicine has failed them, have developed effective protocols to reverse environmental illness.

The Meridian Center in Santa Monica, California, is the home of a team of doctors who have had great success in treating not only environmental illness, but also chronic fatigue syndrome, fibromyalgia, digestive disorders, headaches, infertility, arthritis, and other chronic conditions that baffle conventional doctors. Specializing in reversing the negative health effects of toxic environments, both outside and inside the body, the Center itself was scrupulously designed and outfitted with environmentally friendly materials so it would not become yet another source of toxicity for clients.

Susan Lange, O.M.D., L.Ac., cofounder of the Meridian Center, knows from personal experience how important this is. She spent nearly 12 years figuring out how to recover from environmental illness herself and, in the process, traced its origins to her exposure to numerous toxins, some of which occurred in buildings where she had worked. Specialists in environmental medicine use the term "sick building syndrome" for situations in which the physical environment of a building—its construction materials, furnishings, paints, lighting, ventilation—directly contributes to the ill health of those living or working in it.

In Dr. Lange's case, her first exposure to a "sick building" was in England in the early 1980s. The clinic in which she worked had kerosene gas stoves and small cubicles with no ventilation. "This was a major source of petrochemical poisoning for me," she notes. In 1985, Dr. Lange did postgraduate acupuncture study in China in a hospital that was rife with mold and fungus. "You could actually see the mold running down the walls," she recalls.

Then, in a clinic in Los Angeles where Dr. Lange subsequently worked, the air-conditioning filters had not been cleaned or replaced for years, so the system was venting dirty air and microbial contamination. On reflection, Dr. Lange realized that she may have been carrying petrochemical residues in her system since birth. Dr. Lange's mother lived above a gas station and inhaled diesel fumes every day while she was pregnant with her. "She was throwing up all the time. It was a toxic womb—my cellular terrain [the biochemical condition and vitality of her cells] was damaged at an early age," she says.

Dr. Lange's system was further compromised in her early twenties when she picked up intestinal parasites in India. According to one diagnosis at that time, she had amoebic hepatitis. Years of diarrhea, cramps, and pain ensued. Her doctors gave her a battery of tests, X rays, and conventional drugs such as Flagyl® and cortisone, not understanding that what Dr. Lange most needed was a rebalancing of her intestinal flora with "friendly bacteria," or probiotics.

While the antibiotics were unsuccessful in killing the parasites, they did kill the beneficial microbes, allowing the "unfriendly," pathogenic bacteria to thrive. A friend introduced Dr. Lange to acupuncture and she started receiving treatments. "That helped me survive, but it didn't clear up everything," she comments. (However, it did lead to her studying acupuncture professionally.) Unfortunately, Dr. Lange found her system was too weak to handle the Chinese herbs prescribed for her parasites.

## Using Acupressure to Relieve an Allergy— A Self-Help Approach

Michael Reed Gach, Ph.D., Director of the Acupressure Institute in Berkeley, California, has found that allergic reactions can often be relieved through acupressure—the use of fingertips in place of needles to stimulate acupoints. Dr. Gach explains, "As soon as you begin experiencing an allergic reaction, apply pressure on the point in the center of the webbing of your hand, between your thumb and index finger" (as illustrated).

LI 4

"Gradually apply firm pressure onto the point, angling the pressure toward the bone that connects with the index finger," Dr. Gach instructs. He recommends keeping a constant pressure for at least two minutes while taking slow, deep breaths. Then repeat the process with the same point on your other hand. "This point works like an antihistamine," Dr. Gach further explains. "I have found that this simple technique can often quickly arrest an allergy attack, making it a useful self-help remedy that anyone can use."

> "Sick building syndrome" exists when the physical environment of a building—its construction materials, furnishings, paints, lighting, ventilation—directly contributes to the ill health of those living or working in it.

### Allergic to Her Own House

The combination of environmental influences left Dr. Lange "incredibly ill" and her condition worsened over time. She had frequent heart palpitations and her ability to concentrate on her studies began to wane. She was allergic to about 70% of all foods, and many other substances—gas fumes and perfume—nearly made her faint. "The term 'environmental illness' wasn't in use then," she recalls, "but when I walked into my own house, I felt like passing out."

Fortunately, Dr. Lange found that her system could handle homeopathy, so she used a series of homeopathic remedies to start detoxifying her system of all its poisons, starting with petrochemicals. According to electrodermal screening, these were the key toxins. She used two complex homeopathic remedies, Petrochem Antitox and Mercury Antitox; she also used the classical homeopathic remedy, Sulphur, in doses ranging from 6C to 200C, to help drain toxins and chemicals from her organs. (Dr. Lange cautions that these remedies were prescribed on an individual basis and may not be appropriate for everyone.)

At the beginning, the most she could handle of the detoxification remedies was one drop daily in water (a normal dosage for Mercury Antitox and Petrochem Antitox is ten drops, three times a day). Any more than that and "my heart and head would pound." Gradually, Dr. Lange started feeling better and was able to increase the dosages to five drops a day. She also took a complex homeopathic remedy called *Ribes Nigrum*, which helps the kidneys to drain their toxins. For this, her dosage was two to three drops a day.

Electrodermal screening also indicated that she was seriously allergic to the mercury in her dental fillings. Complicating this was the fact that major dental work performed when she was 16 had misaligned her bite. As she had grown up in Hong Kong and Malaysia, she had received numerous vaccinations for cholera, smallpox, and other tropical infections. These factors weakened her body's "terrain," leaving her vulnerable to illness. "Electrodermal screening enabled me to look back

## Electrodermal Screening

Electrodermal screening is a form of computerized information-gathering, based on physics, not chemistry. A blunt, noninvasive electric probe is placed at specific points on the patient's hands, face, or feet, corresponding to acupuncture points at the beginning or end of energy meridians. Minute electrical discharges from these points serve as information signals about the condition of the body's organs and systems, useful for the physician in evaluation and development of a treatment plan.

through my health history to see how my immune system had been damaged," Dr. Lange says. It also showed her the way to restore her health.

It took three years to build up her system's vitality sufficiently to handle the procedures, but eventually Dr. Lange had her mercury fillings removed and her dental bite corrected. To rebuild her immune system, she received two daily intravenous infusions of vitamin C (up to 10 g) combined with B complex (2 cc) and B12 (500 mg). She also took homeopathic Mercury Antitox to remove the mercury from her tissues. Within three weeks of removing the mercury fillings, her heart palpitations stopped and the chronic diarrhea began to lessen. "On a misery scale of one to ten, I had been a ten, the highest. After this, I went down to a two. That's dramatic."

Next to go were the parasites. Dr. Lange discovered she still had the amoebae from her time in India, along with *Helicobacter pylori* bacteria she had picked up in China, which is associated with stomach ulcers and chronic gastric pain. A combination of Chinese and other herbs (including artemisia, coptis, phellodendron, isitis, grapefruit seed extract, black walnut, and garlic) and an antibiotic eliminated the bacteria and, finally, the amoebae. After the parasites were gone, Dr. Lange began to steadily regain her health.

There was one more factor Dr. Lange had to address in order to fully heal: the psychological and emotional component of her illness. Looking back, Dr. Lange comments: "What kept me going was my commitment to getting well, but my biggest shift came when I faced and let go

## Your Carpets Could Be Making You Ill

Many people who are sensitive to chemicals, highly allergic, or laid low with chronic fatigue syndrome often tell their physicians that they suspect common household items, including carpets, are somehow poisoning them. Often doctors dismiss these associations as purely in the patient's head. Now there is substantial scientific data to support the claims of poisoning. Your carpet may be bad for your health and you may be better off with bare floors.

Rosalind Anderson, Ph.D., of Anderson Laboratories in Dedham, Massachusetts, analyzed the effect of gas emissions on laboratory mice, based on over 300 carpet samples obtained through retail stores, carpet mills, or from patients' homes. All carpets had been in use from 1 week to 12 years; none were older than 40 years. Dr. Anderson performed over 500 different experiments—and the results were disturbing. She found that carpet emissions decreased the breathing rate of mice immediately on contact, from a norm of 280 times per minute to a low of 235 after eight minutes of exposure. When the mice were removed from exposure to the carpet emissions, their respiration rates became normal again. Dr. Anderson next learned that one or more exposures of the mice to the carpet samples produced a range of alarming symptoms, including swollen faces, hemorrhaging beneath the skin surface, altered posture, loss of balance, hyperac-

tivity, tremors, limb paralysis, convulsions, even death. She then analyzed 125 carpet samples for signs of neurotoxicity—that is, emissions that harm brain cells or the nervous system. Dr. Anderson found that 90% produced at least one toxic effect and 60% produced three or more "severe neurotoxic effects" in at least 25% of the mice.

Over 200 different chemicals have been identified in the typical modern carpet, according to Dr. Anderson, and these can produce "diverse toxic effects" in humans, including flu-like symptoms, muscle pain, fatigue, tremors, headaches (lasting up to 16 weeks after exposure), memory loss, and concentration difficulties. When it comes to negative health effects from carpets, "this is not a psychological phenomenon," says Dr. Anderson.*

*Anderson, Rosalind C., Ph.D. "Toxic Emissions from Carpets." *Journal of Nutritional & Environmental Medicine* 5:4 (1995), 375–386.

 For nonallergenic carpets (100% wool, free of chemicals or synthetic materials, almost completely biodegradable, and billed by the manufacturer as "the lowest toxic carpet available"), contact: Environmental Home Center, 1724 Fourth Avenue South, Seattle, WA 98134; tel: (800) 281-9785. Website: www.environmentalhomecenter.com.

of the belief I was carrying that the world is dangerous and everything I put in my body is going to damage me."

## *An Environmentally Friendly Clinic*

A personal, protracted experience with serious illness can be valuable training for a physician. Today, Dr. Lange's patients benefit from her long study of illness from the inside. Dr. Lange put her hard-won knowledge into practice in 1990 when she and her husband, Julian Lange, O.M.D.,

> A doctor's office should not make patients feel sicker spending time there. Being environmentally ill was a large motivation for me in putting the clinic together the way we did. Now that I am well, I am acutely aware of the quality of energy in a building that is necessary for comfort and optimal health.
>
> — *Susan Lange, O.M.D., L.Ac.*

L.Ac., designed, outfitted, and launched the Meridian Center. She knew, and will never forget, that "sick patients require extra-special surroundings because they are so sensitized." A doctor's office should not make patients feel sicker from spending time there, she says. "Being environmentally ill was a large motivation for me in putting the clinic together the way we did. Now that I am well, I am acutely aware of the quality of energy in a building that is necessary for comfort and optimum health."

During her real life tutorial in illness and healing, Dr. Lange came across Bau-biologie, the art and science of the "biological building." Well established in Germany, Bau-biologie is about the impact of building environments on human health and how to use this knowledge to construct environmentally friendly interior spaces that support, not deteriorate, the health of those using them. The Meridian Center, down to the finest detail, is a perfect demonstration of Bau-biologie. Carpets are made of hypoallergenic nylon, free of formaldehyde, moth proofing, stain repellents, pesticides, and other toxic materials typically found in carpets. Formaldehyde, a highly toxic substance, is commonly found in many building materials and furnishings, from wood to upholstery fabrics.

Dr. Lange took great care to avoid using any products containing these or other injurious chemicals. Similarly, the Meridian Center was designed to minimize indoor air pollution, which in

 **Susan Lange, O.M.D., L.Ac.:** The Meridian Center for Personal and Environmental Health, 1411 5th Street, Suite 405, Santa Monica, CA 90401; tel: (310) 395-9525. For more information about **Bau-biologie**, contact: Bau-biologie and Ecology, Inc., 1401A Cleveland Street, Clearwater, FL 33755; tel: (727) 461-4371. Website: http://buildingbiology.net.

many cases can be worse—for its concentration of hazardous chemicals and toxic emissions from common household and workplace products— than outdoor smog and atmospheric pollution. "All aspects of the clinic's

## Inside the Sick Building Syndrome

In the early 1980s, physicians began using the term "sick building syndrome" (SBS) to refer to a host of symptoms produced by low-grade toxic environmental conditions found in living, work, or office spaces. SBS symptoms are numerous: mucous membrane irritation of the eyes, nose, and throat, chest tightness, skin complaints (dryness, itching, abnormal redness), headaches, fatigue, lethargy, coughing, asthma, wheezing, chronic nasal stuffiness, temporary weight loss, infections, and emotional irritability. All of these depress the immune system, rendering the individual susceptible to long-term chronic illness and potentially to a cancer process.

"Indoor air pollution in residences, offices, schools, and other buildings is widely recognized as a serious environmental risk to human health," explains Michael Hodgson, M.D., M.P.H., of the School of Medicine, University of Connecticut Health Center in Farmington. Dr. Hodgson notes that most people in industrialized nations spend more than 90% of their time indoors; that indoor concentrations of pollutants (including toxic chemicals) are often "substantially" higher than found outdoors; and that small children, the elderly, and the infirm are likely to spend all their time indoors, leading to a permanent chronic exposure to low-grade toxic factors.

In most cases, problems with a building's engineering, construction, and ventilation system are the causes. Studies suggest that symptoms occur 50% more frequently in buildings with mechanical ventilation systems. Among 2,000 office workers in Germany with work-related symptoms, there was a 50% higher than average rate of upper respiratory tract infections that were directly traceable to problems with mechanically ventilated buildings, reports Dr. Hodgson. A U.S. study found that 20% of office workers had job-related SBS symptoms, including a subjective sense of being less productive in their work.

Besides ventilation problems, other sources of indoor toxic pollution include volatile organic compounds released from particle-board desks, furniture, carpets, glues, paints, office-machine toners, and perfumes. All contribute to "a complex mixture of very low levels of individual pollutants," states Dr. Hodgson. Bioaerosols are also indoor contaminants; they originate as biological agents from mold spores, allergy-producing microbes, mites, or animal danders; they are then distributed through an indoor space by ventilation, heating, or air-conditioning systems.

Of buildings classified as sources of SBS, one study showed that 70% have inadequate flow of fresh outside air. It also found that 50% to 70% of such buildings have poor distribution of air within the occupied space; 60% have poor filtration of outdoor pollutants; 60% have standing water that fosters biological growths; and 20% have malfunctioning humidifiers.

*Source:* Hodgson, Michael, M.D., M.P.H. "The Medical Evaluation" and "The Sick Building Syndrome" in Effects of the Indoor Environment on Health. Cited in: *Occupational Medicine: State of the Art Reviews* 10:1 (January–March 1995), 167–194.

interior—furniture, walls, paints, ceiling tiles, treatment tables, doors, fabrics, lighting, water, electrical installation, gowns, paper and cleaning products, even the plants—were selected for having the lowest environmental toxicity and for their ability to contribute to, not detract from, human health," says Dr. Lange. "Our facility and Bau-biologie's principles demonstrate that it is possible to use materials that are environmentally safe and easily available."

Staff, patients, and visitors enjoy—indeed, relish—the clinic because "it's so free of the external disturbances experienced in ordinary living environments. The moment patients walk through the door, the healing process begins," she says. "To support the healing of the patient, we need facilities that are designed not to damage the environment, but to bring positive regeneration to it—facilities that are not sick, but that are healing places for the body, mind, spirit, even the planet."

# Ending Nutritional Deficiencies with Supplements

The case stories presented throughout this book show that nutritional deficiencies are often a feature of chronic fatigue syndrome (CFS). Yet, as with most of the factors involved in this disorder, it is difficult to tell which came first, the deficiencies or the immune breakdown of CFS. The immune system and other key physiological systems of the body need proper nutrients in order to maintain health. Without enough or the right kinds of nutrients, these systems cannot function at an optimum level. If the nutritional deficiency becomes chronic, breakdowns in function will occur. In addition, a body whose immune system is continually overactive, as it is in CFS, requires far more nutrients to keep it going than a healthy body does.

Unfortunately, a person with CFS is likely to be receiving fewer nutrients than someone who is healthy, because the various viruses, parasites, fungal overgrowths, and other infections characteristic of CFS interfere with the proper absorption of nutrients. Gastrointestinal disorders further compound this problem, as do poor diet and food allergies. Correcting the underlying problems that contribute to nutritional deficiencies is essential. Until that happens, nutritional supplementation may be wasted. There is no point in introducing into the body what it cannot absorb. Prescribing nutritional supplements without attending to the diet also lessens the likelihood of a successful outcome.

The nutritional testing detailed in chapter 2 can pinpoint a patient's absorption problems and specific deficiencies in vitamins, minerals, amino acids, and essential fatty acids, among others. Test results can then be used as a guideline for designing a therapeutic program, monitoring its effectiveness, and modifying it as needed. Although every person with CFS is different and each program should be tailored to meet individual requirements, there are certain nutritional deficiencies that have been associated with CFS. In addition, there are specific nutrients that are useful for addressing symptoms and areas of dysfunction typical to CFS, such as weakened adrenal glands and an overworked

 Anyone currently under medical care, taking medications, or with a history of specific problems should always consult a physician (preferably one knowledgeable about diet and supplemental nutrients) before making any changes in diet or using supplements.

immune system. As pointed out frequently in this book, restoring depleted immunity is a vital component in treating CFS.

Before we discuss dietary recommendations and useful supplements in detail, let's look at how two alternative medicine physicians employed nutritional supplements to reverse severe CFS.

## Success Story: Back to Work in Three Months

When Elizabeth, 55, developed chronic fatigue syndrome, it became so severe she was disabled for eight months, unable to continue with her job. She sought help from Guillermo Asis, M.D., of Burlington, Massachusetts. Dr. Asis ran tests to see if she had a *Candida albicans*, Epstein-Barr virus, cytomegalovirus, or Coxsackie virus infection, all of which are commonly associated with chronic fatigue syndrome. It turned out that Elizabeth's system registered a high level of Coxsackie; tests also showed that her system was deficient in DHEA, a key adrenal gland hormone.

Dr. Asis started Elizabeth on a daily oral supplement program including a multivitamin formula called Vitality Plus (four times), vitamin C (2,000 mg, twice), magnesium aspartate (400 mg, four times), the antioxidant glutathione (50 mg, twice), DHEA (20 mg on an empty stomach at bedtime), and melatonin (another key hormone that is made in the brain and regulates body cycles) taken in a dosage of 3 mg at bedtime.

 **Guillermo Asis, M.D.**: 83 Cambridge Street, Suite 2C, Burlington, MA 01803; tel: (781) 221-6996.

Next, Dr. Asis began another more intensive supplement program for Elizabeth, in which high doses of selected nutrients were delivered to her body by intravenous (IV) infusion. In this mixture Dr. Asis included vitamin

C (35 g), magnesium (1.2 g), vitamin B5 (500 mg), sodium bicarbonate (615 mg) for a better pH balance (SEE QUICK DEFINITION), and vitamin B complex (1 cc). The advantage of administering vitamin C through IV rather than taking it orally is that it will not produce diarrhea, even at high doses, says Dr. Asis. When vitamin C is ingested orally, the intestines have a set limit on how much of this substance they can absorb at a given time; when bowel tolerance is reached, temporary diarrhea results. Bowel tolerance for vitamin C varies among individuals, but it is probably in the area of 5,000 to 10,000 mg daily for a relatively healthy person.

 The term **pH**, which means "potential hydrogen," represents a scale for the relative acidity or alkalinity of a solution. Acidity is measured as a pH of 0.1 to 6.9, and alkalinity is 7.1 to 14; a pH of 7.0 is considered neutral. The numbers refer to how many hydrogen atoms are present compared to an ideal or standard solution. Normally, blood is slightly alkaline, at 7.35 to 7.45; urine pH can range from 4.8 to 7.5, although normal is closer to 7.0.

Elizabeth received the IV mixture twice weekly while continuing the oral supplements. Within six weeks she was feeling better, Dr. Asis notes. In another six weeks, Elizabeth was able to return to work on a limited basis, gradually building up her strength and the length of her workday.[1]

## Success Story:
## Supplement Prescription Reverses Chronic Fatigue

Marilyn, 47, endured ten years of recurrent colds, sore throats, sinusitis, bronchitis, and asthma. She attributed her chronic health problems to the dampness of her Northern California home. When she began experiencing fatigue and shortness of breath, Marilyn went to two different specialists. Both told her that she had an underfunctioning thyroid gland. Marilyn cut back her hours at work, but her symptoms returned whenever she attempted full-time employment.

Finally, Marilyn and her husband moved to Tucson, Arizona, in the hope that the warm, dry climate might improve her condition. Although the Tucson climate helped with her asthma and bronchitis, Marilyn began experiencing problems with memory and concentration. In addition, her temperature, which was usually slightly below normal at 97.6° F, was elevated at a constant 99° to 100° F. Marilyn was unable to walk or do housework and had to rest after every minor physical exertion. The blood tests she requested from her doctor showed that "nothing was wrong"; even her thyroid was functioning "normally."

> Dr. Dommisse's testing revealed that Marilyn had severe defi-
> ciencies of vitamin B12 and the minerals chromium and man-
> ganese, and that her blood was carrying near-toxic levels of
> copper.

After learning about chronic fatigue syndrome in a health-food store lecture, Marilyn sought out the help of John Dommisse, M.D., a Tucson-based physician who specializes in treating this debilitating illness. Although Marilyn's doctors in California and Arizona had already run general blood tests, Dr. Dommisse tested Marilyn specifically for nutrient and thyroid hormone imbalances. The additional testing revealed that Marilyn had severe deficiencies of vitamin B12 and the minerals chromium and manganese, and that her blood was carrying near-toxic levels of copper.

To get Marilyn's B12 levels back to normal, Dr. Dommisse administered injections of the vitamin (1,000 mcg) once a week for two months. After the initial injection treatment, Marilyn was advised to supplement with B12 lozenges (2,500 mcg twice daily), to be taken under the tongue. Marilyn also took chromium (three tablets at 200 mcg each) and manganese (two tablets at 50 mg each) twice a day. To reduce the copper levels in Marilyn's body, Dr. Dommisse suggested that she only drink and cook with distilled or copper-filtered water.

After a few months on this program, Marilyn reported that her fatigue was reduced by 50%, her temperature had returned to normal, and her chronic colds and sore throats had subsided. In addition, the correction of Marilyn's chromium and manganese deficiencies had contributed to an overall reduction in her appetite and increase in her metabolism. Marilyn dropped 50 pounds of excess weight as a result.

Dr. Dommisse then explored additional causes of Marilyn's fatigue, which was still only 50% improved. He tested her for candidiasis and found Marilyn to have a minor case, but enough to be a problem. For the candidiasis, Dr. Dommisse prescribed 200 mg daily of Nizoral®, a conventional antifungal medication. Dr. Dommisse also suggested that Marilyn treat her candidiasis with a no-sugar, no-white-starch diet, which included supplements of *acidophilus* (1,000 mg, twice daily) and caprylic acid, an anti-*Candida* fatty acid (700 to 800 mg, twice daily).

Seven weeks after beginning this final stage of treatment, Marilyn's

## Improving the Mental Symptoms of CFS

Memory loss and mental confusion are common problems among CFS sufferers, but taking dietary supplements may help reverse these symptoms. Research now suggests that supplementing with the nutrients found in certain brain chemicals can support brain function and improve mental ability. One of these brain chemicals is phosphatidyl-serine (PS), a large lipid molecule also found in trace amounts in lecithin derived from soybeans. PS, when given as a supplement, helps support both membrane functions in nerve cells and cell-to-cell communications. Since the 1970s, 34 clinical studies have demonstrated the effectiveness of PS supplements in improving mental abilities.

A Belgian study of 35 hospitalized patients, all of whom had mild to moderate loss of memory and mental ability, showed that taking PS at the rate of 300 mg per day for six weeks produced improvement in three different brain-function rating scales. In Italy, a study involving 87 patients with moderate brain-function loss linked PS to a strong improvement in attention, concentration, and short-term memory. Study participants also reported feeling less apathetic and withdrawn. In addition, the clinical studies found that PS has a remarkably good safety record, producing only minimal side effects in test subjects.

Lucas Meyer, Inc. has developed a means to produce the PS found in soy lecithin in commercially practical quantities. The PS-containing product—called LECIPS—has been marketed as a dietary supplement geared toward improving brain function. The product's makers recommend an initial dose of 100 to 300 mg daily for one month, followed by a maintenance dose of 100 to 200 mg daily, noting that improvements in mental abilities will fade away if use of the substance is discontinued.

Source: Kidd, Parris M., Ph.D. *Phosphatidyl-serine (PS): A Remarkable Brain Cell Nutrient* (Decatur, IL: Lucas Meyer, 1995). This booklet is available from: Lucas Meyer, Inc., P.O. Box 3218, Decatur, IL 62524; tel: (217) 875-3660.

fatigue had disappeared entirely and it has not returned since. Marilyn no longer suffers from the nasal congestion that caused her to leave Northern California, and her insomnia and shortness of breath have ceased. Even better, Marilyn now has enough energy to exercise daily and has returned to full-time work. "Of all the doctors that treated me in the past six years, all meticulously recorded my symptoms of chronic fatigue," Marilyn says, "but despite the batteries of blood tests and MRI scans, they never tested me for the factors that eventually led to my cure."[3]

## Diet and Nutrition in Chronic Fatigue

The leading nutritional problem in the United States today is "over-consumptive undernutrition," or the eating of too many empty-calorie junk foods, says Jeffrey Bland, Ph.D., a biochemist and nutrition expert based in Gig Harbor, Washington. Although people in the United States consume plenty of food, it is not the right kind of food. Almost two-

> Michael Murray, N.D., naturopathic educator and author of *Encyclopedia of Nutritional Supplements*, says that attention to diet is crucial in reversing CFS. "Your energy level is directly related to the quality of the foods you routinely ingest," he states.

thirds of an average American's diet is made up of fats and refined sugars having low to no nutrient density.

Consequently, the remaining one-third of the average diet must provide the essential nutrients needed to maintain health, and it may or may not consist of high-nutrient-density food. Insufficient nutrient intake weakens overall physiological and mental performance, robs the body of its natural resistance to disease, and leads to premature aging. Chronic nutritional deficiencies can obviously contribute to the domino effect of disorders that characterizes CFS.

Without a healthy diet, nutritional supplementation is like sprinkling a few drops of water on parched earth. Michael Murray, N.D., naturopathic educator and author of *Encyclopedia of Nutritional Supplements*, says that attention to diet is crucial in reversing CFS.[3] "Your energy level is directly related to the quality of the foods you routinely ingest."[4] In his estimation, a healthy diet avoids "empty" foods low in nutrients and high in sugar and fat.

 For more on **food allergies and CFS**, see chapter 9, Addressing the Allergy Connection.

Instead, it concentrates on high-nutrient, high-protein, complex-carbohydrate foods—vegetables, grains, beans, fish, and poultry (care should be taken to avoid mercury toxins in fish and antibiotics in poultry). He advises eliminating caffeine and alcohol. There are many reasons to do so, but perhaps the foremost is to avoid further stress on the adrenal glands and the liver.

Dr. Murray also cautions that, as food allergies may be undermining your nutrient intake, it is important to identify them and take measures to avoid the problem foods. To prevent the development of allergies, don't always eat the same foods, but rather include a variety and rotate what you eat.[5] In addition, Dr. Murray and most alternative medicine physicians recommend drinking eight to ten glasses of pure water daily.

## Nutritional Deficiencies
## and Chronic Fatigue Syndrome

Medical science has long held that healthy adults do not need supplementation if they consume a healthful, varied diet, but the U.S. Department of Agriculture (USDA) has found that a significant percentage of the American population receives well under 70% of the U.S. Recommended Dietary Allowance (RDA) for vitamin A, vitamin C, B complex vitamins, and the essential minerals calcium, magnesium, and iron.[6] A separate study found that most typical diets contained less than 80% of the RDA for calcium, magnesium, iron, zinc, copper, and manganese, and that the people most at risk were young children and women, adolescent to elderly.[7] It is sobering to consider that the situation is even worse than these numbers indicate, because the RDA in itself is judged by many nutritionists to be below the amounts of these nutrients that most individuals actually need.

This is especially true in the face of the numerous factors in modern life that drain us of nutrients and thus raise the levels we require. Even when we eat a healthy diet (which, as stated above, most people in the U.S. don't), the food we are getting is not as nutrient-rich as it once was. Most of the soil in which food is grown in the United States has been depleted by poor farming practices and the use of pesticides. Even organic farming, unless the land was always farmed organically, has to contend with the poor soil produced by decades of conventional farming. Additionally, environmental pollution (both chemical and electromagnetic), stress and other lifestyle patterns, and certain medications create even greater nutrient requirements.

Historically, if patients had no overt symptoms or disease, doctors regarded them as healthy and adequately nourished. Today, doctors and scientists are beginning to recognize mild and moderate nutritional deficiencies, the symptoms of which may often be subtle, overlapping, and varied. For example, the first signs of B-vitamin deficiency may include subtle changes in behavior: an inability to concentrate, insomnia, and mood swings. Other symptoms of nutritional deficiencies can include fatigue, muscle weakness, nervousness, mental exhaustion, confusion, and anemia. It has been reported that marginal deficiencies of vitamins A, C, E, and B6 may also reduce immunocompetence, impairing the body's ability to ward off disease and repair tissues.[8] Do these symptoms sound familiar? All of them are characteristic of CFS.

> Deficiencies in vitamin B12, folic acid, pantothenic acid, vita-
> min C, iron, potassium, and phosphorus have all been impli-
> cated in fatigue. Supplementation with these nutrients has had
> beneficial effects for many people with chronic fatigue.

When nutritional deficiencies are combined with the other elements
of CFS, once again the balance can be tipped toward developing the disorder. Research has clearly linked CFS with deficiencies in magnesium,
essential fatty acids, and the amino acids carnitine and methionine. Further, deficiencies in vitamin B12, folic acid, pantothenic acid, vitamin C,
iron, potassium, zinc, and phosphorus have all been implicated in fatigue.
Supplementation with these nutrients has had beneficial effects for many
people with chronic fatigue.[9] Deficiencies associated with other symptoms of CFS, such as muscle weakness and depression, are discussed in
the following section under the relevant nutrients.

### Nutritional Supplements for Fibromyalgia Relief

Many of the supplements discussed in this chapter are beneficial for treating fibromyalgia, but the following have been found to be especially useful by Chanchal Cabrera, M.N.I.M.H., a clinical herbalist practicing in
Vancouver, British Columbia:

- *Niacinamide.* A form of niacin (vitamin B3); high doses (900 to
  4,000 mg daily in divided doses) of niacinamide are effective in
  reducing musculoskeletal inflammations, but should be taken only
  under a physician's supervision.

- *Lipotropic factors* (substances that remove and prevent fatty
  deposits). A combination of the lipotropic factors phosphatidyl
  choline (lecithin, a neurotransmit-
  ter precursor), inositol (a component of the vitamin B complex),
  and methionine (an amino acid)
  can aid in liver function, helping
  to detoxify the system and correct
  any excessive fat deposits that reduce blood circulation and can
  lead to painful blood clots. Methionine is integral to cartilage, so it

**Chanchal Cabrera, M.N.I.M.H.:**
Gaia Garden Herbal Dispensary, 2672 West Broadway,
Vancouver, B.C., Canada V6K 2G3; tel: (604)
734-4372. Website: www.gaiagarden.com.
The initials M.N.I.M.H. stand for Member of
the National Institute of Medical Herbalists,
a British designation used in Canada to indicate professional status as an herbalist.

can improve the strength of joint tissues. The dosage is one gram of each per day, taken in combination.

- **Vitamin E.** This antioxidant's effective anti-inflammatory action suppresses the breakdown of cartilage while stimulating cartilage growth. A dose of 400 to 1,200 IU a day is recommended.

- **Vitamin C.** This antioxidant nutrient is vital for tissue repair and, when taken in combination with vitamin E, will contribute to the stability of cartilage. The recommended dosage is to bowel tolerance (the amount just under what will cause diarrhea).

- **Eicosapentaenoic acid (EPA).** An essential fatty acid found in most fish oils, EPA is an anti-inflammatory. An effective dosage is 1.8 grams daily.

- **Selenium.** This antioxidant mineral works in combination with vitamin E and inhibits inflammation. Selenium blood levels tend to be low in fibromyalgia sufferers. The recommended dosage is 200 mcg per day.

- **Zinc.** This antioxidant mineral is necessary for tissue repair and may be deficient in people with fibromyalgia. An effective dosage is 25 to 50 mg daily.

- **Magnesium malate.** A lack of magnesium can result in aluminum buildup in the brain, which can, in turn, produce fibromyalgia symptoms. Magnesium (1,000 to 1,500 mg daily) taken in a combination formula with malic acid is an effective supplement.

### Lifestyle Changes and Supplements Can Aid Chronic Fatigue

Julian Whitaker, M.D., author of *Dr. Whitaker's Guide to Natural Healing*, uses a nutritional supplement and lifestyle adjustment program to successfully treat chronic fatigue syndrome. The program "is based on a simple truism of nondrug health care: a multifactorial problem is best addressed with a multifactorial solution," explains Dr. Whitaker. "The Whitaker Wellness Program, on its own, will often lead to complete recovery from chronic fatigue. The major factors that determine your energy levels and the status of your immune system are diet and lifestyle. Once you improve these factors, the rest is easier."

*Start practicing the Whitaker Wellness Program.* Adopt a healthy lifestyle, which means paying attention to nutrition and getting plenty of exercise. Definitely quit using tobacco, alcohol, and recreational drugs.

> The Whitaker Wellness Program, on its own, will often lead to complete recovery from chronic fatigue. The major factors that determine your energy levels and the status of your immune system are diet and lifestyle. Once you improve these factors, the rest is easier.
>
> Julian Whitaker, M.D.

Take a megavitamin/mineral supplement daily so that your intake is well above the RDA. Add to this a strong antioxidant program including vitamins C (3,000 to 8,000 mg daily) and E (1,200 IU daily). Then fortify everything with extra amounts of magnesium (1,000 mg daily), potassium (about 400 mg daily), and essential fatty acids from evening primrose, flaxseed, black currant seed, borage, and fish oils. Finally, eat a diet high in complex carbohydrates and low in fats.

> **Julian Whitaker, M.D.:** Whitaker Wellness Institute®, 4321 Birch Street, Newport Beach, CA 92660; tel: (800) 488-1500. Websites: www.whitakerwellness.com; www.drwhitaker.com. For a subscription to *Dr. Julian Whitaker's Health & Healing,* a monthly newsletter, contact: Health & Healing, 7811 Montrose Road, Potomac, MD 20854; tel: (301) 424-3700.

**Strengthen your immune system vitality** by taking calf thymus extracts (two tablets of ThymuPlex brand, each containing 375 mg of active calf thymus components, twice daily with your meals). The wonder herb echinacea is also a powerful ally here, in dosages of 2 to 4 ml (one to two teaspoons) of tincture three times daily.

**Strengthen your adrenal glands.** Most CFS sufferers have adrenal malfunction due to chronic stress and inadequate nutrition. Useful are oral bovine adrenal extracts (dosage depends on your individual constitution and condition) and Siberian ginseng extract (100 mg three times a day).

### Dietary Guidelines: Why You Need Fats in Your Diet

Nutritional biochemist Patricia Kane, Ph.D., offers the following observations about the importance of having the proper amount of fat in the diet and the dangers of having the wrong kinds:

When your diet no longer supplies the necessary raw materials—many of them derived from fats—for running the body efficiently, lots of things go wrong, and the body and brain start to shut down.

Patricia Kane, Ph.D.

In the interest of staying slim, many people—especially women—reject butter and cream in favor of margarine and hydrogenated (semisolid) fats. This is terribly unfortunate because saturated, hydrogenated fats—a category called trans-fatty acids (TFAs—SEE QUICK DEFINITION), typified by margarine—create havoc in a person's neurochemistry, negatively affecting every system of the body.

At the same time, these inappropriate food choices lead to nutrient depletion because the body is not given the kind of fat it needs from the diet for proper body function. The fats we need are called essential fatty acids. The foods many people choose in their diet are, increasingly, not nutrient-dense—for example, a white-flour bagel or pasta, a salad with non-fat dressing—and therefore fail to provide essential ingredients for body processes.

When your diet no longer supplies the necessary raw materials—many of them derived from fats—for running the body efficiently, lots of things go wrong, and the body and brain start to shut down. Prozac is only a few more wrong meals away. In the contrast between trans-fatty acids and essential fatty acids, you have the cause and cure of depression.

Trans-fats, or hydrogenated manmade fats, were synthesized originally to extend the shelf life of commercial products. But the production of TFAs for human consumption is the most devastating nutritional mistake ever made. In the effort to make foods last longer in the supermarket, all traces of essential fatty acids (such as omega-3s) are obliterated from processed foods, and trans-fats or partially hydrogenated oils take their place.

The absence of omega-3 (SEE QUICK DEFINITION) essential fatty acids in Western diets has contributed to an alarming increase in a number of diseases that appeared only infrequently a hundred years ago. A

**Trans-fatty acids** (TFAs) are chemically and structurally altered hydrogenated vegetable oils (such as margarine), in which the double bonds linking hydrogen atoms are changed from a "cis" form (atoms bonded on the same side of a chain) to a "trans" form (atoms bonded on the opposite sides of a chain), which is considered more stable. The TFA composition of commercially prepared hydrogenated fats varies from 8% to 70% and comprises about 60% of the fat found in processed foods.

It is estimated that Americans consume over 600 million pounds of TFAs annually, in the form of frying fats. TFAs can increase the risk of heart disease by 27% when consumed as at least 12% of total fat intake. TFAs also reduce production of prostaglandins (hormones that act locally to control all cell-to-cell interactions) and interfere with fatty acid metabolism.

**Omega-3 and omega-6 oils** are the two principal types of essential fatty acids—unsaturated fats required in the diet. The numerals "3" and "6" refer to differences in the oil's chemical structure with respect to its chain of carbon atoms and where they are bonded. A balance of these oils in the diet is required for good health. The primary omega-3 oil, called alpha-linolenic acid (ALA), is found in flaxseed (58%), canola, pumpkin seeds and walnuts, and soybeans. Fish oils, such as salmon, cod, and mackerel, contain the other important omega-3 oils, DHA (docosahexaenoic acid) and EPA (eicosapentaenoic acid). Omega-3 oils help reduce the risk of heart disease. The main omega-6 oil, linoleic acid or cis-linoleic acid, is found in most plant and vegetable oils, including safflower (73%), corn, peanut, and sesame. The most therapeutic form of omega-6 oil is gamma-linolenic acid (GLA), found in evening primrose, black currant, and borage oils. Once in the body, omega-3 and omega-6 are converted to prostaglandins: hormone-like substances that regulate many metabolic functions, particularly inflammatory processes.

lack of both the essential fatty acids and the cofactors (such as minerals and vitamins) to handle fat, along with the consumption of trans-fats, is more often the cause of obesity and cardiovascular disease than is eating cholesterol-rich foods. After all, the body needs some cholesterol—it is needed to produce a cascade of crucial hormones including pregnenolone, testosterone, progesterone, estradiol, estrone, and cortisol, among others.

It's not just cholesterol that is needed in the diet. You need fats, too. Like proteins, fats (lipids) are building blocks of the body's essential structures. The membrane of every cell and organelle is a thin envelope of fat that encases and protects the internal biochemical components; within this fatty envelope are thousands of proteins that facilitate communication and transport—acting like gates—across the cell membrane.

Fatty acids strongly influence the *fluidity* of cell membranes, which means the ability of the cell wall to change shape to allow red blood cells through with life-sustaining nutrients. These biomembranes literally control and signal all activities inside and outside the cell; the brain, it's important to know, is 60% lipids. Knowing this, perhaps you can begin to sense the kind of trouble likely to result when there is a disturbance in or deficiency of the right kind of fats in the body. Disturbances in fatty acid metabolism (its energy changes and chemical conversions) are reflected throughout every system of the body, and can manifest in many physical and mental disorders.

Let me express the problem with trans-fatty acids with an image. The more unsaturated the fat, the more it vibrates, and the longer the chemical "tail," the faster the vibration. An unsaturated fat has a "tail" that is extremely vibratory in nature, and this vibration is good. But a saturated fat or trans-fatty acid is rigid and has little movement. A trans-fatty acid sits like cement inside you, shutting everything down such as hormone production, and replacing the good, necessary fats (omega-3s and -6s) with something harmful to health. You can't do anything with a trans-fatty acid except burn it for calories; basically, its activity is to poison your system and generate an abnormal, undesirable biochemistry.

The use of trans-fatty acids shuts down the fatty acid metabolism within the immune, endocrine, and central nervous systems. High-quality fatty acids obtained through the diet are essential for the synthesis of hormones called prostaglandins that control all interactions among cells. Further, your body needs specific fatty acids to maintain the integrity of the gastrointestinal tract lining and the cell walls (to ensure smooth traffic of nutrients and signals across cellular membranes) and to produce hormones and immune system cofactors. Trans-fatty acids must be completely avoided to protect your immune, endocrine, and central nervous systems.

**EDITOR'S NOTE** **Patricia C. Kane, Ph.D.**, is a nutritional biochemist specializing in traumatic brain injury, seizure disorders, autism, and developmental delay. Dr. Kane is the author of *Food Makes the Difference* (1985) and *The Neurochemistry and Neurophysics of Autism* (1996), director of nutritional biochemistry at the Kaplan Institute in Orangevale, California, and director of medical research for Carbon Based Corporation in Incline Village, Nevada. To contact Dr. Kane: 45 Reese Road, P.O. Box 809, Millville, NJ 08332; tel: (888) 320-8338. Website: www.bodybio.com.

## An A to Z Guide to Nutritional Supplements for CFS

The following is a guide to supplements that address the deficiencies often found in CFS as well as the specific disorders characteristic of the illness. Dietary sources of nutrients are listed where appropriate as an additional means of remedying a deficiency.

## Vitamins

The key function of vitamins is to support the activity of the enzymes and coenzymes in the body, but all essential processes are impaired by vitamin deficiency. Vitamins and enzymes work together in the body to maintain all chemical reactions, including energy production.

*Vitamin A.* As one of the primary antioxidants (SEE QUICK DEFINITION), vitamin A protects the body from free-radical damage. It also helps the body ward off disease by: (1) strengthening the immune system through the stimulation of T-cell activity; (2) contributing to the health of the thymus, which is integral to immune health since one of this gland's functions is to activate T cells; and (3) maintaining the health of the skin and mucous linings of the digestive tract, sinuses, lungs, bladder, and other organs that are the first line of defense in keeping disease-causing microorganisms from entering the body. Chronic infection, as in CFS, depletes the body of vitamin A, and a vitamin A deficiency leaves the body more vulnerable to infection, so the cycle of deficiency deepens.

Research indicates that, in addition to increasing immune response, controlled high-dosage supplementation with vitamin A may significantly reduce fatigue.[10] This may be due in part to vitamin A's role in the production of red blood cells, a shortage of which is the condition known as anemia, characterized by fatigue. A person's red blood cell level may not have dropped to the range defined as anemia, but may be in short enough supply to produce fatigue. A compromised immune system obviously contributes to fatigue as well.

An **antioxidant** (meaning "against oxidation") is a natural biochemical substance that protects living cells against damage from harmful free radicals. Antioxidants work against the process of oxidation—the robbing of electrons from substances. If unblocked or left uncontrolled, oxidation can lead to cellular aging, degeneration, arthritis, heart disease, cancer, and other illnesses. Antioxidants in the body react readily with oxygen breakdown products and free radicals, neutralizing them before they can damage the body. Antioxidant nutrients include vitamins A, C, and E, beta carotene, selenium, coenzyme Q10, L-glutathione, superoxide dismutase, catalase, and bioflavonoids such as grape seed extract and pine bark extract (pycnogenol). Plant antioxidants include *Ginkgo biloba* and garlic. When antioxidants are taken in combination the effect is stronger than when they are used individually.

Dietary sources particularly high in vitamin A include liver, chili peppers, carrots, dried apricots, sweet potatoes, and leafy greens.[11] Supplemental dosages of vitamin A for CFS vary, but should not be above 20,000 IU daily without physician supervision, according to Susan Lark, M.D., of Los Altos, California.[12]

*Beta carotene.* Beta carotene, classified as a carotenoid, is the pigment that accounts for much of the color in the plant world and is the dominant pigment in most fruits and vegetables. As an antioxidant and precursor to vitamin A, converted by the body as needed, beta carotene performs the functions of vitamin A. It also has antioxidant and immune-enhancing properties not found in vitamin A.[13] These include increasing the numbers of key immune cells—T, B, and natural killer (NK) cells—as well as macrophage activity (SEE QUICK DEFINITION). Because a decrease in the numbers and function of NK cells is characteristic of CFS,[14] beta carotene supplementation is highly useful for this, in addition to its other immune-supporting abilities. Dr. Murray's dosage for immune enhancement is 25,000 to 300,000 IU daily.[15] As with vitamin A, carrots and sweet potatoes are high in beta carotene.

*Vitamin C (ascorbic acid).* There is now solid evidence that vitamin C, another of the primary antioxidants, is essential for optimal functioning of the immune system.[16] It is vital to the health of white blood cells and their production of antibodies, as well as the manufacture of interferon, which acts as an antiviral. NK cells are only active if they contain relatively large amounts of vitamin C.[17] Vitamin C also reduces pain and inflammation. Further, it is vital to the adrenal glands (located above the kidneys), in which the concentration of vitamin C is the highest in the body.[18] Thus, vitamin C supplementation offers both immune and adrenal support—two critical components in any program to reverse CFS.

Low levels of vitamin C have been linked to fatigue.[19] In a study of 411 dentists and their wives, vitamin C intake and fatigue were inversely related. The low vitamin C users had double the mean number of fatigue symptoms compared to the relatively high vitamin C users.[20] Robert F. Cathcart, M.D., of Los Altos, California, uses massive

 **QUICK DEFINITION**

**Natural killer (NK) cells** are a type of nonspecific, free-ranging immune cell produced in the bone marrow and matured in the thymus gland. NK cells can recognize and quickly destroy virus and cancer cells on first contact. "Armed" with an estimated 100 different biochemical poisons for killing foreign proteins, they can kill target cells without having encountered them previously. As with antibodies, their role is surveillance, to rid the body of aberrant or foreign cells before they can grow and produce cancer or infection.

**Macrophages** are a form of white blood cell (originally produced in the bone marrow and called monocytes) that can literally swallow germs and foreign proteins, then release an enzyme that chemically either damages or kills the substance. The name means "big" (macro) "swallower" or "eater" (phage). Macrophages are the vacuum cleaners and filter feeders of the immune system, ingesting everything that is not normal, healthy tissue, even old body cells.

> In CFS, the mitochondria (the energy factories of cells) are damaged by several or all of the factors associated with the disorder—viruses, bacterial infection, *Candida* overgrowth, allergies, and chemical sensitivities.

doses of vitamin C to treat CFS patients because he terms CFS a "free-radical disease involving damaged mitochondria."

In CFS, the mitochondria (the energy factories of cells) are damaged by several or all of the factors associated with the disorder—viruses, bacterial infection, *Candida* overgrowth, allergies, and chemical sensitivities. "The damaged mitochondria become the major source of free radicals," Dr. Cathcart explains. Further, mitochondria normally refuel vitamin C in its scavenging of free radicals, replacing the electrons vitamin C gives up in the process. Damaged mitochondria are unable to perform this function and the vitamin C is used up after one bout with a free radical. Once again, the vicious cycle of CFS is in operation here. Massive doses of vitamin C are useful, then, both to bolster the immune system and to provide an ongoing supply for free-radical destruction in the face of the mitochondria's inability to refuel the vitamin.[21]

In treating CFS, Murray Susser, M.D., of Santa Monica, California, uses intravenous infusions of vitamin C, along with other vitamins and minerals. As an oral supplement for CFS patients, Michael Murray, N.D., recommends 500 to 9,000 mg a day of vitamin C in divided doses.[22] The foods highest in vitamin C are not citrus fruits, as generally thought, although they do have significant amounts. Red chili peppers have over seven times as much vitamin C as oranges, the leafy greens kale and collard have over three times as much, and broccoli contains over twice as much.[23]

Ester C or esterified vitamin C is a combination of several forms of vitamin C. It has all of the same healthful properties and benefits, but is more quickly absorbed by the body and less seems to be eliminated in the urine as compared to standard vitamin C. Nonacidic, it is also less likely to cause gastrointestinal distress.[24]

**Vitamin E (alpha tocopherol).** The third in the triumvirate of antioxidants formed by vitamins A, C, and E, vitamin E is among the major nutrients required for strong immune response to infection. It is also one of the body's primary agents for protecting cell membranes, including protection against the effects of environmental pollutants. Since chemical toxicity is often a factor in CFS, this is a further reason to include vitamin E in a supplement protocol for the disorder. In addition, vitamin E has antihistamine effects and can stop inflammation.[25] It also improves circulation, which can be of benefit for the muscle pain and weakness associated with CFS and fibromyalgia. For CFS patients, Dr. Murray recommends a dosage of 200 to 400 IU daily.[26] Dietary sources include polyunsaturated vegetable oils, leafy green vegetables, avocados, nuts, seeds, and whole grains.

*Vitamin B Complex.* The B vitamins act as a team to help speed up chemical reactions and support overall energy metabolism. Each assists in the utilization of the others. Since they are essential for red blood cell formation, B-complex deficiency produces anemia (reduced red blood cells), the main symptom of which is fatigue. Fatigue and depression have both been linked to B-vitamin deficiency. Deficiencies of any one or more of the B vitamins also reduce the immune system's ability to fight disease.

Vitamin B1 (thiamin) and vitamin B2 (riboflavin) primarily serve in the maintenance of mucous membranes, formation of red blood cells, and metabolism of carbohydrates, the body's most efficient energy source. Brewer's yeast is an excellent source of both of these vitamins.

Vitamin B3 (niacin) is vital for oxygen transport in the blood, as well as fatty acid and nucleic acid formation. As the primary component of two coenzymes, it is vital to the actions of more than 150 enzymes. Without these enzymatic reactions, our body's energy production would shut down in the blink of an eye. Brewer's yeast is also a good source of B3, as are whole grains, particularly rice.

 B vitamins should be taken in a B-complex form because of their close interrelationship in metabolic processes.

Vitamin B5 (pantothenic acid) is vital for synthesis of hormones and support of the adrenal glands. Pantothenic acid deficiency is cited as a source of fatigue.[27] It is also associated with insomnia and depression. Dietary sources of B5 are brewer's yeast, liver, and soybeans.

Vitamin B6 (pyroxidine) strongly influences the immune and nervous systems. It aids in fat and protein metabolism, DNA/RNA synthesis, hemoglobin function, and tryptophan metabolism (which in turn affects mood and level of alertness).[28] B6 is essential in the production of

# Success Story:
# Vitamins and Exercise Help Reverse Fibromyalgia

Ellen, 54, suffered from chronic low back pain, muscle soreness, general achiness, fatigue, and depression. She endured years of clinical testing and various drug treatments without getting a diagnosis or relief of her symptoms. Frustrated by her lack of progress with conventional doctors, Ellen sought help from Mary Olsen, D.C., a chiropractor based in Huntington, New York. Dr. Olsen identified Ellen's condition as fibromyalgia by testing the 18 trigger points associated with that disorder. Eleven of these points must be sore to the touch to qualify as fibromyalgia, according to the conventional medical definition. In Ellen's case, 16 of the sites were tender.

Dr. Olsen prescribed a three-part treatment program for Ellen. First, she used acupressure on Ellen's trigger points, applying pressure in eight-second intervals and repeating the treatment three times at each site. The trigger points in fibromyalgia are actually muscles in spasm and those near the spine often pull it out of alignment. Dr. Olsen administers acupressure to massage the trigger point, chiropractic to realign the spine, and applied kinesiology (SEE QUICK DEFINITION) to prevent the trigger point from injuring the spine again. Ellen saw Dr. Olsen three times a week until her spine began to respond to treatment, and monthly thereafter.

Second, Dr. Olsen prescribed vitamin supplements specifically tailored to fibromyalgia. From her clinical experience, Dr. Olsen has found that fibromyalgia sufferers tend to have low levels of B vitamins and malic acid. The supplement formula she typically uses for this deficiency includes vitamin B1 (25 mg), vitamin B6 (75 mg), manganese (2.5 mg), and malic acid (300 mg). "In most cases, I notice a dramatic improvement within 48 hours of beginning the vitamin therapy," Dr. Olsen says. Ellen took this formula two to eight times daily, as needed.

Third, Ellen began a moderate exercise program, performing a 10- to 15-minute stretching routine five days a week and walking for 20 minutes three times weekly. The exercise would help raise her serotonin levels, which would, in turn, reduce her fatigue. Dr. Olsen emphasizes that her patients never exercise to the point of pain and this aspect of treatment needs to vary according to the individual. Many people with fibromyalgia are too tired to exercise at all, she says. Dr. Olsen usually waits until the person's condition has improved through vitamin therapy before beginning the exercise program. In Ellen's case, she was able to start exercising relatively quickly.

After one year of treatment, Ellen reported that her low back pain was gone, her muscle aches had subsided, and her energy level had increased considerably. As her condition improved, Ellen began exercising more, which further boosted her energy level. Her increased energy (and relief from pain) also elevated her mood and Ellen no longer suffers from depression.

**Applied kinesiology**, first developed by George Goodheart, D.C., of Detroit, Michigan, is the study of the relationship between muscle dysfunction (weak muscles) and related organ or gland dysfunction. Applied kinesiology employs a simple strength-resistance test on a specific indicator muscle that is related to the organ or part of the body that is being tested. If the muscle tests strong, maintaining its resistance, it indicates health. If it tests weak, it can mean infection or dysfunction. For example, the deltoid muscle in the shoulder is related to the lungs and therefore is a good indicator of any problems there.

**Mary Olsen D.C.:** 42 High Street, Huntington, NY 11743; tel: (516) 421-1248.

prostaglandin E1, which is necessary for normal thymus function and regulation of T cells. Prostaglandin deficiency affects mood and can increase fatigue.[29] Brewer's yeast, whole grains, and sunflower seeds are good dietary sources of this B vitamin.

Vitamin B12 (cobalamin) is virtually absent in vegetable food sources, which means vegetarians are frequently low in this vitamin. It is essential for normal formation of red blood cells and the maintenance of the nervous system and mucous membrane linings (important to prevent pathogens from entering the body). A New Zealand study found that injection of vitamin B12 in CFS patients helped normalize imbalances in their red blood cells.[30] Other research has demonstrated that B12 supplementation appears to improve CFS symptoms.[31]

According to conventional medicine, a person's B12 level is considered normal when it is above 208 picograms per deciliter. However, even when blood tests reveal normal B12 levels, supplementation may be warranted. In a study of 28 people who suffered from fatigue but whose B12 levels tested normal, all 28 felt significantly better after receiving injections of B12 twice a day for two weeks.[32] Vitamin B12 deficiencies have resulted in severe nerve and brain damage when the patients' levels were as high as 300 picograms per deciliter.[33]

The renowned Framingham Heart Study (the health of 5,209 people monitored since 1948) reveals evidence of deficiencies of B12 at levels over 500.[34] According to Jacob Teitelbaum, M.D., author of *From Fatigued to Fantastic: A Manual for Moving Beyond Chronic Fatigue and Fibromyalgia*, the standard for B12 was originally established at the level that prevents anemia, but this amount of B12 does not meet the requirements of the brain and nervous system.

Despite the tendency of conventional medicine to scoff at the efficacy of B12 injections, Dr. Teitelbaum uses them in treating CFS. "In my experience, when their other problems are also treated, many people respond dramatically to B12 injections," he says. "I have found that treating patients with B12, even if their levels are technically normal, often results in marked improvement."[35]

**Folic Acid (folate, folacin).** Part of the B vitamin family, folic acid is essential for blood formation, especially red and white blood cells, and RNA/DNA synthesis. Folic acid deficiency has been linked to fatigue.[36] In a study of 38 patients, researchers found that supplementing with folic acid (10 mg daily) produced a regression of fatigue, lassitude, and depression in two to three months.[37] Leafy green vegetables have high concentrations of folic acid; not surprising when you consider that its name derives from the same root as the word *foliage*. As with the other B-complex vitamins, brewer's yeast is an excellent source of folic acid.

***Biotin.*** Another member of the B vitamin group, biotin is equally essential to food metabolism and the release of energy. A deficiency of biotin produces fatigue, lack of appetite, depression, and muscle pains. Biotin assists in the synthesis of nucleic, amino, and fatty acids. Good food sources for biotin include brewer's yeast, liver, and soybeans.

## Minerals

Some would argue that monitoring mineral deficiencies is even more important than monitoring vitamin deficiencies, as the body doesn't manufacture minerals and they are difficult to liberate from food sources. Like vitamins, minerals are a basic part of all cells. They play an essential role in the body's regulatory functions. The actions of minerals are highly interrelated, to each other and to those of vitamins, hormones, and enzymes. No mineral can function in the body without affecting other functions.

Dosages are not included here for most of the minerals because supplementation is a more delicate process than in the case of antioxidant vitamins, for example. Balancing the minerals with each other is vital and needs to be precisely tailored to meet the individual's imbalances and deficiencies.

***Calcium.*** Necessary for strong bones and teeth, calcium also serves as an essential cofactor in cellular energy production and nerve and heart function. Magnesium is involved in the body's uptake of calcium. As magnesium is one of the most common deficiencies implicated in CFS, calcium is likely to be lacking as well. Low levels of calcium can result in muscle cramps and emotional irritability, two symptoms of CFS and fibromyalgia.

In addition to relaxing blood vessels and calming muscle tension, calcium supplementation can ease stress and anxiety. Given the particularly dependent interaction of the two minerals, calcium and magnesium supplements should be taken in ratio, although calcium is best absorbed at bedtime and magnesium in the morning. Dietary sources of calcium include dairy products, tofu, kelp, leafy green vegetables, and brewer's yeast.

## Nutrients That Can Aid and Hinder Calcium Absorption

The mere fact that you take a calcium supplement or eat a calcium-rich food doesn't mean that your body actually absorbs this essential nutrient. According to Melvyn R. Werbach, M.D., assistant clinical professor at the U.C.L.A. School of Medicine, specific interactions among nutrients can either hinder or aid the absorption of calcium and of any targeted nutrient. Knowledge of nutritional interactions should be regarded "as an essential component of good medical practice," Dr. Werbach urges in his book, *Foundations of Nutritional Medicine,* and not as "an 'alternative' or 'complement' to conventional medicine." Based on his review of a great number of clinical studies, which he summarizes in his book, Dr. Werbach offers the following observations about calcium:

**Bioavailability.** This term indicates the body's ability to process, absorb, retain, and use a nutrient from a dietary or supplemental source. If you are taking a calcium supplement, the most efficient absorption typically occurs in individual doses of 500 mg or less, says Dr. Werbach. You are also

likely to absorb more calcium if you take vitamin D concurrently; you may absorb five times more calcium from milk than from spinach; and some individuals can glean more usable calcium from dairy products than from supplements. If you take a calcium supplement with foods, this increases your absorption by 10%. Late evening is the most effective intake time and calcium in a whole-bone extract tends to be better absorbed than simple calcium salts. Of calcium salts, calcium citrate appears to be among the most bioavailable, but be careful here, because calcium citrate can increase your absorption of dietary aluminum.

**Aiding absorption.** On the positive side, particular nutrients can enhance the absorption or retention of calcium. These include iron, lactose (milk protein), the amino acid lysine (in amounts up to 800 mg, if taken at the same time as a calcium source), potassium, sodium bicarbonate, vitamin D, vitamin B6, and vitamin A. Glucose (simple sugar) can increase calcium absorption by 20% if taken at the same time as a calcium source.

*Chromium.* Many people with CFS suffer from hypoglycemia (low blood sugar). Chromium is beneficial because it stabilizes insulin production, thereby regulating the body's ability to convert and process glucose for energy and thus regulating blood sugar levels. Anything that helps better control blood sugar levels can substantially improve immune function. The United States appears to be a chromium-deficient nation, probably due to our overindulgence in refined grain products.[38]

Chromium is contained in the outer bran portion of grains, so much of it is lost in the production of white flour. In addition, a high intake of white sugar tends to deplete the body of chromium, because our chromium needs increase in proportion to blood sugar levels.[39] In addition to whole grains, brewer's yeast and meat are good sources of chromium. As a supplement, chromium picolinate is the preferred form for those with food sensitivities because it is yeast free. It is also more easily absorbed by the body.

Melvyn Werbach, M.D.

**Hindering absorption.** Other nutrients can decrease the amount of calcium absorbed by the intestines. These include fatty acids, fiber, phytates (found in the bran layer of cereal grains), and uronic acid (found in the fiber content of fruits and vegetables). Oxalates, concentrated in certain leafy green vegetables such as spinach, can block the absorption of calcium if these foods are consumed alone, but not if they are eaten with other calcium-containing foods. A high daily level of zinc supplementation (140 mg) can reduce calcium absorption if, at the same time, a person has an especially low level (200 mg or less) of calcium intake from the diet.

If you are a woman taking estrogen and have a low magnesium intake, calcium supplementation may increase your risk of thrombosis (blood clotting that can lead to a heart attack). Calcium carbonate, such as from ground oyster shells, can produce constipation. Calcium supplements, especially those from natural materials (such as limestone rock), may contain toxic metals, such as lead. In one study of 70 different brands, 25% exceeded lead safety levels, while a second study of one brand of dolomite revealed higher than desirable levels of aluminum, arsenic, cadmium, and lead.

*Germanium.* Among other functions, this element enhances the availability of oxygen to cells, which promotes cell health. Between 20% and 50% of CFS patients given germanium experienced substantial to marked relief of their symptoms.[40] Germanium may accomplish this by stimulating the production of interferon (proteins released by white blood cells), which blocks the spread of viruses and stimulates other immune "workers" in turn.[41] Germanium is not available in food and can only be obtained via a supplement.

*Iodine.* Iodine is part of the structure of the thyroid hormones T3 and T4, which regulate our body's energy usage as well as numerous body functions. Iodine's effects are far reaching, since the metabolism of all the body's cells—except for brain cells—is influenced by thyroid hormones. Iodine deficiency most typically results in hypothyroidism, which is characterized by many of the symptoms of CFS, including fatigue, general weakness, depression, headaches, and memory lapses (see chapter 6). Dietary sources of iodine are cod-liver oil, certain fish, shrimp, kelp, chard, turnip greens, cantaloupe, sunflower seeds, and sea salt.

*Iron.* Iron is essential to red blood cell synthesis, oxygen transport, and energy production through food metabolism. Low iron levels in the blood are commonly paired with anemia and have been linked to fatigue.[42] Once again, testing as normal for iron doesn't necessarily mean that supplementation won't have an effect. In a study of chronically fatigued, but not anemic, women, 66% experienced improvement after iron supplementation.[43] Iron-rich foods include kelp, blackstrap molasses, lecithin, certain nuts and seeds, millet, and parsley.

*Magnesium.* Magnesium is required for ATP synthesis in the body. As you may recall, ATP (SEE QUICK DEFINITION) is our source of energy. Magnesium is a cofactor in more than 300 enzymatic reactions involving energy metabolism and nerve function. Magnesium also aids in the uptake of calcium and in transporting potassium into cells. The daily intake of magnesium in the United States has decreased from 450 to 485 mg daily in the early 1900s to 185 to 235 mg per day currently, probably as a result of magnesium-depleted farming soil and a diet high in processed foods. The RDA is at least 350 mg daily and, as discussed earlier, RDAs are often lower than the optimum level for the body. Obviously, a lot of Americans are walking around with magnesium deficiency.

 **ATP** stands for adenosine triphosphate, a substance found in all cells—particularly muscle—and responsible for energy. When enzymes split ATP, energy is released (12,000 calories/mole of ATP) from the high-energy phosphate bonds. This bond can be instantly split on demand whenever energy is required to run cellular functions; then ATP becomes ADP. When energy is returned, it becomes ATP again. ATP is often called the cell's energy currency because it can be continually spent and remade again in a matter of minutes.

 For more on **thyroid hormones and chronic fatigue**, see chapter 6, Reversing Hidden Thyroid Problems.

Magnesium deficiency results in impaired energy production and has been clearly linked with CFS. Its symptoms resemble the CFS laundry list: tiredness, weakness, muscle pain, nausea, anorexia, learning disability, and personality change. In a study at the University of Southampton in England, 20 CFS patients had lower red blood cell magnesium levels than healthy volunteers. In a companion study, 32 CFS patients had a once-weekly injection of either magnesium or a placebo for six weeks.

Of those receiving the magnesium, 80% had reduced symptoms and improved energy, while less than 20% of those on placebo injections reported improvement. The red blood cell magnesium levels returned to normal in those who had the magnesium injections.[44]

Research has shown that combining magnesium with malic acid, a fruit acid found in apples that is also crucial to the formation of ATP, is useful in the treatment of chronic fatigue syndrome as well as fibromyalgia. In the case of fibromyalgia, low magnesium is what keeps muscles in a state of spasm, so supplementation can aid in relieving this painful symptom. Jay Goldstein, M.D., uses the magnesium/malic acid combination in treating both CFS and fibromyalgia. "Fibromyalgia pain may respond within 48 hours, while fatigue may take about two

 Most physicians recommend that the malic acid/ magnesium supplement be taken on an empty stomach, but some people have reported intestinal problems. If this occurs, the supplement should be taken with food or the dosage reduced.

weeks," he states.[45] Daniel Peterson, M.D., one of the doctors treating patients in the original outbreak of CFS in Incline Village, Nevada, has found that 40% of CFS patients benefit from taking magnesium and malic acid.[46]

A study by Guy D. Abraham, M.D., and Jorge D. Flechas, M.D., showed positive results for the reversal of fibromyalgia with magnesium and malic acid supplementation. Fifteen patients with fibromyalgia who took magnesium (300 to 600 mg daily) and malic acid (1,200 to 2,400 mg daily) experienced subjective improvement in their symptoms within the first 48 hours. Over an eight-week period of supplementation, their degree of muscle tenderness and pain dropped from 19.6 to 6.5, according to medical scores.[47]

Dietary sources of magnesium include tofu, kelp, leafy green vegetables, whole grains, nuts, seeds, raisins, dried figs, and blackstrap molasses.

**Manganese.** Manganese is an important catalyst and cofactor in many enzymatic processes and reactions, including energy metabolism, regulation of blood sugar, and thyroid hormone functions.[48] It is part of the main antioxidant enzyme, superoxide dismutase (SOD), and there is some evidence that it may help to counteract the immune-suppressive effects of stress hormones (corticosteroids), which have been shown to be elevated in people with CFS. Manganese may also increase the binding ability and other activities of white blood cells.[49]

Manganese can be found in whole grains, leafy green vegetables, dried fruit, and nuts.

**Phosphorus.** A member of the nitrogen family, this element occurs in combined form in phosphate, which plays a major role in energy production and activation of B vitamins. Phosphorus is also a component of RNA/DNA, bones, and teeth. Research has shown that phosphorus deficiency can produce fatigue.[50] High-protein foods like milk, cheese, meat, and fish are also high in phosphorus.

**Potassium.** Potassium is a primary electrolyte (SEE QUICK DEFINITION), important in controlling pH (acid/base) and water balance. It plays a role in nerve function and helps maintain cell integrity by regulating the transfer of nutrients into the cells. Potassium supports the adrenal glands, which is important for CFS sufferers, as these glands are often severely impaired from a protracted period of functioning in a continual state of stress response. Fatigue and muscular weakness are the most common symptoms of potassium deficiency.[51] A review of studies involving a total of nearly 3,000 patients found that 75% to 91% of those treated with potassium and magnesium aspartates (1 g of each salt daily) experienced "pronounced relief of fatigue," usually after four to five days.[52]

Potassium is found in fruits, vegetables, whole grains, nuts, and seeds. According to Dr. Susser, it is important to balance potassium intake with salt intake and the ratio should be greater than five (potassium) to one (sodium).[53]

 **Electrolytes** are substances in the blood, tissue fluids, intracellular fluids, or urine that conduct an electrical charge, either plus or minus. Examples include acids, bases, and salts, such as potassium, magnesium, phosphate, sulfate, bicarbonate, sodium, chloride, and calcium. Electrolytes provide inorganic chemicals for cellular reactions and control mechanisms, such as the conduction of electrochemical impulses to nerves and muscles. Electrolytes are also needed for key enzymatic reactions involved in metabolism, or the release of energy from food.

**Selenium.** Selenium is an important constituent of the antioxidant enzyme system (glutathione peroxidase) that protects tissues against free radical damage. Selenium works synergistically with vitamin E, meaning that the two nutrients mutually reinforce the body's immune defenses. A deficiency in selenium can depress immune function.[54] Studies have shown that supplementation with selenium enhances immune function by increasing the ability of lymphocytes and NK cells to rid the body of harmful microorganisms.[55] Dietary sources of selenium are wheat germ, Brazil nuts, bran, and red Swiss chard.

*Zinc.* This mineral is a cofactor in numerous enzymatic processes and reactions crucial for healthy body function. Like selenium, zinc supports many aspects of the immune system. It is necessary for the free radical–quenching activity of the enzyme superoxide dismutase (SOD). A deficiency of zinc can lead to depressed activity of NK and other immune cells.[56] B cells use up zinc when they make antibodies, so someone who has been fighting infection for a prolonged period, as in CFS, is likely to be deficient in zinc.

Declining levels of zinc are implicated in the shrinkage of the thymus gland (an endocrine gland located behind the sternum), which occurs with age. Zinc supplementation can help restore the thymus and thus bolster the immune system. Research links zinc deficiency with fatigue[57] and indicates that supplementing with zinc improves muscle strength and reduces muscle fatigue.[58] Oysters contain high concentrations of zinc. Whole-grain wheat, wheat germ, and pumpkin seeds are also good food sources.

## Additional Supplements

The following nutritional supplements are also helpful in the treatment of CFS:

*Amino Acids.* Amino acids are the building blocks of protein. Since amino acids work as a team and in ratio to each other, it is important to identify specific deficiencies and design a precise supplement program based on the results. Amino acid deficiencies and imbalances are common in CFS. Carnitine[59] and methionine[60] seem to be the ones most implicated.

Carnitine is vital to mitochondrial energy production. Low carnitine levels have been found in CFS patients.[61] In addition, a more severe deficiency correlates with a greater degree of fatigue.[62] Carnitine deficiency may also account for the muscle pain and weakness and the post-exercise exhaustion typical of CFS.[63]

Among its other functions, methionine helps the liver to detoxify. Given the probable overload on the liver due to an elevated level of chemical toxins in a person with CFS, supplementation with methionine can assist the liver in its detoxification function. Methionine also aids in reducing the body's uptake of mercury, thereby freeing immune cells to focus on the viruses and other opportunistic infections involved in CFS. Mercury dental fillings can deplete methionine through the continual need they present for detoxification.

This is also true of glutathione, another amino acid that aids in detoxification. Glutathione reduces free-radical damage to cells, prevents depletion of other antioxidants, and activates certain immune cells. "The ability of cells to maintain an adequate glutathione status is critical to our health," states Jay Lombard, M.D., author of *The Brain Wellness Plan: Breakthrough Medical, Nutritional, and Immune-Boosting Therapies.* To raise glutathione levels, Dr. Lombard recommends a combination of N-acetyl cysteine or NAC (an amino acid precursor of glutathione; 1 g daily on an empty stomach), lipoic acid (a vitamin-like substance necessary for ATP production; 200 mg daily with food), and selenium (no more than 200 mcg daily with food).[64] Shari Lieberman, Ph.D., C.N.S., a clinical nutritionist based in New York City, considers glutathione a must for people with environmental sensitivities whose detoxification organs and systems have been overloaded and are in need of support. "Glutathione is a powerful antioxidant that works inside our cells. It is also used in many of the body's detoxification mechanisms," Dr. Lieberman says.

For more on **glutathione**, see chapter 4, Restoring Immune Vitality.

*Chlorella.* Chlorella (*Chlorella pyrenoidosa*, a freshwater single-celled green algae) has numerous benefits for CFS sufferers. For one, it is a first-string detoxifying agent, capable of removing alcohol from the liver and heavy metals (such as cadmium and mercury), certain pesticides, herbicides, and polychlorbiphenyls (PCBs) from the body's tissues. Since chemical and heavy metal toxicity is often a factor in CFS, supplementing with chlorella can be a useful part of treatment.

Second, chlorella contains 60% protein, including all the essential amino acids, as well as high levels of beta carotene and chlorophyll. This has clear benefits for the nutrient-depleted state of most people with CFS. Third, chlorella can absorb toxins from the intestines, help relieve chronic constipation, favorably alter the bacterial flora content of the bowel, and eliminate intestinal gas.

Chlorella can assist in reversing the digestive disorders common to CFS. In addition, both scientific documentation and reliable anecdotal reports indicate that chlorella is effective in helping to reduce the symptoms of viral and bacterial infections, low blood sugar, and anemia,

## A Guide to Taking Supplements

Nutritional experts Jeffrey Bland, Ph.D., and Lindsey Berkson, D.C., offer these recommendations and advisories to follow when taking nutritional supplements:

- Nutritional supplements should be taken with meals to promote increased absorption. Fat-soluble vitamins (such as vitamin A, beta carotene, vitamin E, and the essential fatty acids linoleic and alpha-linolenic acid) should be taken during the day with the meal that contains the most fat.
- Amino acid supplements should be taken on an empty stomach at least an hour before or after a meal; take them with fruit juice to help promote absorption. When taking an increased dosage of an isolated amino acid, be sure to supplement with an amino-acid blend.
- If you become nauseated when you take tablet supplements, consider taking a liquid form, diluted in a beverage.
- If you become nauseated or ill within an hour after taking nutritional supplements, consider the need for a bowel cleanse or rejuvenation program prior to beginning a course of nutritional supplementation.
- If you are taking high doses, do not take the supplements all at one time, but divide them into smaller doses taken throughout the day.
- Take digestive enzymes with meals to assist digestion. If you are taking pancreatic enzymes for other therapeutic reasons, be sure to take them on an empty stomach between meals.
- Take mineral supplements away from the highest-fiber meals of the day; fiber can decrease mineral absorption.
- When taking an increased dosage of an isolated B vitamin, be sure to supplement with a B complex.
- When taking nutrients, be sure to take adequate amounts of liquid to mix with digestive juices and prevent side effects.

among other disorders. Because the presence of multiple infections is the symptomatic centerpiece of CFS and the other two conditions frequently present as well, chlorella has obvious application in these areas.

Chlorella's far-reaching effects may be due to its ability to increase albumin levels in the body. Albumin, continually secreted by the liver, is the most abundant protein found in the blood. It acts as a major natural antioxidant, con-

 For more on **chlorella in mercury detoxification**, see chapter 7, Eliminating Heavy Metal Toxicity.

tributing an estimated 80% of all neutralizing activity against free radicals in the blood that would otherwise damage cells and tissues. Strengthening the immune system is an important feature in any CFS treatment program.

***Coenzyme Q10.*** Coenzyme Q10 (coQ10), also known as ubiquinone, is vital to the mitochondria and thus to energy production. A powerful antioxidant, it also improves oxygenation and helps to prevent toxicity.

In the event of a coQ10 deficiency, common among CFS sufferers, ATP production is seriously impaired. CoQ10 is found in every plant and animal cell.

The fact that vegetarians tend to have almost double the blood levels of coQ10 compared to meat eaters seems to indicate that plants have a higher percentage, but food sources don't deliver high amounts of coQ10 and supplementation is therefore the best way to derive therapeutic benefits.[65] Supplementing with coQ10 has been shown to improve symptoms of CFS.[66] A general dosage for CFS is 25 to 50 mg three to four times daily; for fibromyalgia, 30 to 200 mg per day.[67]

 **Essential fatty acids (EFAs)** are unsaturated fats required in the diet. Omega-3 and omega-6 oils are the two principal types. The primary omega-3 oil is called alpha-linolenic acid (ALA) and is found in flaxseed (58%), canola, pumpkin seeds and walnuts, and soybeans. Fish oils, such as salmon, cod, and mackerel, contain the other important omega-3 oils, DHA (docosahexaenoic acid) and EPA (eicosapentaenoic acid). Linoleic acid or cis-linoleic acid is the main omega-6 oil and is found in most plants and vegetable oils, including safflower (73%), corn, peanut, and sesame. The most therapeutic form of omega-6 oil is gamma-linolenic acid (GLA), found in evening primrose, black currant, and borage oils. Once in the body, omega-3 and omega-6 are converted to prostaglandins, hormone-like substances that regulate many metabolic functions, particularly inflammatory processes.

 Alternative practitioners sometimes recommend dosages higher than those currently considered safe by conventional medicine. The scientific literature and numerous clinical trials generally support these elevated dosages for short periods of time, but they should always be taken with medical supervision.

*Essential Fatty Acids.* Essential fatty acids (EFAs) (SEE QUICK DEFINITION) are vitamin-like compounds that cannot be made in the body and must be ingested through the foods you eat. Without EFAs, your organs cannot manufacture prostaglandins—substances that are key regulators of immune, digestive, cardiovascular, and reproductive functions. Furthermore, cell membranes consist mainly of lipids (fats) that are highly susceptible to free-radical damage. EFAs help to protect against this damage. EFAs also aid in reducing the release of serotonin; elevated brain serotonin levels may be a factor in CFS and help to explain the severe fatigue. Research has found that too much serotonin is as detrimental as too little.

Research suggests a link between CFS and low levels of essential fatty acids.[68] A study of 63 patients with post-viral fatigue syndrome who also had low EFA levels found that three months of supplementation with a combination of evening primrose oil and fish oil resulted in normal EFA levels and highly significant improvement in all the individual symptoms, including fatigue, aches and pains, and depression.[69] Evening primrose oil contains GLA (gamma-linolenic acid), a particularly powerful EFA. For CFS patients, Dr. Murray suggests flaxseed oil, one tablespoon per day.[70]

Dr. Lieberman has found that EFA supplementation (three to six capsules daily of high-potency fish oil) is particularly useful for people with fibromyalgia. "It works like a natural cortisone to decrease inflammation," she reports. Sometimes she adds GLA (one or two 240–300 mg capsules daily), but not in the form of evening primrose oil because, according to her, the latter also contains an acid that is pro-inflammatory.

*Quercetin.* A bioflavonoid found in fruits and vegetables, quercetin is known as a vitamin C "helper," which means it enhances the beneficial activities of vitamin C by increasing its absorption. As an antioxidant, quercetin provides the body with protection against environmental stresses that can result in allergies. It also inhibits the release of histamine, the substance that produces the symptoms of an allergic reaction. Further, quercetin is an effective antiviral. All of these functions are beneficial for CFS. Commercially, quercetin can be found in blue-green algae.

## How Nutrients Work Together

Vitamins and minerals help regulate the conversion of food to energy in the body and can be separated into two general categories: energy nutrients, which are principally involved in the conversion of food to energy; and protector nutrients, which help defend against damaging toxins derived from drugs, alcohol, radiation, environmental pollutants, or the body's own enzyme processes.

"The B complex vitamins and magnesium are examples of energy nutrients," says nutritionist Jeffrey Bland, Ph.D., "for they activate specific metabolic facilitators called enzymes, which control digestion and the absorption and use of proteins, fats, and carbohydrates. These nutrients often work as a team, their mutual presence enhancing each other's function."

In the process of converting food to energy, free radicals are produced that can damage the body and set the stage for degenerative diseases. Protector nutrients—such as vitamin E, beta carotene, vitamin C, and the minerals zinc, copper, manganese, and selenium—play a critical role in preventing or delaying these degenerative processes. Vitamins A, C, and E work together as a team, protecting against breakdown and helping each other maintain adequate tissue levels.

Lindsey Berkson, D.C., of Santa Fe, New Mexico, notes that vitamins and minerals are what make the chemical and electrical circuitry of the body work, and that the body's functioning is therefore profoundly affected by how nutrients work either together or against each other. Nutrients can help each other or inhibit each other when taken simultaneously. For example, iron is best absorbed when taken separately from pancreatic enzymes and should also not be taken with vitamin E, says Dr. Berkson. There are also certain nutrients that can help "potentiate" the other nutrients; for example, vitamin C taken with iron facilitates the maximum absorption of the iron.

# eleven

# Healing Psychological and Emotional Factors

In chapter 1, Jesse Stoff, M.D., spoke of learning the "lessons of the disease." Why did *this* person get *this* illness at *this* time? Holistic physicians ask such questions because they realize that illness is more than a matter of imbalanced physiology. There are always psychological and emotional aspects to every health problem and unless these are thoroughly addressed, no cure will ever be complete and lasting. This chapter focuses on how a person's ways of thinking, acting, and being can cause or contribute to CFS and other illnesses, and keep these conditions in place.

Lifestyle choices, including how one thinks and acts, can contribute to chronic fatigue. For example, a lifestyle of high-paced overachievement or workaholism characterizes the lives of many CFS sufferers prior to becoming sick. For some people, dealing with unremitting fatigue is the only way they will ever take the time to focus on their internal world. Alternative medicine competently addresses the psychological and emotional side of all illnesses, including chronic fatigue, recognizing the uniquely individual factors in each patient. While not all chronic fatigue patients have the same psychological make-up, all of them do have psychological issues that play a contributing role in their illness, and these mental and emotional factors constantly interact with their physiological condition.

Let's begin by looking at a case that brings together a number of the components discussed throughout this book. Enzyme, hormonal, and

> Holistic physicians realize that illness is more than a matter of imbalanced physiology. There are always psychological and emotional aspects to every health problem and unless these are thoroughly addressed, no cure will ever be complete and lasting.

nutrient deficiencies, as well as allergies, all contributed to Michelle's fibromyalgia, but psychological and emotional factors were as significant as the physical imbalances in creating her illness. Norman Levin, M.D., of Aldie, Virginia, who is board certified in internal medicine, rheumatology, and chelation therapy, explains how mental-emotional factors must be addressed to successfully reverse a chronic condition such as fibromyalgia.

## Success Story:
## Michelle Stops Carrying the Weight of the World

Before seeing me, Michelle, 39, had suffered from severe muscle pain for about two months. On the surface, it seemed ironic that a woman as physically active as Michelle should develop the classic symptoms of fibromyalgia. Michelle taught a full-time schedule of aerobics classes, and ran around constantly to keep up with her two young children. She was the kind of person who tried to do and be everything for everybody. As we discovered, this attitude was at the core of her muscle aches.

When a person has problems with muscle spasms or muscle irritability, often there is an absolute or relative deficiency of magnesium in the body. As a general rule, I will give the Meyers' Cocktail (SEE QUICK DEFINITION) to patients with fibromyalgia or muscle spasms to get sufficient magnesium into their systems. Often, a standard blood test for magnesium levels does not

 **QUICK DEFINITION** The **Meyers' Cocktail** is an intravenous vitamin and mineral protocol developed in the 1970s by John Meyers, M.D., a physician at Johns Hopkins University in Baltimore, Maryland. It contains magnesium chloride hexahydrate (5 cc given), calcium gluconate (2.5 cc), vitamin B2 (1,000 mcg/cc; 1 cc given), vitamin B5 (100 mg/cc; 1 cc given), vitamin B6 (250 mg/cc; 1 cc given), the entire vitamin B complex (100 mg/cc; 1 cc given), and vitamin C (222 mg/cc; 6 cc given). The solution is slowly injected over a 5- to 15-minute period. The "Cocktail" is indicated for patients with chronic fatigue, depression, muscle spasm, asthma, hives, allergic rhinitis, congestive heart failure, angina, ischemic vascular disease, acute infections, and senile dementia.

> Michelle was the kind of person who tried to do and be everything for everybody. As we discovered, this attitude was at the core of her muscle aches.　　　　　— *Norman Levin, M.D.*

reveal true magnesium status. First, a regular blood test does not necessarily tell you the amount of magnesium available in the body because most of it is stored inside the cells. Second, even ascertaining how much magnesium exists in the cells (intracellularly) is not the final answer, because the reading could be normal yet the patient may respond favorably to extra doses of magnesium (as was the case with Michelle).

In addition to considering magnesium supplementation, it is often advisable to run a delayed allergy hypersensitivity test on a person with fibromyalgia symptoms. Frequently, there are hidden food or substance allergies that can aggravate the symptoms, although the reaction may not take place until hours—12 hours is not uncommon—after eating the food, thereby displacing our attention from the allergen itself. For example, you could eat wheat and have a migraine headache the next day, or have some corn and experience an arthritis flare-up 24 hours later. In addition, you may think you're on a healthy diet but you may, in fact, be allergic to one of the "healthy" foods you're eating. For instance, drinking organic carrot juice may contribute to your physical symptoms if you're allergic to carrots.

Michelle's allergy test indicated she was reactive to most dairy products (Romano cheese, yogurt, and whole butter, in particular), tuna fish, raspberries, cherries, coffee, food additives and preservatives (MSG, saccharine, sodium benzoate), and environmental chemicals such as cleaning products, benzene, and trichloroethylene. As a first measure, Michelle began avoiding these substances.

 For more about **magnesium deficiency**, see chapter 10, Ending Nutritional Deficiencies with Supplements. For more about **allergies**, see chapter 9, Addressing the Allergy Connection. For more about the **Comprehensive Digestive Stool Analysis**, see chapter 2, Testing. For more about **enzymes**, see chapter 8, Replenishing Enzyme Deficiencies.

Next, we used a laboratory test called the Comprehensive Digestive Stool Analysis to see how her digestion and intestines were working. The results indicated large amounts of residual fats and vegetable fibers, which told us that Michelle had a nutrient malabsorption problem. I put her on a digestive enzyme formula called Digestin that contains the primary enzymes for each food group (fats, proteins, carbohydrates, and fibers), hydrochloric acid (the stomach's principal digestive juice), and ox bile (to aid the small intestine in its digestive processes).

Concurrently, I put Michelle on several other nutrients and formulations. She took esterified vitamin C to bowel tolerance (the point just before diarrhea); the ester form is better absorbed. She took Fibroplex to provide nutrients for muscle energy. Specifically, this formula contains magnesium, malic acid, manganese, and vitamins B1 and B6. Providing magnesium and malic acid in adequate amounts often produces favorable benefits for fibromyalgia, possibly by removing aluminum from the body. In addition, Michelle took a supergreens concentrate called Greens Plus twice daily as a powder added to water or juice. The purpose here was to provide a full natural nutrient array in organic form that could be easily assimilated by the body. The product contains a large amount of chlorophyll, which is a natural, easily absorbed source of magnesium. Michelle also took vitamin B12 as a capsule that dissolves and is absorbed under the tongue. She responded better to B12 when it could enter her body without having to pass through her digestive tract.

After checking Michelle's DHEA (SEE QUICK DEFINITION) levels, which tested low, I started her on 5 mg daily of this hormone. I had her slowly increase her DHEA intake until she achieved the maximum benefit and before she started experiencing adverse side effects (in her case, 25 mg daily). Most people tolerate DHEA well but, because it is a precursor hormone, in the bodies of some women it can turn into other hormones, such as estrogen or testosterone. This can lead to side effects of abnormal bleeding, breast tenderness or swelling, acne, or unusual hair growth. I also had Michelle take 5 mg of the hormone melatonin (widely used to rebalance disturbed sleep/wake cycles) at bedtime to aid her sleeping, which was a major problem for her. Finally, Michelle consulted a chiropractor who used a deep-muscle massage technique called myotherapy (SEE QUICK DEFINITION) to release "trigger points" in her musculature. These are specific points on the body known to carry and concentrate stress; releasing them through massage is an effective contribution to overall pain reduction.

After about four weeks of following this program (including the once-weekly Meyers' Cocktail), Michelle reported considerable gains. Her digestion was improved, she was coping better with stress, and she felt more at peace with herself and in greater control of her life. She told me, "I feel like I have more energy. I feel less shaky, the muscle spasms aren't as bad, and I'm starting to get a little perspective on my condition." The perspective Michelle was gaining had to do with insight into why she had fibromyalgia. She was highly motivated to get well, willing to do the hard psychological inner work and to make the life changes such insight required. In a sense, she had to, because she had reached the point where the pain was so severe she could no longer function. Pain had forced her to cut back on her aerobics classes and teach only the much less demanding water aerobics. Then she had had to give that up as well.

When I urged her to ask herself about the message of her condition, Michelle began to see that she always strove to be the super mom, super wife, super teacher, and super performer in every situation or relationship. Her striving wasn't egotistical, but came out of her caring and industriousness. Michelle saw how everybody leaned on her and how, because she felt this was her role, she could never say no—and it was too much. Michelle understood how she had developed severe, almost total body pain that forced her to stop in her tracks. She saw what she had been doing and appreciated that she could no longer do it—nor did she want to. Finally, Michelle realized that it was okay to say no and to ask for help.

Not everyone with fibromyalgia will fit this pattern, but there is a certain general trend to the psychological factors involved in chronic muscle pain of this type. A person feels burdened and overwhelmed, as if everybody is leaning

 **DHEA** (dehydroepiandrosterone) is naturally produced by the human adrenal glands and gonads, with optimal levels occurring around age 20 for women and age 25 for men. After those ages, DHEA levels gradually decline so that 80-year-olds produce only a fraction of the DHEA they did when they were 20. As an antioxidant, a hormone regulator, and the building block from which estrogen and testosterone are produced, DHEA is vital to health. Low DHEA levels have been associated with cancer, diabetes, multiple sclerosis, hypertension, obesity, AIDS, heart disease, Alzheimer's, and immune dysfunction illnesses. Test subjects using supplemental DHEA reported improved sleeping patterns, better memory, an improved ability to cope with stress, decreased joint pain, increases in lean muscle, and decreases in body fat. No serious side effects have been reported to date, although acne, oily skin, facial hair growth on women, deepening of the voice, irritability, insomnia, and fatigue have been reported with high DHEA doses.

**Myotherapy** is a technique of pain relief developed by physical fitness and exercise therapy expert Bonnie Prudden. The myotherapist applies deep manual pressure, usually with the fingertips on the skin, for five to seven seconds, to precise sites of muscular pain, called "trigger points." Prudden found that this technique can relieve pain for about 90% of all muscle-related pain conditions, making it unnecessary to use painkilling injections.

 For more information about **Ester C**, see chapter 10, Ending Nutritional Deficiencies with Supplements.

Not everyone with fibromyalgia will fit the same pattern, but there is a certain general trend to the psychological factors involved in chronic muscle pain. A person feels burdened and overwhelmed, as if everybody is leaning on their body, as if they are carrying the world's weight on their shoulders.

— *Norman Levin, M.D.*

**Norman Levin, M.D.**

on their body, as if they are carrying the world's weight on their shoulders. So the "weight" goes to the muscles, which eventually complain, using the body language of aches and spasms. As the nutrients, dietary restrictions, and psychological work took effect over the next several months, Michelle recovered almost completely. Now she has returned to her active schedule and to teaching aerobics full time; in fact, she is an instructor for other people with fibromyalgia.

The successful reversal of chronic pain, such as fibromyalgia, may certainly require the use of multiple nutrients, enzymes, hormones, and dietary changes, but you must also examine the patient's state of mind and life conditions. Rather than a patient asking "Why did this illness happen to me?"—which is the common complaint—the better question might be "Why is this illness happening at all?" Often when patients probe their own life circumstances—to see how they feel about what is happening—the "Why?" behind the illness becomes clear and the condition usually clears up more quickly and thoroughly than expected.

 **Norman Levin, M.D.**: P.O. Box 107, Route 50 West, 39070 John Mosby Highway, Aldie, VA 22001; tel: (703) 260-3484.

## Lifestyle Choices and Personality Characteristics in CFS

If the emotion of fibromyalgia is often one of "carrying the weight of the world on your shoulders," the mindset underlying chronic fatigue syndrome might be expressed by the belief: you're only okay if you're producing. This is a generalization of the psychological state underlying a complex health condition, and of course each patient has their own

> Every single person I have seen with CFS was an overachiever.
>
> — *Shari Lieberman, Ph.D., C.N.S.*

particular cluster of emotional issues that may be contributing to their illness. Yet numerous practitioners experienced in treating CFS have noted that people who develop the syndrome tend to be overachievers.

"Every single person I have seen with CFS was an overachiever," states Shari Lieberman, Ph.D., C.N.S., a nutritional specialist in New York City. "These were people who, when they got flu or another sickness, refused to give in to it, didn't rest enough, and quickly went back to a full schedule of work and exercise. These people are go-getters. The common thread is that their CFS was precipitated by an illness in which they didn't take care of themselves enough."

W. John Diamond, M.D., of Reno, Nevada, also observes that all of his patients with chronic fatigue syndrome are overachievers. His medical practice—which includes homeopathy, a therapy that emphasizes the psychological side of illness—has schooled him in looking for these factors. The self-image of these chronic fatigue patients is "locked into or associated with their personal productivity," he says. Driven by the pressure to succeed, their bodies eventually break down. "As a physician, I have to go backward into my patients' histories to trace the whole issue," says Dr. Diamond. "Invariably, I find that my chronic fatigue syndrome patients have terrible life skills and poor habits. That kind of insulting treatment of their system adds up and the body finally says, 'no more.'"

Jacob Teitelbaum, M.D., concurs that CFS sufferers tend to be type-A personalities. These are people who are accomplishment-oriented, driven, operating on deadlines, usually anxious—the term is often used to describe people prone to heart attacks. Such people often live in what Dr. Teitelbaum calls "role entrapment" before they become ill. "Role-entrapped people were taught that they have to be the perfect spouse or the perfect parent or the perfect employee. The 'superwoman' complex is a good example. CFIDS can be your body's way of getting out of the roles in which you are trapped," he explains.[1] In addition to the psychic discomfort of attempting to fulfill someone else's idea of what you should be, trying to live up to these roles creates a tremendous amount of stress in people's lives. A high stress level is a common feature in those who get CFS.

> Role-entrapped people were taught that they have to be the perfect spouse or the perfect parent or the perfect employee. The "superwoman" complex is a good example. Chronic fatigue can be your body's way of getting out of the roles in which you are trapped.
> — *Jacob Teitelbaum, M.D.*

Dr. Stoff defines stress as "the internal state that results when the capacity to adapt to what is has been exceeded."[2] When this condition persists, the immune system is weakened and the body becomes vulnerable to breakdown. "Excessive stress is like putting the welcome mat out for the first 'evil' germ (be it EBV, cytomegalovirus, or Coxsackie virus) that feels like setting up camp," says Dr. Stoff.[3]

Operating at an ongoing high stress level also overloads the adrenal glands, which then leads to fatigue, as the adrenals are integral to energy production. As mentioned previously, CFS patients tend to have high levels of cortisol (one of the adrenal hormones), indicating that the adrenal glands are overworking. Clearly, taking steps to reduce the stress in your life is an important part of reversing the patterns that contributed to your CFS. Maoshing Ni, D.O.M., Ph.D., L.Ac., a practitioner of traditional Chinese medicine who has treated many people with CFS, sums up the process involved: "I describe my patients as people who, before treatment, were gulping coffee. After treatment, they learn how to sip tea."

Your illness may have forced you out of your previously stressful mode of living, but it is important when you begin to recover through the various methods covered in this book that you do not resume your old habits. A first step might be to find out what you want to do in your life; how you want to spend your time. It is vital to the healing process that patients begin to get to know themselves better, says Dr. Stoff. "Self-awareness will reveal many harmful patterns and make them healthier. It is not merely an intellectual exercise," he states.

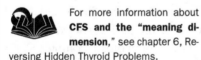 For more information about **CFS and the "meaning dimension,"** see chapter 6, Reversing Hidden Thyroid Problems.

This is what Dr. Stoff means by learning the lessons of your disease. It's also what Dr. Teitelbaum has in mind when he says: "Although you likely view your illness as an enemy, you should let it become your ally."[4] Making it an ally by doing the hard internal work of sorting through the emotional and psychological com-

## Stressed Out—A Pervasive Western Problem

Although the concept of being "stressed out" or "under constant stress" may be commonly discussed today, the role stress plays as a contributing factor in many diseases is still underappreciated. Estimates suggest that as much as 70% to 80% of all visits to physicians' offices are for stress-related problems. Chronic stress directly affects the immune system and, if not effectively dealt with, can seriously compromise health.

Stress is a pervasive problem among Americans, according to a 1996 poll of corporate executives. For example, 44% of employees polled said their work load is excessive compared to 37% in 1988; 43% are bothered by excessive job pressure; and 55% worry considerably about their company's future; 25% of both men and women feel stressed out at work every day, another 12% feel it almost every day, and another 38% feel it once to several days a week.[a]

Research in psychoneuroimmunology, or PNI, has shown that the immune and nervous systems are linked by extensive networks of nerve endings in the spleen, bone marrow, lymph nodes, and thymus gland (a primary source of T cells). At the same time, receptors for a variety of chemical messengers—catecholamines, prostaglandins, thyroid hormone, growth hormone, sex hormones, serotonin, and endorphins—have been found on the surfaces of white blood cells. Such connections serve to integrate the activities of the immune, hormonal, and nervous systems, enabling the mind and emotional states to influence the body's resistance to disease.[b]

Stress can be defined as a reaction to any stimulus or interference that upsets normal functioning and disturbs mental or physical health. It can be brought on by internal conditions, such as illness, pain, emotional conflict, or psychological problems, or by external circumstances, such as bereavement, financial problems, loss of job or spouse, or relocation. Stress, when it becomes chronic, is often unrecognized by the person whose body is experiencing it; one begins to accept it as a fact of life, without being aware of how it is actually compromising all bodily function and laying the foundation for illness.

More specifically, research confirms that high levels of emotional stress increase one's susceptibility to illness. Unrelieved, chronic stress begins taxing and eventually weakening, even suppressing, the immune system. Stress can also lead to hormonal imbalances, which, in turn, interfere with immune function. Of all the body's systems, stress damages immune function the most. It does so by overly activating the sympathetic part of the autonomic nervous system, the part that controls the "fight-or-flight" response and initiates adrenaline and cortisol release.

---

[a]Schellhardt, Timothy D. "Company Memo to Stressed-Out Employees: 'Deal With It.'" *The Wall Street Journal* (October 2, 1996).
[b]Marx, J. L. "The Immune System 'Belongs to the Body.'" *Science* 277 (1985), 1190–1192.

---

ponents of your illness will, when combined with the treatments for the physical factors involved, result in lasting recovery.

## Using Homeopathy to Provoke Emotional Healing

Homeopathic treatment of CFS and other chronic illnesses begins by eliminating the immediate symptoms, then progresses to the older,

**Homeopathy** was founded in the early 1800s by German physician Samuel Hahnemann. Today, an estimated 500 million people worldwide receive homeopathic treatment; in Britain, homeopathy enjoys royal patronage. Homeopathy is now practiced according to two differing concepts. In classical homeopathy, only one single-component remedy is prescribed at a time in a potency specifically adjusted to the patient; the physician waits to see the results before prescribing anything further. In complex homeopathy, a prescription involves multiple substances given at the same time, usually in low potencies.

underlying "layers" of the condition. One of these layers may be unresolved emotions the patient has been suppressing, often for many years. An emotional imbalance of this kind has as strong an impact as a physical malady on the overall health of the body. Homeopathic remedies help the patient release the stored emotions. If all the layers of an illness are not addressed, healing is incomplete and, as mentioned above, relapse or the development of a different disease or disorder is likely.

In the following section, W. John Diamond, M.D., a physician specializing in homeopathy (SEE QUICK DEFINITION) and other alternative modalities, describes a multilayered case of CFS and the homeopathic treatment of each layer, including the emotional component of the illness.

### Success Story:
### Reversing a 14-Year Episode of Chronic Fatigue

When Rebecca, 38, first came to me, she had already seen eight conventional physicians for her multifaceted condition. She had chronic fatigue; depression; joint, muscle, and low back pain; migraine headaches; and severe pelvic and anal pains. Often her knees hurt and her legs would feel heavy. According to standard laboratory tests, Rebecca had a low white blood cell count, indicating her immune system was seriously weakened; it also showed she had a high level of Epstein-Barr virus, which is often the case in CFS patients.

Rebecca had used three different antidepressants but none had lifted her depression. Earlier, a physician had put her on Synthroid, a standard drug for inflammation of the thyroid gland (thyroiditis). Rebecca also felt claustrophobic, had frequent panic attacks, was afraid of new medications, was chronically constipated, and had, in her own words, "no energy." Rebecca had been on antibiotics since she was 20 for pelvic inflammatory disease, but they failed to resolve this problem. She told me she had pain in her pelvis "all the time."

Here is how Rebecca described her state: "When I get a bad pain attack in my back or pelvis, it comes over me in waves and I need to go and hide away in my bedroom and just get under the covers and rest. Sometimes

## Controlled Exercise Can Help Chronic Fatigue

Postexercise exhaustion is on the CDC's list of chronic fatigue syndrome symptoms. Many people with CFS experience a worsening of their symptoms after exercise. However, according to a study published in the *British Medical Journal*, graded (or gradually increasing) exercise can actually produce lasting benefit for some CFS patients. The study of 66 people with CFS consisted of three groups: (1) participants in a graded exercise program; (2) a control group of flexibility training and relaxation therapy instead; and (3) 22 control subjects who "crossed over" into the exercise program after the first 12 weeks of the study.

The graded exercise consisted mainly of walking, but some cycling or swimming if desired, and the sessions initially lasted between 5 and 15 minutes, increasing at the rate of 1 or 2 minutes per week to a maximum of 30 minutes. If patients experienced increased fatigue, they were advised to continue at the same level of exercise for an extra week. This allowed their bodies to adjust to the increase in aerobic activity.

Of the 29 patients in the exercise group, 16 (55%) considered themselves "much" or "very much" better than at the start of the trial, compared to 8 out of 30 (29%) in the control group. In the crossover group, 12 out of 22 (55%) rated themselves as better following the exercise phase. Follow-up interviews revealed that the benefits of graded exercise appeared to continue even after the program had ended, with 68% reporting they still felt better three months after the study ended.

Researcher Peter D. White, M.D., speculates that graded exercise—not simple exercise by itself—may work by functioning as a type of behavior therapy. "Graded exercise can reduce the anxiety and apprehension understandably felt by many CFS patients, who have learned that unstructured exercise tends to cause relapses of their condition," Dr. White says. "By making the exercise graded and agreed upon by the patient, he or she is able to feel more in control."*

---

*White, Peter D., et al. "Randomized Controlled Trial of Graded Exercise in Patients with Chronic Fatigue Syndrome." *British Medical Journal* 314 (June 7, 1997), 1647–1652.

it's for days. The energy just ebbs out of me. When I have no energy, my pelvis aches and throbs. I have to sit down to stop the pain. It feels like my uterus will just about drop out of me." Further, she had memory and concentration problems, craved salty foods, was usually hot and sweaty while she slept, and woke frequently at night only to stare emptily at the bedroom wall just as she had done as a child. She told me that all aspects of her problem worsened at the age of 24, which, I later learned, was when she got married to a man who already had three young children.

I asked her about her childhood. "It was terrible," she said. Both parents had been alcoholics and addicted to drugs. Her two older brothers were heavy drinkers and had sexually abused her. Rebecca said her mother hated her because she was competing for her husband's affections. Rebecca's mother repeatedly told her she was a "worthless child," that she was "a nothing, less than a dog."

## Massage Therapy Can Reduce the Pain of Fibromyalgia

Twenty-one of 26 fibromyalgia patients experienced reduced pain and general improvement after receiving massage therapy. The study discovered a relationship between a fibromyalgia patient's degree of pain and an increase in blood levels of myoglobin (the oxygen-carrying protein of the muscle tissue). The pain may be the outcome of myoglobin leaking from the muscles. Along with the pain reduction after massage, there was a gradual decline in the high levels of myoglobin in the patients' blood.

Source: Scandinavian Journal of Rheumatology 15:2 (1986), 174–178.

Beginning at age six, Rebecca became a surrogate mother for the household, since her mother was chronically drunk. Rebecca did all the chores around the house. Meanwhile, her father was drunk most of the time and often violent. Her parents argued and fought frequently; when they did, Rebecca would retreat to her bedroom and stare at the wall. In sum, she was extremely passive, quiet, and depressed as a child.

At 18, she had an abortion, about which she felt exceedingly guilty, and she moved out of the family house. She began drinking steadily and drifted around until she married at the age of 24. She moved to another town with her husband and his children. Consider what she did here: Rebecca duplicated the situation she had lived with as a child. She became the surrogate mother again, which was, truly, the last thing she wanted to do. Eventually her biology decided this arrangement was not what she needed and shut her down with a mass of symptoms.

*Fine-Tuning the Diagnosis With Electrodermal Screening.* As part of my medical practice, I regularly use electrodermal screening (EDS—SEE QUICK DEFINITION) to identify hidden energy blockages in the body. It is also an effective way to get beyond times when a patient prefers not to admit a fact from their history or perhaps literally does not remember it; at such times, these hidden facts may be the key to a case. My electrodermal evaluation of Rebecca showed highly inflammatory conditions in her tonsils and pharynx.

A "normal" EDS reading is about 50, but for Rebecca the needle hovered between 70 and 80. It also indicated trouble in her spleen, liver, kidneys, intestines, and uterus. In some instances there was a sudden change in the read-

 **Electrodermal screening** is a form of computerized information gathering, based on physics, not chemistry. A blunt, noninvasive electric probe is placed at specific points on the patient's hands, face, or feet, corresponding to acupuncture points at the beginning or end of energy meridians. Minute electrical discharges from these points serve as information signals about the condition of the body's organs and systems, useful for the physician in evaluation and development of a treatment plan.

> The first time you see a patient, you need to give remedies that will get the physiological system working properly again, removing from the body all the obstacles to healing. Then you can give a single remedy and the body will respond.
>
> — *W. John Diamond, M.D.*

John Diamond, M.D.

ings, from a high to a low value; in the electrodermal screening world, we call this an "indicator drop" and it is a bad sign. It suggests that the organ is leaking energy and may be undergoing severe degeneration, starting at an energy level and moving into a more tangible deterioration.

On the basis of all the evidence I collected about her symptom picture, it seemed clear to me that there was a strong link between her history of childhood sexual abuse and her chronic pelvic problems. In my approach to homeopathy, the first time you see a patient, you need to give remedies that will get the physiological system working properly again. This means removing from the body all the obstacles to healing. Then, according to classical homeopathy, you can give a single remedy and the body will respond by healing completely.

***Removing the Obstacles to Healing.*** I prepared a remedy program for Rebecca consisting of six components. My prescribing philosophy in this case was to give her the strongest remedies possible. Her immune system needed major stimulation after 14 years of not working correctly. First, I gave her a homeopathic nosode (SEE QUICK DEFINITION) of Epstein-Barr virus (EBV) at a strength of 200C, which she would take once weekly for a month. This would help her body start to eliminate the high levels of EBV in her tonsils, liver, and kidneys. Second, I gave Rebecca a nosode called Viricin to be taken once daily. This broad-based formula contains all the main viruses including EBV but at a low potency. I wanted to be sure to catch all the virus problems.

 A **homeopathic nosode** is a super-diluted remedy made as an energy imprint from a disease product, such as bacteria, tuberculosis, measles, bowel infection, influenza, and about 200 other substances. The nosode, which contains no physical trace of the disease, stimulates the body to remove all "taints" or residues of a particular disease that it holds, whether it was inherited or contracted. Only qualified homeopaths may administer a nosode.

Third, Rebecca took *Rehmannia* 6, a remedy composed of Chinese herbs, to address the energy imbalance in her kidneys as evidenced by her night sweats. She took three tablets, three times daily. Fourth, I prescribed a homeopathic formula for detoxification. This was a combination of three low-dose "drainage" remedies (SEE QUICK DEFINITION), called Liquiessences, for the lymph, kidneys, and liver in potencies of 1X and 2X (one and two successive dilutions and successions or vigorous shaking). Rebecca took these drops three times daily.

Fifth, I selected a single homeopathic remedy called *Sepia* 12C, according to classical homeopathic prescribing. Rebecca took *Sepia* once daily. This remedy comes from squid ink; its oceanic origins (and other psychological and physiological factors) perfectly matched Rebecca's condition—even her choice of words, such as "waves" and energy "ebbs." In fact, her expression that her uterus felt as if it might "fall out" is typical of the type of images that consistently are presented by patients needing *Sepia*. The sense of her uterus falling out, the sexual abuse, the abortion, and the subsequent guilt are all connected. It was as if, on a psychological or metaphorical level, Rebecca wanted to get rid of her uterus, to push it out so the experience would be gone from her life along with the organ that bore its memory.

 **Drainage remedies** comprise low-potency homeopathic substances and tinctures (alcohol extractions) of both Chinese and Western herbs. The concept of drainage derives from French homeopaths who were interested in applying homeopathy at a grosser, physiological level rather than at the level of "mentals" (psychological, emotional, and spiritual factors). Drainage remedies encourage the lymphatic system, liver, kidneys, blood, tissues, intercellular spaces, fat, and skin to eliminate, or "drain," their toxins, thus keeping them from circulating in the body or being deposited in other tissue. The best-known drainage remedies are *Solidago* and *Berberis* for the kidney; *Taraxacum, Silymarin,* and *Carduus* for the liver; *Hydrastis* as a general drainage; and *Myosotis* for the lymphatic system.

Sixth, I addressed her chronic constipation and years of excessive antibiotic intake by giving her Multiflora, a "friendly bacteria" or probiotics product. This blend contains *acidophilus* and *bifidus* cultures and fructo-oligosaccharides (which are helpful "fast food" for the beneficial bacteria). She took two capsules, three times daily to start restoring the normal population levels and balance of intestinal microflora previously destroyed by all the antibiotics.

*Helping the Patient Confront the Past.* Rebecca left my office with these six remedies and instructions to take them all concurrently. I didn't hear from her for a month. When she called, her report was highly encouraging. Her pelvic pain had worsened the first several days on the remedies and was followed by a copious vaginal discharge of, in her

> The day after she took the *Staphysagria*, Rebecca's anger welled up so strongly that she was mad at everyone in her life—husband, children, and parents. She took an angle iron and smashed up her garage door until all her anger was discharged. From that moment, her remaining pelvic pain disappeared and has not returned.

words, a "smelly yellow liquid." This went on for three days, but when it stopped, she felt "so much better."

A temporary worsening of symptoms followed by an often powerful discharge, then rapid improvement, is typical of how homeopathic remedies work. I interpreted the discharge as her body's way of getting rid of what was ailing in her pelvis. In a sense, her body materialized all the emotional toxins (from parental abandonment, sexual abuse, and other traumatic factors from her personal history) and forcibly expelled them from her body.

It was understandable, therefore, that during the period of her vaginal discharge Rebecca was exhausted. As soon as it was finished, her energy began increasing daily until she estimated her energy level was 80% improved. After a week, she was sleeping better and her constipation gave way to normal, daily bowel motions. She stopped feeling cold and stopped craving salt; her panic attacks disappeared and she was no longer fearful about taking new medicines. (Initially, Rebecca had been highly resistant to the remedies and I had to persuade her that it was in her best interest to take them.)

She reported that emotionally she felt remarkably better and that the pain had receded from her anus and pelvis and was localized over the bladder and uterus. Overall, the pain had decreased by 50% but, for me, this wasn't good enough. I was left with a woman whose physical symptom picture had markedly improved yet she still had 50% pain in her pelvis. Using electrodermal screening, I found that there was no longer any evidence of Epstein-Barr virus anywhere in her system and the only organ carrying any imbalance was her uterus.

To address this underlying imbalance, I gave her a single homeopathic

**W. John Diamond, M.D.**: Triad Medical Center, 9436 Double R B1, Reno, NV 89502; tel: (775) 829-2277.

remedy called *Staphysagria* (larkspur seeds) at a medium strength of 200C. This remedy often helps break open a condition of internalized anger. Rebecca came to my office a month later with good and surprising news. The day after she took the *Staphysagria*, her anger welled up so strongly that she was mad at everyone in her life—husband, children, and parents. She telephoned the latter and directly confronted them with their neglect and abuse of her as a child. She had avoided them for years before this moment. Then she took an angle iron and smashed up her garage door until all her anger was discharged. From that moment, the remaining pelvic pain disappeared and has not returned.

## Success Story:
## Resolving the Emotional Core of Chronic Fatigue

Deeply suppressed grief can be as debilitating as the unexpressed anger that was the central emotion contributing to Rebecca's illness. The following case illustrates the role of both grief and anger in long-standing CFS and, again, how homeopathy can assist in releasing the stored emotions.

Homeopath Judith A. Lewis, R.N, N.D., of Mill Valley, California, consulted with Rhonda, 43, who worked part-time as an editor. She had suffered from chronic fatigue syndrome, genital herpes, and chronic allergies for nearly 15 years, and from an underactive thyroid (hypothyroidism) for eight years. Rhonda had previously consulted nearly two dozen practitioners of alternative medicine and had been put on various herbal treatments, intestinal cleansers, and allergy elimination diets. She had received multiple remedy homeopathic medicines and undergone extensive psychotherapy, and was currently taking a conventional drug for her thyroid imbalance.

As a younger person, Rhonda had been athletic and excelled in her studies; as an adult, she was a perfectionist and hard worker, but prone to depression, with a defeatist attitude. She was impatient and overly self-critical, reports Dr. Lewis. Her 25 physical symptoms included sleep-

> The result [of these experiences] was deeply suppressed grief and anger. To release and clarify these strong emotions, Dr. Lewis gave Rhonda *Naturum Muriaticum* 30C. During the next month, Rhonda's buried emotions began to surface and be released, and her overall mental state improved.

ing a great deal, allergies, bloating, constipation, a feeling of body-wide toxicity, frequent headaches, a diminished libido, sluggish digestion, and recurrent bouts of genital herpes about every six weeks.

To start the treatment, Dr. Lewis recommended Rhonda take *Nux Vomica* 12X (homeopathic poison nut), two daily for ten days. This remedy would clear away the confusing energy picture in Rhonda's system, produced by having received so many different herbs and homeopathic mixes over the years. *Nux Vomica* would also help to drain toxins from Rhonda's liver. Dr. Lewis also suggested that Rhonda start a supplement program including kelp herbal extract (one teaspoon, three times daily), vitamin A (10,000 IU daily), vitamin C (6 to 10 g daily), vitamin E (400 IU daily), and a balanced vitamin B complex pill daily. In addition, every day Rhonda was to drink an herbal tea made of dandelion, burdock, ginger, and red clover.

One month after beginning this program, Dr. Lewis gave Rhonda a single dose of *Carcinosin* 200C. This is a nosode made from homeopathically potentized cancer cells. The purpose here, Dr. Lewis explains, is to remove the energy residue (called "miasm"—SEE QUICK DEFINITION) of a strong family history of cancer; it would otherwise remain in her system as a subtle but persistent interference in her complete healing.

During Dr. Lewis's lengthy initial interview with her, Rhonda revealed that she had experienced three deaths in close succession shortly before she

 **QUICK DEFINITION**

A **homeopathic miasm**, as originally described by Samuel Hahnemann, the nineteenth-century German founder of homeopathy, is a subtle taint or energy residue of previous illness, which recurs over generations. As an inherited predisposition for chronic disease that is far more subtle than anything genetic, miasms are broad-focused, predisposing individuals and families to specific illnesses, such as tuberculosis or cancer. According to Hahnemann, three miasms underlie all chronic illness and parallel broad stages in the history of human experience with primary disease states. They are the *Psoric* miasm (from *psora*, meaning "itch"), the *Syphilitic* miasm (deriving from syphilis), and the *Sycotic* miasm (arising as a residue of gonorrhea). Some homeopaths add a fourth *Cancer* miasm, and a fifth *Petroleum* miasm.

> This case shows clearly how a powerful but unaddressed emotional experience can set in motion a complicated and chronic illness pattern. When you release the triggering emotion, then the body is able to start eliminating the secondary physical symptoms.

became sick. Two close family members and a family pet had died suddenly; in addition, Rhonda had had a shocking near-death experience. The result was deeply suppressed grief and anger, observes Dr. Lewis. To release and clarify these strong emotions, Dr. Lewis gave Rhonda *Naturum Muriaticum* 30C (homeopathic common salt). During the next month, Rhonda's buried emotions began to surface and be released, and her overall mental state improved.

Her digestive problems had worsened, however. In a subsequent follow-up interview, Rhonda revealed that she had contracted severe dysentery while traveling abroad. Dr. Lewis believed that this microbial contamination was still upsetting Rhonda's digestion, so she prescribed one dose of *Bacillus* No. 7 (a homeopathic bowel nosode) to remove all energy taints of this infection. At this point, Rhonda had considerable emotional upheaval; some symptoms had improved but many had relapsed, which is typical of the healing process in homeopathy, says Dr. Lewis.

During the fifth month of treatment, Dr. Lewis gave Rhonda a single stronger dose of *Naturum Muriaticum*, and during the sixth month, she further increased the strength of the single dose. During this period, Rhonda experienced several outbursts of grief and anger. "This was a sign of progress because emotions lie deeper than the physical symptoms," says Dr. Lewis. At the end of this period, Rhonda's thyroid was back to normal and she discontinued her thyroid medication after having been dependent on it for six years. In addition, she was no longer experiencing herpes outbreaks.

Rhonda reported herself to be 85% improved and "liberated from chronic fatigue after 15 years." Her energy levels felt normal again and she was able to work almost full-time. Rhonda initiated new social contacts and began a new relationship, also for the first time in 15 years. All her digestive and allergy problems had disappeared; her sleeping patterns were normal again; and as far as her mental state and bodily functions were concerned, Rhonda's chronic fatigue was entirely an experi-

## Releasing the Trapped Emotions Underlying Fibromyalgia

Alternative medicine practitioner Christiane Northrup, M.D., author of *Health Wisdom for Women*, believes that fibromyalgia has a strong emotional element. Negative feelings of despair and resentment, from job stress, family problems, or even childhood memories, get "trapped" in the muscles and constrict them. To release trapped emotions, Dr. Northrup recommends the following steps, which she says can often produce good results in three to six weeks:*

- **Exercise:** Even though it seems you can't move your muscles, you must keep moving every day; your pain will actually diminish as you build a consistent exercise program.
- **Rest and Relax:** Sleep 8 to 10 hours nightly; go to bed before 10 p.m. and get up at the same time every morning.
- **Meditate:** Even 15 minutes a day will help balance your brain chemicals, or neurotransmitters.
- **Balance the Prostaglandins:** Keep your prostaglandin hormone levels in balance by eating no more than 500 calories per meal; keep your diet low in refined carbohydrates and fats, and moderate in protein.

- **Increase Your Serotonin:** Use blue-green algae in a progressive, four-week supplementation program to enhance levels of this important neurotransmitter. First week: Take two Cell-Tech digestive enzymes with Alpha Sun or Omega Sun blue-green algae capsules before breakfast and lunch. Also take two capsules of acidophilus with algae, 30 minutes before breakfast. Second week: Add to this one capsule of Alpha Sun and Omega Sun before breakfast. Third week: Continue this while increasing the algae intake to two to four capsules, three times daily with meals. Fourth week: Continue with this regimen, increasing the algae if necessary. This will increase your serotonin levels and have an anti-depressant effect.
- **Use Supplements:** Take magnesium (300 to 600 mg daily); malic acid (1,200 mg daily, divided into three doses, building to 2,400 mg if pain persists after two weeks); all the B vitamins (100 mg each, daily); and manganese (10 to 20 mg).

*Northrup, Christiane, M.D. *Health Wisdom for Women* 2:5 (1995), 3–5.

ence of the past. "This case shows clearly how a powerful but unaddressed emotional experience can set in motion a complicated and chronic illness pattern," observes Dr. Lewis. "When you release the triggering emotion, then the body is able to start eliminating the secondary physical symptoms."

## Lifting the Depression Associated with Chronic Fatigue

Most people with CFS, fibromyalgia, and environmental illness suffer from depression. The impact of these debilitating disorders on one's life is enough in itself to induce depression, but there are numerous biochemical factors that may also be causing the persistently low feelings.

These include hormonal imbalances, nutritional deficiencies, hypoglycemia (low blood sugar), allergies and sensitivities, chemical or heavy metal toxicity, and viral or fungal infections.[5] Note that all of these factors have been discussed earlier in this book as agents that help cause chronic fatigue. Observe the continuous cycle of illness. The factors that create CFS produce depression as well, and this, in turn, suppresses immune function. Then, the more compromised the immunity becomes, the worse the deficiencies and imbalances; this then leads to a deepening of the depression and the cycle continues.

Evidence indicates that depression is an outcome rather than a precipitating factor in CFS, but some in the conventional medical establishment still view CFS as a psychogenic or psychosomatic ailment (having mental as opposed to physical origins) and believe the depression associated with it is a sign of these origins. However, even the U.S. Centers for Disease Control and Prevention (CDC) now acknowledges that most CFS patients report their depression and anxiety as starting *after* the onset of the illness. On this basis, the CDC is willing to concede that these symptoms are "secondary reactions to CFS."[6]

For **antidepressant herbs**, see chapter 12, Treating Chronic Fatigue with Herbs.

The fact that people with CFS led very active lives before getting sick supports this conclusion, since depression is characterized by low energy and a sense of immobilization. In addition, the depression of CFS tends to lift as the person begins to feel better. "A reactive depression to the extreme fatigue of CFS should not be surprising," says Leon Chaitow, N.D., D.O. "Those with CFS have often been suffering debilitating symptoms for a number of years, barely acknowledged by the medical establishment, and have been offered little appropriate treatment other than a 'chin up' attitude and handfuls of antidepressants."

However, just as unresolved emotions may be contributing to CFS, they may be a factor in the depression experienced in the illness as well. The following section demonstrates how deep depression and the associated CFS can be reversed with traditional Chinese medicine (TCM).

**Marie Hoshimi-Wilkes, N.D., Ph.D., O.M.D.:** Oriental Medicine Plus, 120 West Chestnut, Las Cruces, NM 88005; tel: (505) 647-8077.

Marie Hoshimi-Wilkes, Ph.D., N.D., O.M.D., of Las Cruces, New Mexico, describes how emotional and psychological factors are often a source of physical imbalances and how she uses TCM to address these elements:

## Healing Depression Without Prozac

An estimated 12 million people worldwide (six million Americans) take Prozac for depression, resulting in annual sales of $2 billion for Eli Lilly and Company, Prozac's maker. Why further enrich this drug company when safer, inexpensive alternatives exist to successfully elevate your mood? According to naturopathic physician and educator Michael T. Murray, N.D., lifestyle, dietary, and psychological therapies can serve as natural antidepressants and keep you Prozac free.

- **Lifestyle.** First, make sure your depression does not have an organic, physiological cause, such as diabetes, cancer, or heavy metal toxicity, or is not due to a food allergy or overuse of prescription drugs. Then know that it is highly beneficial to create a mental attitude that is positive and optimistic, says Dr. Murray. Set achievement goals, practice affirmation. Quit smoking, reduce or eliminate your intake of caffeine and alcohol, exercise regularly, practice a relaxation and stress reduction exercise every day for at least ten minutes, and laugh more.

- **Dietary.** Nutrient imbalances or deficiencies can contribute to chronic depression, says Dr. Murray. "Correcting an underlying nutritional deficiency can restore normal mental function and relieve depression," he adds. Among Dr. Murray's recommendations: reduce your fat intake; eat at least five daily servings of fresh fruits and vegetables; minimize your consumption of refined sugars and salt; eat much more fiber and complex carbohydrates (whole grains); and keep your protein intake moderate.

- **Supplements.** Start correcting the nutritional foundation of your health with a daily high-potency multiple vitamin and mineral formula, says Dr. Murray. In addition, he suggests taking daily folic acid (800 mcg), vitamin B12 (800 mcg), vitamin B6 (50 to 100 mg), and flaxseed oil.

- **Herbs.** As an additional antidepressant support, Dr. Murray recommends using *Ginkgo biloba*. For people over 50, take 80 mg, three times daily, with addition folic acid (1,200 mcg). For people under 50, take St. John's wort extract, 300 mg, three times daily.

- **Amino Acids.** Deficiencies or imbalances in the body's levels of amino acids, which are essential protein building blocks, can also contribute to depression. Dr. Murray suggests 2,000 mg of D- or L-phenylalanine, or 1,000 mg of L-tyrosine, taken once daily, before breakfast.

- **Insomnia.** Depression often brings a disruption of normal sleeping rhythms. Helpful here are melatonin (3 mg) before bedtime; valerian herbal extract (150–300 mg) taken 30 minutes before bedtime; or GABA (gamma aminobutyric acid, an amino acid derivative), taken at 200 to 400 mg, 30 minutes before bedtime.

"Adopting these guidelines is all that the majority of people with depression will need to do to elevate their mood," says Dr. Murray.

Source: Murray, Michael T., N.D. *Natural Alternatives to Prozac* (New York: William Morrow, 1996).

## *Success Story: Resolving Depression Related to CFS*

The statement from Chinese medicine that over 90% of all diseases have a psychological and emotional origin continually influences my work. I believe you cannot possibly heal somebody through Chinese medicine without working through a great deal of their psychological and emotional issues. As soon as you start getting the body well, these deeper causes of the physical symptoms will begin to surface.

You have to work on them, because otherwise they will come back up into the body again and produce more symptoms. I use acupuncture, moxibustion (SEE QUICK DEFINITION), herbs, counseling, even flower essences and color therapy, to give the patient enough strength to start looking at the deeper problems with clarity. Chronic fatigue syndrome, from my perspective, is about deep-seated emotions—deeply repressed feelings of anger, even self-hatred—that have finally affected the immune and digestive systems, producing a host of symptoms, as the case of Elaine illustrates.

 In **moxibustion**, a dried herb called moxa (usually mugwort) is burned over the skin at a specific acupuncture point. The moxa may be attached to a special acupuncture needle or in a free-standing cone set on a slice of ginger; its slow burning provides a penetrating heat. The purpose is to warm the blood and *qi* (vital life force energy flowing through the body's energy pathways), particularly when a patient's energy picture is cold or damp.

Elaine, 45, came to me with deep depression and extreme exhaustion. She had low energy, no concentration, bad memory, fevers, sweat, chills, poor sleep, dizziness, cold extremities, high blood pressure, respiratory problems, irregular periods, and back, neck, and muscle pain. She was defensive and ready to cry, even at innocuous remarks. She had been previously treated for a chronic bladder and kidney obstruction, and was still sporadically unable to urinate. Elaine had suffered these chronic symptoms for four years.

In Chinese medicine terms, she had kidney *yang* deficiency, which means she didn't have enough *yang*, or active, fiery energy in her kidneys, leaving her sluggish, passive, inactive, fearful, tired, holding water, and with no willpower. During her first 90-minute session, I inserted needles on all the organ points on her back, especially her kidney points, then followed this with moxibustion to strengthen her *qi*, or vital body energy. I also made suggestions as the needles remained in place: "Elaine, I'm working on your kidneys now, so let's release fear and anxiety. It's safe to release fear." This had immediate effects.

Elaine knew she had deeply buried emotions, but didn't know how to process them. All the time I was treating her physically, I was also working with the emotional and psychological energies associated with the physical symptoms. Her back went into spasms and ripples as she started coming in contact with these old painful feelings made available through the needles, such as sexual abuse by her uncle, grief over the death of a malformed infant, deep guilt taken on from her dead mother,

## Nutritional Deficiencies Associated with Depression

Nutritional biochemist Patricia Kane, Ph.D., of Millville, New Jersey, has observed distinct nutritional deficiencies among patients diagnosed with depression. Dr. Kane cites the case of Sylvia, 29, who had suffered a prolonged depression lasting for three years. Initially, she had complained of chronic fatigue and mood swings; later, she reported digestive difficulties and food allergies, and although she had avoided conventional drugs, she was on the verge of taking Prozac.

A comprehensive blood test revealed the nutritional, or biochemical, side of Sylvia's depression. It showed she had either a deficiency or an excess of 31 substances, indicating "a deeply imbalanced biochemistry," says Dr. Kane. "Most generally stated, Sylvia's blood status was an 80% match with the known 'disease pattern' for depression. Further, Sylvia's blood nutrient status deviated by 31% from the healthy norm." For the most part, Sylvia was 10% deficient in many key nutrients. Basically, owing to her dietary choices (low in natural fat, high in synthetic fats, or trans-fatty acids), Sylvia didn't have enough of the essential raw materials for her body to produce the hormones, proteins, and other substances necessary for a healthy physiology, Dr. Kane explains.

"Most often, a depressed person will have lower than average amounts of five substances: blood urea nitrogen, chloride, cholesterol, potassium, and uric acid." Sylvia's pattern matched four out of five of these criteria: her blood urea nitrogen (nitrogen in urea form in the urine) was 33% low; cholesterol 80%; potassium 33%; and uric acid (a crystalline acid from nitrogen metabolism) 64%; her chloride was high at 57% above the norm. Usually, high chlorides are correlated with epilepsy or high anxiety, while low chlorides are often found with depression. Three other markers consistently associated with depression were also low in Sylvia's blood chemistry: iron, creatinine, and albumin.

 **Patricia C. Kane, Ph.D.:** 45 Reese Road, P.O. Box 809, Millville, NJ 08332; tel: (888) 320-8338. Website: www.bodybio.com.

---

profound sadness over the fact she had never known her father. She was also now in a marriage that had been abusive for years; before seeing me, she had resigned herself to living with it.

After the first session, Elaine's spirits lifted and she was able to have a sense of humor and objectivity about her condition. I gave her five flower remedies (see below) to take hourly to help further lift her mood; they were Self Heal, California pitcher plant, St. John's wort, Scotch broom, and fuchsia. After her second session, I prescribed a mixture of Chinese herbs to improve her energy, to help the bladder and kidney problem, and to tone her digestion. These included *Fo-ti*, to nourish and detoxify the blood; *fructus Lycii*, to help liver and kidney energy; *fu-shen*, for calming the spirit; *dong quai*, to build up the blood; aconite, to bring up *yang* energy; and astragalus, for the night sweats; plus cinnamon,

> It all comes down to what we say in alternative medicine: you have to treat the whole person of body, mind, and spirit. You cannot just treat the body or the spirit alone, because they're part of the same system.
>
> —*Marie Hoshimi-Wilkes, N.D., Ph.D., M.D.*

licorice, and diascoria. She took these twice a day, in liquid form, for about three months; I modified the mix according to her symptoms.

I also employed color therapy at each session, using a German-made Vegalux color generator to project different colors (through little flashlights at the tips of fiber optic tubes) onto her skin. Color therapy is a soothing, energy-building adjunct to acupuncture. For example, I used orange on her lower abdomen for endocrine insufficiency, and blue and yellow on her feet to release stress and prenatal feelings. I left the colors in place for 40 minutes a session.

*Doing the Deep Work.* As the needles, moxibustion, flowers, color, and herbs built up her energy, Elaine began to have a lot of emotional releases and psychological insights, which surprised and encouraged her. She is a good patient, willing to do the hard work of healing.

During her second session, Elaine said it was as if an animal were trying to eat her up from the inside, devouring all her energy. Another time she said she felt she had a "hole" in her body (or what I might call an energy field) out of which energy kept leaking. All this time she had been making drawings of volcanoes that could only blow steam and lava out their sides, not their tops. In a later session, we focused on her so-called victimhood. I said to her: "Why don't you make your own heart affirmation while I'm treating you. Give me words that tell me who you truly are, not the victimized person you think you are."

After six treatments, Elaine had enough energy to resume doing things she couldn't do for years and to confront the fact that her marriage was not satisfactory. This is what her healing was about: having the energy to face her life issues and bad marriage and to make the necessary changes. It means now, after only eight sessions spread over three months, she's strong enough to move courageously to take control of her life again.

Elaine is about 70% cured and I'm confident the treatment is working, as her energy is steadily improving. Elaine's illness was probably brewing for seven years before she came to me, and for about three years before all the symptoms started. Her newborn child's death seven years earlier may have triggered it all, producing a deep sadness and feeling of futility. The body follows these emotional clues and begins to weaken. Then as the person starts to get physically well, these old, buried issues start to come up again and must be dealt with as part of the healing process. It all comes down to what we say in alternative medicine: you have to treat the whole person of body, mind, and spirit. You cannot just treat the body or the spirit alone, because they're part of the same system.

## How Homeopathy Can Help Fibromyalgia

In a double-blind trial, 24 patients with fibromyalgia experienced "statistically significant" improvement after taking one of three homeopathic remedies indicated for their particular condition and individual make-up: *Arnica* (mountain daisy), for muscle fatigue, characterized by aches, pains, and exhaustion; *Bryonia* (wild hops), typically used in cases of arthritis and rheumatism; and *Rhus tox* (poison ivy), often the first remedy administered when there is stiffness and pain.[a] Another study confirmed these results.[b]

[a]*British Homeopathic Journal* 75:3 (1986), 142–147.
[b]*British Medical Journal* 299 (1989), 365–366.

## Healing the Emotions Using Flower Essences

Flower essences comprise subtle liquid preparations made from the fresh blossoms of flowers, plants, bushes, even trees, to address emotional, psychological, and spiritual issues underlying physical and medical problems. The approach was pioneered by British physician and renowned homeopath Edward Bach, M.B., B.S., M.R.C.S., L.R.C.P., D.H.P., in the 1930s, when he introduced the 38 Bach® Flower Remedies, based on English plants. Today, an estimated 20 different brands of flower remedies—based on plants native to many landscapes, from Australia to India to Alaska—offer about 1,500 different blends for a diverse range of psychological conditions.

Dr. Bach based his revolutionary belief upon his personal observations of patients whose physical illnesses seemed to be predisposed by negative psychological or emotional states, such as fear, anxiety, insecurity, jealousy, shyness, poor self-image, anger, and resentment. Today, numerous studies conducted at major universities and medical centers have verified Dr. Bach's early conviction, revealing a definite connection between negative emotional and mental states and a reduction of the body's natural resistance to disease.

The Bach Flower Remedies, renamed the Bach Flower Essences in

America, remain the most popular form of flower essences among alternative medical practitioners, having been proven effective for over 70 years. All flower essences are noninvasive and sold over the counter. They are taken orally or rubbed topically on pulse points along the body; because they are nontoxic, nonaddictive, and without side effects, they can be used without professional guidance. "The essences do not interact or interfere with medications or supplements and are totally complementary to other healing modalities," explains Alicia Sirkin, B.F.R.P., an internationally known Bach Foundation registered practitioner, educator, and expert on the Bach essences. "They even seem to make other modalities work better, a claim made by Dr. Bach himself and later confirmed by therapists in other fields."

In the following account, Sirkin relates how Bach Flower Essences were able to help one of her clients recover from fibromyalgia.

## Success Story:
## Fibromyalgia Relieved by Using Bach Flower Essences

Conventional medicine considers fibromyalgia incurable. When Juliana first came to see me, she had endured years of allopathic treatment with little relief from the almost constant pain of this chronic disease. On March 19, 1999, Juliana contacted me after hearing me speak on the radio. Her discomfort was more than she could handle, she told me, and she was willing to try anything that might help. As a Bach Flower Essence Practitioner, I told her that we gently deal with emotional imbalances, not physical ailments, but that I would try to help her use this complementary healing modality to bring emotional relief during her physical distress. Imagine our mutual delight, then, when after using the essences for only a couple of weeks, her physical symptoms began to disappear.

Juliana was 37 years old, a slim, attractive mother of five-year-old twins. But she had trouble enjoying family life because of constant pain and exhaustion. When she arrived at my office, she seemed pleasant and soft-spoken, yet somewhat anxious as she told me that she had had headaches all her life. She was also struggling with sleeplessness, depression, nervousness, panic attacks, and constant exhaustion, all while trying to raise her family and tend to her parents, who were also living in her household. Pain would wake her two to three times a night. She was taking St. John's wort for depression.

Along with her health, her personal freedom and family life were deteriorating. "I was really irritable with my mom and dad for anything, and with the kids," she said. "I would get really upset over anything." Ordinary daily activities like driving also caused her great distress and pain. "The tension from the headaches pulled my muscles so much that it was painful to stretch my arms or to turn my head. I would do an aerobics class and get a strong headache. Eventually I stopped exercising completely because I didn't even have the energy to go."

Juliana didn't know what was wrong with her. One doctor told her she had tension headaches; another, muscle spasms. Subjecting herself to many tests and treatments, Juliana still didn't get a clear answer, or a cure.

Her primary care physician prescribed a type of aspirin with codeine, then Valium®, but her pain returned. After three days on a higher dose, still in pain, she decided to stop taking the drug because it didn't seem to help. She was then referred to an orthopedic physician, who reported a narrowing of the spaces in the cervical spine. But an MRI came back negative for abnormalities. For pain relief and muscle spasms, the doctor performed an infiltration of the spine with pain medication and corticosteroids. Juliana didn't like taking the steroid shots because she knew it wasn't a cure.

Going from doctor to doctor to try to find a cure, with minimal results, Juliana said, "I felt afraid because I didn't know what was going on with me. I didn't know if the problems were from allergies, or age, or my hormone system. I thought it could be my thyroid or too much stress." When she went back to her primary care physician, he decided she was suffering from fibromyalgia.

I explained to Juliana that when positive states of mind are restored, the physical body responds—sometimes quite dramatically. Troublesome feelings such as fear, frustration, loss, anger, anxiety, sadness, depression, and hopelessness often chronically surround a physical illness and hamper healing—undermining the ability to feel in control of the outcome.

Bach Flower Essences are homeopathically prepared liquids. They work on an energetic level to gently release negative mental and emotional states, thereby strengthening our ability to cope. Additionally, it is not uncommon for clients to report unexpected relief from physical symptoms such as chronic pain, overweight, and nervous or addictive habits. As a Bach Flower Essence Practitioner, my first step was to help Juliana identify the states of mind contributing to her difficulties in life.

Bach Flower Essence therapy starts with a client/practitioner dialogue about the client's immediate interests and difficulties. The consultation dialogue process is essential to the correct choice of flowers, since each essence is specific to a particular mental or emotional state of imbalance.

Gentle to the psyche, the process has an inherent simplicity. It looks only at what is consciously experienced in the moment. Initial sessions often last an hour, with subsequent visits commonly being shorter.

Ongoing use of the Bach Flower Essences commonly results in what I call "peeling the layers of the onion." Layer by layer, as a client's state of mind becomes comfortable, hidden emotional traumas or unresolved issues from the past are gently revealed. Peace of mind is then restored with the appropriate flower essences. In this natural process, long-standing wounds can be healed at the client's pace.

In the course of one session, Juliana confided, "If something really bothers me from the past, I keep it inside. If I don't talk about it, I get the headaches and stress. I feel like it's reflected in my physical body." Quite often an individual cannot distinguish, or is not in touch with, specific out-of-balance emotions creating their distress. When this happens, I help clients clearly identify which unwanted emotions, attitudes, thoughts, and personality traits are hampering their happiness, success, inner peace, and joy of life.

As I guide our conversation, I carefully note clients' exact words and phrases, always looking for keywords that will secure indications for specific beneficial flower essences. Some clients feel that they need support for 15 to 20 different emotional states (with varying degrees of intensity) at the same time. When this happens, we begin a prioritization process, leaving out less urgent negative emotional states, to arrive at a combination formula of up to six or seven essences.

Each one of us acts and reacts to our ailments in a different way. We may withdraw, or become fearful, angry, or resentful. Or perhaps we may feel like a victim, or that we deserve our sickness. The way we react toward illness or difficult life challenges determines the flower essences we choose. For this reason, no two combination formulas are alike for the same illness. We consider the client's personality, rather than their disease. By listening closely, I have learned that each client, on some level, holds the key to his or her emotional imbalances.

In selecting Juliana's remedies, I asked her to describe the greatest challenges she was experiencing. As she discussed unwanted emotional states such as anxiety and depression, I asked, "Do you know why you are feeling like this?" Juliana explained anxiously that she was planning a vacation trip to visit relatives in South America. At this point, she was already very fragile and dreading the trip. This clearly pointed to the essence "Olive," the indication for which is great physical, mental, or emotional exhaustion.

Juliana also wasn't able to say "no" to her family regarding the trip. She perceived her parents as very strong-willed. Weak-willed in their presence, she had been unable to set boundaries and confront them when necessary to be true to herself and her own needs. After more questioning, I saw that she fit into the caregiver, nurturer personality type—gentle and overanxious to please others. To restore strength to this personality type and help empower her identity, the essence "Centaury" was strongly indicated.

Juliana said she is usually very nervous about the safety and well-being of her family members. It had been a persistent problem. Here, the essence "Red Chestnut" was indicated, chosen to release the fear that something terrible could happen to loved ones when one imagines the worst-case scenario.

As there was a whole constellation of fears, we reviewed the other fear essences. Juliana told me she has panic attacks when she travels. She always thinks she's in danger without being able to identify the cause. "Aspen" can be used for sudden panic attacks of unknown origin. To calm her feelings of terror and panic, "Rock Rose" was indicated to help restore courage and a balanced state of mind. "Mimulus," for restoring courage when there are known fears, was also considered.

In addition, there was a pattern of chronic overstriving for perfection, which contributed greatly to her nervousness. If she planned a trip, it had to be "perfect." I could see she was putting a lot of pressure on herself to perform. After my inquiry, she agreed that she is also very strict with herself in her daily routines. "Rock Water" was chosen for her perfectionism, strict self-discipline, and the tension this can create. "Pine" was also considered because she blamed herself when she didn't achieve her goals.

Juliana said she recently felt depressed due to a setback in her health ("Gentian"). She is impatient ("Impatiens" restores patience) and is occasionally afraid she'll lose control of her mind ("Cherry Plum" reestablishes sanity and control of the mind).

Another major complaint was having too many thoughts racing around in her head, which often resulted in sleeplessness ("White Chestnut" quiets the mind). When asked what kinds of persistent thoughts she had, she said, "I always think about the past." ("Honeysuckle" puts the past in perspective, releasing emotional triggers and bringing one's focus back to the present.) To help Juliana change the pattern of her recurrent symptoms, "Chestnut Bud" was considered to help her learn from her experiences and not repeat mistakes.

Additionally, since childhood, Juliana had been plagued by indecision, vacillating between choices, resulting in confusion ("Scleranthus" to help make quick decisions with clarity). The combination formula Rescue Remedy was also indicated, due to Juliana's major stresses.

From the 16 single flower essences that were considered, we prioritized seven. We agreed that the most important problems for her to address at the moment would be helped by Centaury, Honeysuckle, White Chestnut, Red Chestnut, Scleranthus, Chestnut Bud, and Rescue Remedy, which is a special combination formula of five essences indicated for any kind of trauma, available as a single remedy. Rescue Remedy counts as one essence when combining as many as six or seven essences in a one-ounce treatment bottle for a personal formula.

Juliana was faithful to the dosage requirements and her response was quick. In two and a half weeks, when we next spoke, she had almost finished this formula. Little by little the headaches were going away, she felt calm and relaxed, and although she had a little bit of discomfort in the neck, she slept better. This was major progress. She said she hadn't felt the need to return to her physician.

Later, when recounting her experience, she told me, "When I first saw you I wasn't going to the gym at all, but I really wanted to work out. I wasn't sure if the drops were working. The first time I started working out again, I got such a strong headache that I was afraid that I might faint and crash while driving home. I called my husband for help, but I did make it home. Upon arriving home I put four drops of the formula under my tongue and the headache started to go away in about 15 seconds. By the time my husband arrived 20 minutes later, the headache was gone. That was the first time I realized that the drops worked on me. It was amazing! I felt so wonderful. I held that bottle like a baby. Then I started to take the drops four times a day every day. My husband, who had been skeptical, said, 'If it's really working, don't stop.'"

Juliana followed a fairly typical process when, in a later session, she said, "It gave me hope. Something inside told me that it would work for me. From the first day, I felt different, but I wasn't sure. As the days passed I felt better. But then when that day came at the gym, I knew they were working."

Juliana did take the trip to South America. She said, "I used to take Valium because I was scared to go on the plane. So I took the Rescue Remedy and I felt really relaxed. I wasn't afraid."

After three months of treatment, Juliana's life had radically changed. She reported feeling 80% better and began taking a yoga class. She said her headaches and the stiff neck were gone. She was no longer taking any painkillers or anti-depressants. She was thrilled to be gaining freedom from her pain. In the past, Juliana used tranquilizers to help her sleep. Now, without medication, she reported sleeping better and feeling energetic upon awakening.

While Juliana was taking the essences, she did not institute any new form of therapy or medication. After three months, she said, "I started to take vitamins and do yoga. I prayed every day. I watch what I eat. I try to avoid things that can give me discomfort or tension and avoid arguments. Or if I feel like I'm going to be in a situation that will turn into an argument, I'll take my drops."

After four months on Bach Flower Essence therapy, Juliana reported doing shoulder stands in yoga class, walking with intermittent jogging three times a week, and sleeping through the whole night without pain. She stopped taking St. John's wort. Her tiredness, dizziness, impatience, and depression are gone.

During our fifth consultation session, Juliana also recognized the need to improve her ability to relate in a harmonious way to her family. Due to her excellent progress, three of the original essences were no longer needed, which made room to add three new ones—a classic example of the "peeling" effect.

Now Juliana reports new confidence. "I don't have any problem with my parents," she says. "I care about them, but I don't worry. I feel more harmony, more closeness."

Juliana continues to make improvement. Her fearful state is greatly minimized. Her panic attacks are a thing of the past, and she now has energy to do the things she enjoys. "Now I take my life more easily," she reports. "I think more about it. I don't worry too much. I don't know how to explain it but I'm happier. A lot more joy. And I'm not afraid—and I was afraid of everything. Now I feel that life is life. No matter what comes, we have to take things easy and not worry about it, to just enjoy life. I'm happier."

The **Dr. Edward Bach Centre** in England provides information and referrals to registered practitioners. Mailing address: Mount Vernon, Bakers Lane, Sotwell, Oxon, OX10 0PZ, UK. Tel: +44 (0) 1491 834678; fax: +44 (0) 1491 825022. E-Mail: mail@bach-centre.com; Website: www.bachcentre.com. Bach Flower Essences are trademarks of Bach Flower Remedies Ltd., Oxfordshire, England. **Alicia Sirkin** is one of only 40 Bach Foundation Registered Practitioners (B.F.R.P.) in the United States. Mailing address: P.O. Box 33-0841, Miami, FL 33233-0841; tel: (888) 875-6753; e-mail alicia@flowerhealing.com. Website: www.flowerhealing.com.

# twelve

# Treating Chronic Fatigue with Herbs

Herbal medicine can be of great assistance in the treatment of chronic fatigue syndrome. Herbs can help strengthen weakened body systems and relieve symptoms, ranging from uncomfortable to debilitating, produced by this weakness. Herbs are a practical and desirable therapy because they provide their benefits without the side effects so frequently experienced with conventional drugs. Each herb has one or more specific healing properties, an advantage enabling the skilled herbalist to design a treatment program targeting specific ailments or imbalances. For example, ginseng is useful in chronic fatigue because it is both an adaptogenic herb, meaning it increases resistance to stress by supporting the adrenal glands, and a tonic, meaning it builds overall vital energy by nurturing and enlivening the entire system.

Although there are no universal remedies, particularly for a complex condition such as chronic fatigue, there are a number of herbs that have proven useful for the syndrome. Many alternative medicine physicians have developed herbal protocols that have been effective for their CFS patients. For example, Susan M. Lark, M.D., author of *The Chronic Fatigue Self Help Book*, recommends ginkgo, Siberian ginseng, oatstraw, ginger, licorice, and dandelion root to improve energy levels and combat depression in CFS sufferers. Those who have the accompanying symptoms of anxiety and insomnia should look into passionflower, chamomile, hops, and valerian root, she says. To support a faltering

304

> Using herbal medicines as the primary therapeutic modality, Dr. van Benschoten sees a response in 85% to 90% of his patients. "The time necessary to completely resolve the situation can vary from as short as 4 to 6 weeks to as long as 12 to 18 months," he reports.

immune system—always a factor in chronic fatigue sufferers—Dr. Lark relies on garlic, echinacea, and goldenseal.[1] However, before starting any program, you should consult a qualified herbalist to ensure that the herbs you take meet your individual needs.

As another example, Matt van Benschoten, O.M.D., M.A., C.A., of Reseda, California, uses herbal medicine to treat the viral infections and immune suppression found in CFS patients. "The initial therapy has to be focused on antiviral measures," he says. "Once that's accomplished and the virus is well eliminated, you can begin to address some of the secondary factors that cause the weakness in the immune system, such as stress-induced weakness, problems in the intestinal tract, heavy metal poisoning (such as dental mercury), and low-level pesticide poisoning." Prescriptions are individualized for each patient, he says.

Using herbal medicines as the primary therapeutic modality, Dr. van Benschoten sees a response in 85% to 90% of his patients. "The time necessary to completely resolve the situation can vary from as short as four to six

## Herbs That Can Help Chronic Fatigue

- **Immune-Building:** astragalus, echinacea, garlic, ginger, ginkgo, ginseng, goldenseal, nettle
- **Adrenal Support:** ginseng, licorice
- **Antimicrobial:** astragalus, echinacea, garlic, ginger, goldenseal, licorice, St. John's wort
- **Fatigue:** ginseng, oatstraw
- **Brain Function:** ginkgo, ginseng
- **Sleep Disorders:** chamomile, hops, passionflower, St. John's wort, valerian
- **Joint and Muscle Pain:** cayenne, chamomile, nettle, peppermint, valerian
- **Allergies:** chamomile, ephedra, milk thistle
- **Digestive Disorders:** astragalus, cayenne, chamomile, dandelion, ginger, goldenseal, licorice, peppermint
- **Anxiety:** chamomile, hops, kava-kava, passionflower, valerian
- **Depression:** oatstraw, St. John's wort

weeks to as long as 12 to 18 months," he says, "depending upon the duration of the illness and other accompanying health problems."

## Success Story:
## Cayenne Contributes to Fibromyalgia Relief

The following case highlights how herbs (in this case, cayenne) can occupy a central role in the treatment program for fibromyalgia.

Henrietta, 42, had consulted seven doctors over a two-year period before receiving the correct diagnosis—post-traumatic fibromyalgia—and successful treatment by chiropractor Dennis Zinner, D.C., of San Francisco, California. The stress of those two years "amplified her syndrome," Dr. Zinner says. In addition to constant pain and lack of proper sleep, that time was made more difficult by "the missed diagnosis, the stress of facing a work layoff, and the worry that other people think your symptoms are all mind-derived."

In Dr. Zinner's assessment, Henrietta's post-traumatic fibromyalgia resulted from a work-related injury to her left shoulder at age 40, with subsequent lower back pain. When she was 15, Henrietta sustained two bone fractures in her lower back from a car accident; at age 34, her family physician diagnosed osteoarthritis in her lower back; at 41, she sprained her wrist, and at 42, she had surgery for breast cancer.

At the time she began treatment with Dr. Zinner, Henrietta complained of left shoulder pain, neck pain leading to severe headaches, constant severe pain in her lower back, hips, and feet, ankle swelling, and general physical impairment affecting sitting, walking, and job performance. In addition, she had generalized fatigue, morning stiffness, depressive episodes, irritable bowel syndrome, and nonrestful sleep. Henrietta had discomfort in all 18 of the tender point sites common to fibromyalgia, and her conditions worsened under stress. "With new studies, we are discovering that fibromyalgia is a neuromuscular problem in which, for reasons we do not yet know, the muscles stay in contraction and do not relax," explains Dr. Zinner.

The first step in Dr. Zinner's treatment plan for Henrietta was to apply a microcurrent probe at each of the 18 tender point sites on her body, three times weekly. Second, he applied deep heat (for 15 minutes) to Henrietta's two most painful sites to decrease muscle spasm. At home, Henrietta repeated the procedure using a moist heating pad. Third, Dr. Zinner instructed Henrietta to massage capsaicin cream into her sore points four times daily. Capsaicin is a pungent alkaloid of cayenne pepper that has a warming effect on the body. Fourth, for her sleeping disorders, Dr. Zinner prescribed the hormone melatonin (6 mg, taken 30 minutes before bedtime). He also made chiropractic adjustments, as needed, to areas related to the location of the 18 tender spots. Dr. Zinner further advised Henrietta to do regular aerobic exercise followed by heat treatment such as a whirlpool.

Dr. Zinner notes that the use of capsaicin has two benefits. First, it dissolves the sensation of pain. Second, capsaicin usefully depletes bodily reserves of substance P (SEE QUICK DEFINITION), believed to be overabundant in patients with fibromyalgia. Substance P intensifies and perhaps prolongs muscle inflammation and pain. In other words, too much Substance P may be a factor that prevents fibromyalgia from going away. Research has shown that capsaicin can be effective in the treatment of fibromyalgia. The Medical College of Wisconsin in Milwaukee treated 45 people suffering from primary fibromyalgia with capsaicin (0.025%) cream for four weeks. The patients reported less tenderness in the spots treated and a significant increase in their grip strength.[2]

**Substance P** is a naturally occurring polypeptide (several amino acids bonded together) that is normally present in small amounts in the nervous system and intestines. It stimulates the expansion and contraction of smooth muscles, both in the intestines and elsewhere. It is also involved in the secretion of saliva and the functioning of the peripheral and central nervous system, notably for the role it plays in the pain response.

Substance P is released in response to injuries to tissues and muscles, and is overabundant in patients with fibromyalgia and chronic muscle pain. This overabundance stimulates the release of histamine, causing tissue swelling and inflammation, smooth muscle contraction, and pain transmission. Substance P also suppresses serotonin, a neurotransmitter that conducts nerve "messages." Under healthy conditions, serotonin inhibits the overabundance of Substance P, thus providing relief from chronic muscle pain.

**Dennis Zinner, D.C.:** 2320 Sutter Street, San Francisco, CA 94115; (415) 885-5563.

After six months of regular therapy, Henrietta reported a change in her pain from "constant severe" to "constant slight to moderate" with only occasional severe episodes. Her improvement continued under Dr. Zinner's fourfold program. "Henrietta's outcome was good. She is back to living her life," says Dr. Zinner. "She has returned to school full-time to get a degree in child development and she works part-time at the school. She sees me every three months for a treatment but she is managing her infrequent episodes of pain."[3]

# Glossary of Herbs That Can Help Ease Chronic Fatigue Syndrome

The following are some of the many herbs that can help alleviate the numerous symptoms of chronic fatigue, such as extreme debilitating fatigue, joint and muscle pain, memory problems and poor concentration, depression, anxiety, allergies, gastrointestinal complaints, and sleep disorders. Antimicrobial herbs (antivirals, antifungals, and antibiotics) and herbs that strengthen the immune system, provide adrenal support, or aid the liver in its toxin-filtering function are also described.

## Astragalus (Astragalus membranaceus)

A medicinal staple in Chinese medicine, astragalus is an energy tonic known for its healing abilities in chronic conditions in which weakness is a major factor. It exerts a potent influence on the immune system, increasing the production of white blood cells (important immune "workers"). It also aids the immune system by acting as an antiviral and antibacterial agent.[4] In addition, it facilitates digestion. Its system-wide strengthening abilities have led many alternative medicine physicians to include astragalus in their herbal protocol for CFS.

## Cayenne (Capsicum annuum)

Cayenne or red pepper is an effective systemic stimulant, meaning it invigorates the physiological activities of the body. It is especially helpful for the circulatory and digestive systems, stimulating blood flow and strengthening the heartbeat and metabolic rate.[5] It is used to treat insufficient peripheral circulation, characterized by cold hands and feet, frequently a symptom of CFS. It also helps ward off colds.[6] Externally, it is used for muscle and joint pain.[7]

Chamomile

## Chamomile (German or wild, Matricaria recutita; Roman, Anthemis nobilis)

The flower of the chamomile plant produces a calming effect, easing anxiety and reducing tension.[8] It can thus be helpful with overall anxiety, sleep disorders, and muscle tension. Its calming property has a beneficial effect on the gastrointestinal system as well. In addition, it stimulates digestive secretions, so it can improve digestive function. In Europe, chamomile is recognized as a digestive aid, a mild sedative, and an anti-inflammatory, notably in antibacterial oral hygiene and skin preparations.[9] Its anti-inflammatory properties also reduce allergic response. In Germany, chamomile is licensed as an over-the-counter drug for internal use against gastrointestinal spasms and inflammatory diseases of the gastrointestinal tract.

## Dandelion (Taraxacum officinale)

As both a liver and digestive tonic, as well as a blood cleanser and diuretic (urine-increasing agent), dandelion can aid in detoxification of the body.[10] The liver is a filter for toxins and, as such, serves as one of the body's main detoxification mechanisms. As testimony to dandelion's powerful influence on the liver, severe hepatitis has been reversed by dandelion tea along with dietary restrictions in as short a period as a week.[11]

Chemical or heavy metal toxicity is frequently involved in chronic fatigue syndrome; dandelion can help cleanse the body of these toxins and support the liver in its toxin-eliminating function. As a digestive tonic, dandelion may also help clear up the gastrointestinal complaints associated with CFS.

## Echinacea (Echinacea angustifolia)

Often called purple coneflower, echinacea refers to several species of plants that are generally found in the Great Plains region of North America, where it was the most widely used medicinal plant of the Native Americans in that area. They used echinacea for its external wound-healing and anti-inflammatory properties. Echinacea is widely used in Europe and becoming more well known in the United States for its immune-stimulating properties; most popularly, for its ability to help relieve flu and the common cold.

Echinacea

Over 180 over-the-counter echinacea products are marketed in Germany alone, including extracts and fresh-squeezed juices from both the roots and leaves of echinacea.[12] The German government has approved oral dosage of echinacea for use in recurrent infections of the respiratory and urinary tracts, progressive systemic disorders such as tuberculosis, leukosis (abnormal growth of white blood cells), connective tissue disease, multiple sclerosis, and, when applied topically, for surface wounds with a poor tendency to heal. Liquid echinacea preparations have been shown to have immune-stimulating properties when administered both orally and parenterally (denoting any medication route other than the intestine, e.g., intravenously).

Specifically, echinacea increases the number of leukocytes (white

Due to its widely demonstrated immune-enhancing qualities, echinacea is a standard ingredient in many doctors' herbal regimens for CFS. Combining equal parts of tinctures of echinacea, goldenseal, and myrrh results in an even more powerful immune booster.

blood cells) and splenocytes (white blood cells of the spleen) and enhances the activity of granulocytes (granular white blood cells) and phagocytes (cells that have the ability to ingest and destroy substances such as bacteria, protozoa, and cell debris).[13]

Due to its widely demonstrated immune-enhancing qualities, echinacea is a standard ingredient in many doctors' herbal regimens for CFS. Combining equal parts of tinctures of echinacea, goldenseal, and myrrh results in an even more powerful immune booster. The recommended dosage is one teaspoonful of this blend three times a day.

### Ephedra or Ma-huang (Ephedra sinica)

Ephedra, also known as *ma-huang*, is a medicinal plant that has been cultivated for over 5,000 years in China, where it was used for asthma and hay fever–like conditions. The stems of the plant contain two primary alkaloids, ephedrine and pseudoephedrine, which are primary ingredients in conventional over-the-counter decongestant and bronchial drugs. Ephedrine has a marked peripheral vasoconstricting (causing constriction of the blood vessels) action. Pseudoephedrine is a bronchodilator (able to dilate the bronchial air passages), approved for use in asthma and certain allergy medicines.

*Ma-huang* and its extracts are found in a number of herbal formulas that are designed to increase energy and reduce appetite. Both ephedrine and pseudoephedrine have properties that stimulate the central nervous system (CNS), ephedrine being more active. The CNS activity of these alkaloids has been characterized as being stronger than caffeine and weaker than methamphetamine (a

**CAUTION** In December 2003, the FDA announced a national ban on the herbal dietary supplement ephedra, used as an adrenaline-like stimulant for weight loss. Ephedra as administered by practitioners of traditional Chinese medicine will be exempted from the ban, as it has been used safely for over 5,000 years to treat allergies and respiratory conditions. CFS sufferers should consult a qualified practitioner before taking ephedra and it should be used with caution or avoided by those with high blood pressure, diabetes, glaucoma, and related conditions for which hypertensives are contraindicated.

central nervous system stimulant). Ephedra can be useful in the treatment of CFS for both its antiallergy and its energy-stimulating abilities.

## Garlic *(Allium sativum)*

Garlic is probably the most well-recognized medicinal herb. It is used in traditional medical practices all over the world and its applications are as varied as its geographical distribution. The chemistry and pharmacology of garlic is well studied; over 1,000 research papers have been published in the past 25 years.

Garlic and its preparations are known for their antibiotic, antifungal, and antiviral activity; for use in clearing congested lungs and for coughs, bronchitis, and sinus congestion; as a preventive measure for flus and the common cold; and for intestinal worms, dysentery, certain ulcers, gout, and rheumatism.[14] Garlic has shown an ability to aid certain immune functions, particularly for increasing natural killer cell (SEE QUICK DEFINITION) activity.[15] Studies indicate general benefits from almost any form of garlic, be it raw garlic, dried garlic, garlic oil, or a prepared commercial product.[16]

 **Natural killer (NK) cells** are a type of nonspecific, free-ranging immune cells produced in the bone marrow and matured in the thymus gland. NK cells can recognize and quickly destroy viral and cancer cells on first contact. "Armed" with an estimated 100 different biochemicals for killing foreign proteins, NK cells can kill target cells without having previously encountered them. As with antibodies, their role is one of surveillance, to rid the body of aberrant or foreign cells before they can grow and produce cancer or infection.

## Ginger *(Zingiber officinalis)*

In addition to its popular food-flavoring qualities, ginger is widely used as a medicinal herb in traditional Chinese and Ayurvedic medicines; it is often added to herbal formulas to increase digestion and the activity of other herbs. Ginger helps combat respiratory infections, improves circulation, aids the body in releasing toxins by promoting sweating, and

Garlic, Ginger, Ginkgo

> Ginkgo is an antioxidant and also improves blood circulation, particularly to the brain.[17] Ginkgo is known for its ability to improve cognitive function by increasing capillary circulation and thus facilitating greater oxygen flow to brain cells.

eases intestinal complaints. All of these functions are useful in the treatment of CFS.

### Ginkgo (Ginkgo biloba)

The ginkgo is the oldest living species of tree on earth. Its leaves contain compounds called ginkgolides, which are the biochemical substances responsible for ginkgo extract's healing properties. Ginkgo is an antioxidant and also improves blood circulation, particularly to the brain.[17] Ginkgo is known for its ability to improve cognitive function by increasing capillary circulation and thus facilitating greater oxygen flow to brain cells. In Germany, it is licensed for the treatment of cerebral dysfunction, including the following symptoms: difficulty in memory, dizziness, tinnitus, headaches, and emotional instability coupled with anxiety.

At least three volumes of technical papers on the chemistry, pharmacology, and clinical studies of *Ginkgo biloba* extract have been published.[18] In a 1995 study, Alzheimer's patients received either 80 mg of ginkgo extract or a placebo three times daily. Among the patients taking ginkgo, significant improvement in cognitive function was noticed. Memory and attention span increased in the first month of supplementation. Another study of ginkgo, involving people over the age of 50, showed that 40 mg taken three times daily for 12 weeks significantly improved overall cognitive function in individuals with mild to moderate memory impairment.[19]

Ginseng

### Ginseng

Ginseng has an ancient history and as such has generated much folklore about its actions and uses. Common varieties are Oriental ginseng (*Panax ginseng*) and American ginseng (*Panax quinquefolius*). The genus name *Panax* is derived from the Latin word *panacea*, meaning "cure all." Many of the claims that surround ginseng are exaggerated, but it is clearly an important remedy, receiving attention from researchers around the world.[20] Ginseng has many healing properties that are useful in the treatment of CFS.

One of the oldest general tonics from traditional Chinese medicine, ginseng sharpens mental abilities, concentration, and alertness, improves stamina, and delays the onset of fatigue after physical exercise.[21] It is a powerful adaptogen[22] (SEE QUICK DEFINITION), aiding the body to cope with stress, primarily through effects upon the functioning of the adrenal glands.[23] Ginseng has antioxidant,[24] antihepatotoxic (liver-protecting),[25] and hypoglycemic[26] effects.

Ginseng's main application is with weak, debilitated, stressed, or elderly people, for whom its therapeutic properties can be especially helpful.[27] In addition, ginseng may lower blood cholesterol[28] and stimulate a range of immune system[29] and endocrine responses.[30] If ginseng is abused, however, serious side effects can occur, including headaches, skin problems, and other reactions. For this reason, the proper dosage for the individual should be determined and respected.

Another variety of ginseng—Siberian ginseng or eleuthero (*Eleutherococcus senticosus*)—has a very low toxicity.

 **Adaptogens** are substances that provide a nonspecific effect on the entire body by increasing resistance to stress and toxins (physical, chemical, or biological) and promoting a balancing or normalizing condition. The key function of adaptogens is support for the adrenal glands, which are located near the kidneys and activated in response to stress. Chronic stress can overwhelm the adrenals, leading to symptoms including fatigue, reduced immune function, and poor blood sugar metabolism. Adaptogens help reinvigorate and support the adrenals, enabling the body to deal more effectively with stress. In addition to adrenal support, adaptogens enhance central nervous system activity, provide protection for the liver, act as antioxidants, and increase stamina.

Copious clinical and laboratory research has been conducted on Siberian ginseng in the former Soviet Union. Initial findings from controlled experiments indicate that Siberian ginseng produces a dramatic reduction of total disease occurrence, especially in diseases related to environmental stress.[31] There is a long list of illnesses that improve with the use of this herb, including chronic fatigue, chronic gastritis, diabetes, and atherosclerosis (hardening of the arteries).

### Goldenseal *(Hydrastis canadensis)*

One of the most widely used American herbs, goldenseal is considered to be a tonic remedy that stimulates immune response and is itself directly antimicrobial. In addition, because of its bitter effects, goldenseal can help in many digestive problems, from peptic ulcers to colitis.[32] Its bit-

Goldenseal, Hops, Licorice, Milk Thistle

ter stimulation helps in loss of appetite, and the alkaloids it contains promote production and secretion of digestive juices.

Goldenseal's antimicrobial properties are due to berberine.[33] This alkaloid, found in a number of other herbs as well, has marked antimicrobial activity. Its inhibiting effects have been demonstrated against bacteria, protozoa, and fungi, including *Staphylococcus*, *Streptococcus*, *Candida albicans*, and *Giardia lamblia*,[34] which are often implicated in CFS. Berberine has also been shown to activate macrophages (cells that digest cell debris and other waste matter in the blood).[35]

### Hops *(Humulus lupulus)*

Hops has been used as a bittering and preservative agent in brewing for centuries. In Germany, hops is licensed for use in states of unrest and anxiety as well as for sleep disorders, due to its calming and sleep-inducing properties. European medicinal plant researchers have approved the use of hops for such conditions as nervous tension, excitability, restlessness, and sleep disturbances, and as an aid to stimulate appetite. Unlike other types of sedatives, there are neither dependence nor withdrawal symptoms reported with the use of hops, nor are there any reports of adverse side effects.[36]

### Kava-Kava *(Piper methysticum)*

An extract of the kava-kava plant (a slow-growing bushy perennial) acts as a natural tranquilizer. According to E. Lehmann, M.D., and colleagues, when 29 patients with diagnosed anxiety (including panic disorder and general tension) took kava-kava at the rate of 100 mg three times daily for four weeks, and were then evaluated using three standard psychological profiles of anxiety, all measures were significantly lower. No side effects or adverse reactions occurred, and benefits were noted as early as the first and second weeks.[37]

In another study of 101 people, 100 mg of kava-kava extract taken

> In a study of 101 people, 100 mg of kava-kava extract taken three times daily produced significant improvement in anxiety and tension. The effects were noted from the eighth week of supplementation.

three times daily produced significant improvement in anxiety and tension of nonpsychotic origin. The effects were noted from the eighth week of supplementation. Specifically, 20% of those taking kava-kava were rated "very much improved" according to a standard anxiety scale, while only 10.5% of the placebo group received a similar rating. After 24 weeks of taking the herbal extract, the percentages were 53.1% of the kava group and 30.2% of those taking a placebo.[38]

## Licorice *(Glycyrrhiza glabra)*

Licorice is another traditional herbal remedy with an ancient history. Modern research has shown it to have beneficial effects on the endocrine system, adrenal glands, and liver. It is also a systemic anti-inflammatory.[39] Constituents of this herb, called triterpenes, are metabolized in the body into molecules that have a similar structure to the adrenal cortex hormones, which is possibly the basis for licorice's anti-inflammatory action and its effectiveness in cases of adrenal insufficiency.[40]

As overworked adrenal glands are characteristic of CFS, licorice has obvious application. In addition, glycyrrhizin, one of the triterpenes, inhibits liver cell injury from chemicals, another benefit for CFS sufferers.[41] Glycyrrhizin prevents the growth of several viruses, inactivating herpes simplex virus particles irreversibly.[42] Licorice is used as a treatment for digestive problems such as gastritis, peptic ulceration, and abdominal colic. It is also effective for bronchitis, coughs, and other bronchial problems.

The *Quarterly Review of Natural Medicine* cited a case report of successfully treating chronic fatigue syndrome with licorice dissolved in milk (2.5 gm per 500 ml daily). The logic behind using licorice for CFS is sound, accord-

 There is a small possibility of affecting electrolyte balance with extended use of large doses of licorice. It can cause retention of sodium, thus raising blood pressure. The whole herb has constituents that counter this, but it is best to avoid licorice in cases of hypertension or kidney disease, or during pregnancy. It is important to clarify here that the kind of licorice effective in CFS patients is licorice root, which contains glycyrrhizic and glycyrrhetinic acids, not the deglycyrrhizinated form of licorice from which these acids have been removed.

ing to the article. Glucocorticoid levels are often low in CFS patients and licorice can reverse this deficiency. The authors of the article recommend following up initial licorice treatment with Oriental ginseng and eleuthero as long-term adrenal support.[43]

### Milk Thistle (Silybum marianum)

Historically this herb has been used in Europe as a liver tonic. In addition, it is an antihistamine and an anti-inflammatory, and therefore inhibits allergic response. A wealth of laboratory and clinical research on this herb is revealing exciting data about reversal of toxic liver damage, as well as protection from potential hepatotoxic agents such as chemicals.[44] These properties are of use in the case of CFS for improvement of liver function, to help the body deal with toxic overload, and to ease the allergies which usually accompany the syndrome.

Nettle

### Nettle (Urtica dioica)

Nettle is one of the most widely used herbs in the Western world. Throughout Europe it is employed as a general tonic and detoxifying remedy. It is both a circulatory and immune stimulant. A lectin (plant protein) found in the plant's leaf promotes lymphocyte production.[45] Traditional use of nettle in the treatment of allergic rhinitis (hayfever) is gaining research support.[46] Fresh nettle has been used as a safe diuretic (urine-increasing agent), and thus is helpful in assisting the body in flushing toxins.[47] Again, all of these healing abilities have application to CFS.

### Noni (Morinda citrifolia)

Among the lay healers of Tahiti, the reputation of the noni fruit as a medicinal food ranks high. The plant itself is found throughout French Polynesia and can grow as high as 20 feet, bearing noni fruits the size of potatoes. In Malaysia, it is known as mengkudu and is used for urinary problems, coughs, and painful menstruation, while in the Caribbean, people know it as the Pain Killer Tree. People throughout the region have long used the noni fruit as a dietary staple.

Anecdotal reports suggest that juice from this fruit can be significantly helpful in numerous health conditions, such as chronic fatigue syndrome, hypertension, wounds and infections, ulcers, skin rashes, digestive disorders, PMS, colds, influenza, arthritis, and cancer. Mitchell Tate, director of the Center for Lifestyle Disease in St. George, Utah, reports using noni to prevent sore throats and bacterial infections after his family was exposed to strep infection. Tate further reports that while researching noni at the University of Honolulu in Hawaii (noni also grows in Hawaii), he found that "a significant amount of research had been done on the plant and that most of it substantiated claims by the Tahitians."

Noni

One laboratory study showed that noni was effective as an antiseptic against nine types of infectious bacteria. As bacterial infection can be an underlying factor in CFS, this finding has obvious implications for CFS treatment. However, the application of Tahitian noni to CFS is more wide-reaching. According to a testimonial published in the *Health News*, Colleen Abbott, 55, had suffered with chronic fatigue syndrome for 20 years. A variety of nutritional supplements had improved her symptoms but not eliminated them. A recent accident injured her back, leaving her in pain, almost immobile, and on painkillers. Colleen reports that after taking noni for three days, she was able to "get up, walk, and climb stairs without crawling." Her sleep improved, her pain and most of her CFS symptoms went away, and instead of needing chiropractic adjustments twice daily, she had them only once a month.

"The mechanism by which noni juice accomplishes these dramatic results may be that it acts indirectly by enhancing the immune system involving macrophages and/or lymphocytes," according to researcher A. Hirazumi, Ph.D.[48] Studies by R. M. Heinicke, Ph.D., at the University of Hawaii, suggest that the active ingredient in noni is xeronine, a digestive enzyme similar to bromelain in pineapple. Dr. Heinicke emphasizes that noni must be consumed on an empty stomach, preferably upon rising in the morning, for the enzyme to become activated by the intestines. Dr. Heinicke believes that, once activated, xeronine helps to repair damaged cells by regulating the rigidity and shape of particular proteins comprising those cells. "Since these proteins

For more information about **noni**, contact: American Nutraceuticals, 1920 Northgate Boulevard, Suite A5, Sarasota, FL 34234; tel: (941) 351-9334.

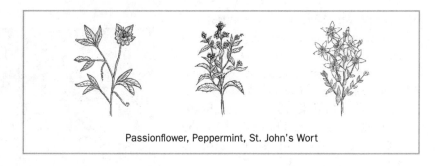

Passionflower, Peppermint, St. John's Wort

have different functions within the cells, this explains how the administration of noni juice causes a wide range of physiological responses," states Dr. Heinicke.

### Oatstraw, Oats (Avena sativa)

Traditionally, oatstraw has been used to help patients recover from exhaustion and depression, and it has been widely recognized as an excellent nerve tonic. Oatstraw (which is the whole oat plant including the ripe grain) contains saponins and alkaloids that stimulate and restore the nervous system. Oatstraw is also capable of providing key nutrients, including calcium, that feed a compromised nervous system. Oatstraw is sold dried and as capsules, concentrated drops, tinctures, and extracts.[49]

### Passionflower (Passiflora incarnata)

Passionflower has enjoyed a tradition of use for its mildly sedative properties. In Germany, passionflower is approved as an over-the-counter drug for states of "nervous unrest."[50] It is often added to other calming herbs, usually valerian and hawthorn. Passionflower and hawthorn are often used together as antispasmodics for digestive spasms in cases of gastritis and colitis. It also increases circulation to the peripheries[51] and can therefore be helpful with the CFS symptom of cold hands and feet. Pharmacological studies attest to the antispasmodic, sedative, anxiety-allaying, and hypotensive (blood pressure–lowering) activity of passionflower extracts.[52] For the anxiety and digestive problems associated with CFS, this can be an effective herb.

### Peppermint (Mentha piperita)

Peppermint has been a popular folk remedy for digestive disorders for over 200 years and is currently one of the most economically significant aromatic food/medicine crops produced in the United States.[53] Its ben-

> In 23 separate clinical trials involving 1,757 patients with depression, taking between 500 and 900 mg daily of St. John's wort extract was three times more effective than a placebo and as effective as standard antidepressants such as Prozac and Zoloft.

efits to digestive problems come from peppermint oil's relaxing effect on the smooth muscles of the bowel. It can aid in conditions from gastrointestinal cramps to irritable bowel syndrome. Peppermint oil and menthol are common ingredients in over-the-counter external pain-relieving balms and liniments. In Germany, this combination is approved for external use for muscle and nerve pain.[54]

### St. John's Wort (Hypericum perforatum)

A remedy long used as an anti-inflammatory, wound healer, mild sedative, and pain reliever, St. John's wort has recently attracted medical attention. Traditionally used to treat neuralgia, anxiety, tension, and similar problems, it is now increasingly being recommended in the treatment of depression.[55] Recent research has also suggested an antimicrobial role for this herb in viral infections from influenza to HIV.[56]

In Germany, St. John's wort is widely prescribed for depression. Research supports this application: in 23 separate clinical trials involving 1,757 patients who reported mild to moderately severe depression, taking between 500 and 900 mg daily of St. John's wort extract (containing 0.75% to 2.7% hypericin, the active component of the herb) was three times more effective than a placebo and as effective as standard antidepressants such as Prozac and Zoloft®. In addition, St. John's wort produced mild side effects in only 19% of users compared to 52.8% of those taking the conventional medications who experienced mild to severe side effects. The herb produced no toxic reactions or unfavorable interactions with other drugs. The researchers noted that it generally takes two to four weeks of steady use before the mood-elevating benefits of St. John's wort take effect.[57]

Christopher Hobbs, L.Ac., founder of the American School of Herbalism, has found St. John's wort useful in sleep disorders as well. He credits this to the same action behind the herb's antidepressant properties; that is, it maintains serotonin levels in the brain. Serotonin is a neurotransmitter (essential brain chemical) that influences mood and helps produce sleep. Dr. Hobbs also suggests adrenal-supporting herbs because compromised adrenal glands result in hormonal imbalances that can disturb sleep.[58] (See previous descriptions for ginseng and licorice.)

Valerian

### Valerian (Valeriana officinalis)

The odorous root of valerian has been used in European traditional medicine as a natural tranquillizer for centuries. In Germany, valerian root and its teas and extracts are approved as over-the-counter medicines for "states of excitation" and "difficulty in falling asleep owing to nervousness."[59] A scientific team representing the European community has reviewed the scientific research on valerian and concluded that it is a safe nighttime sleep aid. These scientists also found that there are no major adverse reactions associated with the use of valerian and, unlike barbiturates and other conventional drugs for insomnia, valerian does not have a synergy with alcohol, meaning it is not dangerous to mix the two—as is the case with the conventional medications.[60] Possessing warming qualities, valerian is also effective in easing muscle pain when applied topically.[61] Dr. Hobbs recommends a valerian-hops preparation as a daytime sedative because it will not interfere with or slow reflexive responses[62]—again, unlike conventional pharmaceuticals.

## Herbs Can Be Used in Many Forms

As a result of an herbal-medicine renaissance, herbs and herbal products are now available not only in natural foods stores, but also in grocery stores, drug stores, and gourmet food stores. Herbs come in many forms, including:

**Whole Herbs.** Whole herbs are plants or plant parts that are dried and then either cut or powdered. They can be used as teas or other products.

**Teas.** Teas come in either loose or teabag form. When steeped in boiled water for a few minutes, the fragrant, aromatic flavor and the herbs' medicinal properties are released.

**Capsules and Tablets.** One of the fastest-growing markets in herbal medicine in the past 15 to 20 years has been capsules and tablets. These

# How to Use Herbs to Help Reverse Chronic Fatigue

**For the acute infectious stage of CFS, Michael T. Murray, N.D., typically recommends:**

- Echinacea, goldenseal, and licorice; three times a day of each in the following dosages:

  - as dried root (or tea), 1 to 2 g

  - as freeze-dried root, 500 to 1,000 mg

  - as tincture (1:5), 4 to 6 ml or 1½ teaspoons

  - as fluid extract (1:10), 0.5 to 2.0 ml or ¼ to ½ teaspoon

  - as powdered solid extract (4:1), 250 to 500 mg

    Note: Dr. Murray warns that if licorice is to be used for a long time, it is necessary to increase the intake of potassium-rich foods.

- Pokeweed (*Phytolacca decandra/Phytolacca americana*), dried root, 100 to 400 mg three times daily

- Wild indigo (*Baptisia tinctoria*), dried root, 0.5 to 1.0 g three times daily

**For the chronic phase of CFS, Joseph Pizzorno, N.D., typically recommends:**

- Goldenseal and licorice, three times a day in the same dosages as used by Dr. Murray above

- Astragalus, dried root, 5 to 15 g three times daily

- Siberian ginseng, three times daily in the following dosages:

  - as dried root (or tea), 2 to 4 g

  - as fluid extract (1:1), 2 to 4 ml or ½ to 1 teaspoon

  - as solid extract (20:1), 100 to 200 mg

**For the recovery phase of CFS, Dr. Pizzorno typically recommends:**

- *Panax ginseng* in the following dosages:

  - as dried root, 1.5 to 2.0 g three times daily

  - as fluid extract, equivalent to 25 to 50 mg daily of ginsenosides (the biologically active ingredient)

- Siberian ginseng, three times daily in dosages as above

---

offer consumers convenience and, in some cases, the bonus of not having to taste the herbs, many of which have undesirable flavor profiles: from intensely bitter (such as goldenseal root), due to the presence of certain alkaloids, to highly astringent (such as oak bark), due to the presence of tannins.

*Extracts and Tinctures.* These offer the advantage of a high concentration in low weight and volume. They are also quickly assimilated by the body in comparison to tablets. Extracts and tinctures almost always contain alcohol. The alcohol is used for two reasons: as a solvent to extract the non-water-soluble compounds from an herb and as a preservative to maintain shelf life. Properly made extracts and tinctures have a virtually indefinite shelf life. Tinctures usually contain more

## Herbal Remedies for Fibromyalgia

According to Chanchal Cabrera, M.N.I. M.H., a clinical herbalist practicing in Vancouver, British Columbia, the following formula treats the symptoms of inflammation and helps ease the pain associated with fibromyalgia, while boosting the immune system. The blend should be taken three times a day, 1 tsp each time. However, before beginning any herbal protocol, Cabrera urges you to consult a qualified herbalist, as no single standard formula works for everyone.

Blend equal parts of:

- Echinacea—immune tonic
- *Cimicifuga racemosa* (black cohosh)—anti-inflammatory
- *Harpagophytum procumbens* (devil's claw)—anti-inflammatory
- *Glycyrrhiza glabra* (licorice)— adrenal tonic and anti-inflammatory
- *Taraxacum officinale* (dandelion)— used to treat all liver conditions; aids in toxin removal
- *Apium graveolens* (celery)— removes acid wastes

 **Chanchal Cabrera, M.N.I. M.H.:** Gaia Garden Herbal Dispensary, 2672 West Broadway, Vancouver, B.C., Canada V6K 2G3; tel: (604) 734-4372. Website: www.gaiagarden.com.

alcohol than extracts (sometimes 70% to 80% alcohol) depending on the particular herb and manufacturer.

***Essential Oils.*** Essential oils are usually distilled from various parts of medicinal and aromatic plants. Some oils, however, like those from lemon, orange, and other citrus fruits, are expressed directly from fruit peels. Essential oils are highly concentrated, with one or two drops often constituting an adequate dosage. Thus, they are to be used carefully and sparingly when employed internally. Some oils may irritate the skin and should be diluted in fatty oils or water before topical application. Notable exceptions are eucalyptus and tea tree oils, which can be applied directly to the skin without concern about irritation.

***Salves, Balms, and Ointments.*** For thousands of years, humans have used plants to treat skin irritations, wounds, and insect and snake bites. Today, a number of herbal salves, balms, and ointments, usually with a vegetable oil or petroleum jelly base, are sold in the United States and Europe to treat a variety of conditions. These products often contain aloe, marigold, chamomile, St. John's wort, comfrey, or gotu kola.

## How to Make an Herbal Tea

Loose teas are usually steeped in hot water: 3 to 5 minutes for leaves and flowers (this method is called infusion), or 15 to 20 minutes at a rolling boil for denser materials like root and bark (called a decoction).

## Infusions

Infusions are the simplest method of preparing an herb tea; either fresh or dried herbs may be used. Due to the higher water content of the fresh herb, three parts fresh herb replace one part of the dried herb. To make an infusion:

Put about one teaspoon of the dried herb or herb mixture for each cup into a teapot. Add boiling water and cover. Let steep for 5 to 10 minutes. Infusions may be taken hot, cold, or iced. They may also be sweetened.

Infusions are most appropriate for plant parts such as leaves, flowers, or green stems where the medicinal properties are easily accessible. To infuse bark, root, seeds, or resin, it is best to powder them first to break down some of their cell walls before adding them to the water. Seeds like fennel and anise should be slightly bruised to release the volatile oils from the cells. Any aromatic herb should be infused in a pot that has a well-fitting lid, to reduce loss of the volatile oil through evaporation.

## Decoctions

For hard and woody herbs (such as ginger root and cinnamon bark), it is best to make a decoction rather than an infusion, to ensure that the soluble contents of the herb actually reach the water. Roots, wood, bark, nuts, and certain seeds are hard and their cell walls are strong, requiring more heat to release them. These herbs need to be boiled in the water. To make a decoction:

Put one teaspoon of dried herb or three teaspoons of fresh material for each cup of water into a pot or saucepan. Dried herbs should be powdered or broken into small pieces, while fresh material should be cut into small pieces.

Add the appropriate amount of water to the herbs.

Bring to a boil and simmer for 10 to 15 minutes.

When using a woody herb that contains a lot of volatile oil, it is best to make sure that it is powdered as finely as possible and then used in an infusion to ensure that the oils do not boil away. Decoctions can be used in the same way as an infusion.

 To locate an herbal practitioner in your area, contact: American Herbalists' Guild, 1931 Gaddis Road, Canton, GA 30115; tel: (770) 751-6021. Website: www.americanherbalist.com.

# thirteen

# Lipid Replacement Therapy

*Combating Chronic Fatigue and Fibromyalgia Pain with a Comprehensive Approach to Integrative Health*

While we may not yet understand all we need to know about chronic fatigue syndrome and fibromyalgia, by looking at the basic mechanism of cellular energy, it is possible to reverse these conditions, according to Tony Jimenez, M.D., medical director for the Rapha Clinic in Tijuana, Mexico, and a leading authority on clinical applications as they relate to cellular health and chronic degenerative disease. Though trained as a conventional physician, Dr. Jimenez feels strongly that there are better treatment protocols available to treat chronic conditions such as CFS and fibromyalgia, beyond what conventional medicine has to offer. In this chapter he explains how he treats both disorders by using an innovative integrative approach.

## Addressing CFS and Fibromyalgia at the Cellular Level

After years of misunderstanding and enigmatic diagnoses of fibromyalgia and chronic fatigue syndrome, conventional medical treatment still does not produce satisfying results for the thousands who continue to suffer from these conditions. Pain and fatigue have so many negative avenues of influence, yet positive cellular energy creation has but a few avenues to effect a positive change.

As modern medicine seeks complicated conclusions to fundamental concerns, people continue to develop and suffer from the debilitation

Tony Jimenez, M.D.

> The use of the term *syndrome* may help modern medicine, with its myriad of specialties and its evolution of compensation, but it is of little comfort to patients suffering from pain and fatigue.
>
> —*Tony Jimenez, M.D.*

of fibromyalgia and CFS. I contend that the most basic biochemical action—the lack of cellular energy function and protection—is the source of the disorder. I also contend that the sufferers of these disorders can find relief through an innovative treatment program that we call lipid replacement therapy.

## Why We Use the Term Syndrome

The more we learn in medicine, the more confused we become. Rather than risk our patients seeing us as confused, we classify our research in grades, or classes, of understanding. A syndrome is one such classification. According to the *American Heritage Dictionary of the English Language, Fourth Edition*, a syndrome is defined as "a group of symptoms that collectively indicate or characterize a disease, psychological disorder, or other abnormal condition." This is a safe way for the medical profession to look at a newer set of circumstances that cause people to feel less than healthy.

It is important to realize that in medicine, something is defined as a syndrome because there is only an indication or a characterization of an illness; it cannot be defined as an illness because the medical profession would then have to work around the clock to meet the public demand for a cure. If we do not know what causes a problem, we cannot define its cure to the satisfaction of our scholars, insurance companies, and skeptics. To give ourselves more time, we classify it in a more enigmatic sense. This may keep the suffering patient in confusion, but it keeps the medical industry safe.

The use of the term *syndrome* may help modern medicine, with its myriad of specialties and its evolution of compensation, but it is of little comfort to patients suffering from pain and fatigue. For example, for years researchers suggested that both CFS and fibromyalgia were diseases of psychological origin. It seems it is easier to treat these illnesses this way, even though innovative researchers were suggesting for years that the problem rested in several other areas of physiology, including nutrition, biochemical breakdown, hormonal imbalance, and fat disposition. Only recently have innovative physicians followed a more holistic path in diagnosing and treating CFS and fibromyalgia.

Eventually we will discover a true diagnosis and prognosis; until then, practitioners and patients will read all they can about the disorder, seek explanation and comfort from fellow sufferers, and speak of these conditions as syndromes and enigmatic "diseases of modern living."

## Looking Back to Move Ahead in Treatment

Fatigue and pain are nothing new. Chronic fatigue and fibromyalgia are not new, either. In fact, the only thing new about these so-called "diseases of modern living" is their names—which bring comfort to no one except those commanded to explain it. There is also a school of thought that suggests that the two disorders are really one disorder. Let's consider both.

Chronic fatigue immune deficiency syndrome (CFIDS) is a term used to describe a number of disorders that are characterized by severe and sometimes debilitating fatigue. This disorder was described as "muscular rheumatism" in the early 1800s; in 1824, a physician in Edinburgh described specific tender points, now recognized as a specific symptom of fibromyalgia. In 1880, a psychiatrist described and wrote about a disorder that he termed *neurasthenia*. This disorder consisted of a collection of symptoms such as fatigue, widespread pain, and psychological disturbance. Sounds a lot like a syndrome, doesn't it?

It wasn't until 1904 that Sir William Gowers introduced the term *fibrositis*, or inflammation, into the medical literature to identify patients with muscular rheumatism who also had specific tender points. In 1913, a physician by the name of Dr. Luff wrote about the symptoms of fibrositis in the *British Medical Journal*. He noted that symptoms seemed to worsen during periods of lowered barometric pressure; interestingly, today patients with CFS and fibromyalgia frequently mention rain and temperature fluctuations as exacerbating their symptoms. The term *fibromyalgia* (muscle pain) was introduced in 1976 to replace fibrositis, but it wasn't until 1987 that the American Medical Association recognized fibromyalgia as a true illness and cause of severe disability. Yet, we still see the illness classified as a syndrome in texts, clinical reports, and popular media. Similarly, the CDC continues to classify CFS as a syndrome in the information it provides about its diagnosis and treatment. (Generally speaking, in order to receive a diagnosis of chronic fatigue syndrome, a patient must satisfy two criteria. They must have chronic fatigue for six months or longer with other medical conditions excluded by clinical diagnosis; and, concurrently, they must have four or more of the following symptoms: substantial impairment in short-term memory or concentration; sore throat; tender lymph nodes; muscle pain; multi-joint pain without swelling or redness; headaches of a new type, pattern, or severity; unrefreshing sleep; and postexertional malaise lasting more than 24 hours.)

The establishment of a separate diagnosis for fibromyalgia came in 1990. The unique presence of tender points or bumpy lesions led to the classification of fibromyalgia as rheumatic in origin. The American College of Rheumatology published these criteria in the *Report of the Multicenter Criteria Committee*, which stated that the classification of fibromyalgia depended upon the presence of widespread pain for at least three months in combination with tenderness of 11 or more of the 18 specific tender point sites. Pain was noted in all four quadrants of the body (pain on the left and right side of body as well as above and below the waist) in 97.6% of patients with fibromyalgia and in 69.1% of all control patients.

Individuals afflicted with these "syndromes" experience a wide variety of symptoms—most notably, persistent, debilitating fatigue. Very often, the exhaustion is so severe that simple physical tasks become impossible. Indeed, in many cases, the quality of life is so severely impacted that it limits the person's ability to work. If you are reading this book, chances are you know exactly what I am talking about.

Because there is so much confusion surrounding the diagnosis of these disorders—and because both conditions present themselves as a collection of symptoms that can easily mimic other illnesses, making proper diagnosis difficult—CFS and fibromyalgia can easily be overlooked for many years. Even so, a recent study determined that as many as 2% of all Americans suffer from a CFS-like condition. Health-care providers have seen CFS in people of all ages, races, and socioeconomic classes, yet the prevalent race of those affected is Caucasian and it is diagnosed two to four times more often in females than in males. This may be because more women are known to report symptoms to their physicians, however.

Additionally, in the United States, there are an estimated four to eight million people aged 18 and over afflicted with fibromyalgia. The overall prevalence rate is 2% to 4% for the general population and has been found to increase with age. While adults and children of both sexes are affected, the majority is female, aged 25 to 50.

A study using the Quality of Well-being Scale gauged the level of wellness in 594 patients diagnosed with chronic diseases. This scale measured a patient's level of functioning in three major areas—mobility, physical activity, and social activity—and assessed the presence of a wide variety of symptoms. While these symptoms may not always interrupt daily function, the quality of life for these patients can be lowered by the mere presence of these symptoms. These patients had significantly lower scores compared with patients diagnosed with advanced cancer, rheumatoid, arthritis, and chronic obstructive pulmonary disease. In essence, the pain and fatigue characterized in the syndromes are greater than the quality-of-life symptoms for most other major debilitating diseases of the modern world. Though the likeness of the two disorders is close, the distinguishing characteristic is the pain that sufferers of fibromyalgia must endure. Fibromyalgia is a chronic, systemic disorder characterized by musculoskeletal pain; specific tender points; neurological symptoms such as numbness, tingling, and burning; irritable bowel syndrome; insomnia and sleep disturbances; depression; soft-tissue tenderness; enlarged lymph nodes and flu-like symptoms; headaches; sensitivity to cold; visual problems; difficulty concentrating; shooting pain; and severe fatigue. In considering such a wide variety of symptoms, it is easy to see why these patients are often misdiagnosed with other disorders or simply not diagnosed at all.

## Causes of the Syndromes Must Precede the Treatment

If our concept of syndrome versus disease holds true, we can only accept theories of the cause of the syndromes. Indeed, there is the lack of a single explanation for the disorders that has so labeled them. The general lack of knowledge of the cause of the conditions only leads researchers to speculate—theorize—the causes. CFS may come on gradually or suddenly. Many people report their symptoms beginning after an infection like a cold, an intestinal condition, or a bout with a severe viral infection, such as mononucleosis, although fatigue is a symptom of all these disorders. The key distinction is time. If the fatigue remains long afterward (more than six months), the person may have CFS. For others, CFS emerges more slowly over time, with no obvious event preceding the fatigue, although patients frequently report that the illness developed during a stressful period in their life.

Fibromyalgia, by contrast, usually appears after a traumatic event resulting in physical injury and/or emotional trauma. These events can include viral or bacterial infections, exposure to environmental toxins, medical operations, medications, nutritional deficiencies, and excessive dietary fat. Fibromyalgia often begins with an early phase after the precipitating event occurs. During this phase, patients often report one or two symptoms such as irritable bowel syndrome, numbness and tingling, blurry vision, concentration problems, headaches, and unexplainable fatigue, but have no visible lesions or tender points.

Patients in the prefibromyalgia phase often go undiagnosed due to the lessened severity of the symptoms. Poor diet, poor sleep and work habits, caffeine and alcohol abuse, lack of exercise, and emotional stress, coupled with a trigger event, may predispose certain people to develop fibromyalgia. The person may also possess a certain genetic make-up that does not allow for successful adaptation to exposure to the outside world.

# Cellular Dysfunction Causing Fatigue and Pain

To fully explain my treatment program for both CFS and fibromyalgia, it is important to understand some basic concepts of human biology and biochemistry. What follows is an overview of the concept of cellular influence on fibromyalgia and chronic fatigue that explains how to recognize the biological reasons for the causes of these disorders, the role of cellular energy in this causation, and how studies about this cause and effect relate specifically to sufferers of fibromyalgia and CFS.

### *A Short Lesson on the Cell and Energy Function*

The human cell is our fundamental source of energy. Before we can discuss energy function, it is important to understand the make-up of the cell and its importance to the body. The human body has over 75 trillion cells. Each one is its own working entity, but works together with the cells around it to produce an action, as part of a gland, organ, system, or function within the body.

Each cell also has a brain, known as a nucleus, which houses the important information for the cell and its genetic characteristics, known as DNA. The cells also contain other materials, including the mitochondria—the cell's energy-producing engine. The cell and the mitochondria are encased in two membranes—inner and outer—by a fatty substance known as a lipid or, more specifically, a phospholipid. The outer membrane is fairly smooth, but the inner membrane is highly convoluted, forming folds called cristae. The cristae greatly increase the inner membrane's surface area. It is on these cristae that food (sugar,

> It is especially important to the body that the mitochondria are well protected, are fed properly, and have optimal communication between the mitochondria and its components, and that this protection exists between the cells. When there is a breakdown in this protection and communication, energy production is compromised and muscle fatigue results. Multiply this breakdown to a systemic level and the whole body becomes fatigued.

enzymes, and micronutrients) is combined with oxygen to produce adenosine triphosphate (ATP)—the primary energy source for the cell.

Phospholipids, glycolipids, cholesterol, and proteins make up the phospholipid membranes encasing the cell and mitochondria. Phospholipids control what enters and leaves. By allowing in oxygen and food, the phospholipid "communicates" to the enzymes, which results in the creation of ATP, our basic energy source. The principal constituents of the phospholipid layer—the cholesterol, glycolipids, and fat-derivatives such as phosphatidylcholine and phosphatidyl-serine—are key to the effective use of nutrients and oxygen within the energy-producing engine of the mitochondria.

Different types of cells require different activities and make-up within the cell itself. Since we are focused on fatigue, let's focus on muscle cells. While similar in structure to other cells, muscle cells have fibers that contract, called actin and myosin. Some muscle cells contract voluntarily; others, such as heart muscle cells, operate in an involuntary manner. It takes a lot of energy for muscle cells to operate, so they contain more mitochondria. For this reason, it is especially important to the body that the mitochondria are well protected, are fed properly, and have optimal communication between the mitochondria and its components, and that this protection exists between the cells. When there is a breakdown in this protection and communication, energy production is compromised and muscle fatigue results. Multiply this breakdown to a systemic level and the whole body becomes fatigued.

### Degeneration and Free Radical Activity within the Cell

All of the deficiencies noted above set the stage for chronic, degenerative conditions that only increase in severity with time. It is a well-known fact that our cells are subjected to oxidative stress from the moment we are born. Our ability to fight this stress depends in part on our lifestyles and habits. Oxidative stress results in the formation of free radicals— highly unstable, unpaired electrons, toxic to all living cell membranes. They most notably attack the vital phospholipids, which house the enzymes that produce ATP, the major fuel for the body.

The normal processes of energy generation by these enzyme complexes, as well as the killing of abnormal cells by the immune system, result in the production of free radicals. If the stability of phospholipids is compromised, the enzyme complexes will be less efficient in producing energy and will actually generate more free radicals, and symptoms of fatigue will occur. Since these enzyme complexes are located next to the mitochondrial DNA, there is ample opportunity for the DNA to be damaged by the free radicals.

All cells contain cellular antioxidants to help combat this type of damage by stabilizing the free radicals, but if an individual is depleted nutritionally and exposed to overwhelming environmental stress, these antioxidants will be depleted very quickly. It should also be noted that there are individuals who produce fewer antioxidants due to their genetic make-up. As these natural defense systems are depleted, damage accumulates and can result in mutational changes to the DNA as well as deletions. Mutational changes can result in an abnormal protein being produced, which can be even more toxic to the body.

As I mentioned earlier, oxidative stress to the phospholipids in the cell membrane can cause a loss of stability. This most notably affects the proteins embedded within the membrane, because their ability to move and communicate with other proteins depends on the fluidity of the membrane. Membrane damage, specifically to the phospholipids, will result in loss of these vital lipids and/or changes in the fluidity of the fat, which decreases the mobility of the proteins. As a result, cellular communication is decreased or eliminated.

The cell reacts to this type of stress by producing chemical messengers, which initiate a cascade of events that will promote conditions of inflammation and chronic disease. Oxidative stress by free radicals can also puncture cell membranes, leaving the cells vulnerable to viral and bacterial invasion, which will overburden the immune system by damaging specialized killer cells.

The free-radical theory first proposed by Dr. Denham Harman has become the foundation of the explanation for the development of chronic, degenerative disease and aging. The burden from the daily stress

> If we consume the antioxidant nutrients to protect our cell's membranes, they will communicate better, protect the cell and the cell's DNA, and preserve the function of energy production throughout the life of the cell and, thus, throughout the life of the body. As a result, fatigue will not be an issue.
>
> —*Tony Jimenez, M.D.*

of our environment, poor nutrition, and lifestyle can be counteracted by effectively improving these parameters to reduce toxicity and by supplying what the body needs nutritionally to increase antioxidant defense. In essence, if we consume the antioxidant nutrients to protect our cell's membranes, they will communicate better, protect the cell and the cell's DNA, and preserve the function of energy production throughout the life of the cell and, thus, throughout the life of the body. As a result, fatigue will not be an issue.

### *Mycoplasma Infections*

Mycoplasmas are simple parasitic organisms lacking cell walls, which steal nutrients from healthy cells for their own survival. These small bacterial organisms can invade and disrupt several different types of human cells. They are termed parasitic in nature due to their opportunistic action. Their survival depends on the successful incorporation of lipids (fats), amino acids, and vitamins from healthy cells. Mycoplasmas, the smallest organisms known to science, lack the genetic material for synthesis of these important molecules.

Once the organism has initiated the invasion of a normal, healthy cell, it begins to steal lipids from the cell membrane and mitochondrial membrane. In turn, once this membrane becomes weakened, the energy-producing enzymes leak out, leading to a decline in energy production that results in chronic fatigue. These organisms are also capable of incorporating much of the cell's surface receptors into their own structure. The immune system responds to these abnormal cells by producing pro-inflammatory cytokines (SEE QUICK DEFINITION) such as Interleukin-1, 2, and 6.

Mycoplasmas are considered pleomorphic, due to their ability to change shape, and they possess a very fluid lipid outer surface that enables them to bend and squeeze through tight spaces. It is this ability that makes them undetectable by normal laboratory blood tests and increases the chances for contamination of hospital filters and vaccines. The lack of a reliable laboratory test for these organisms led, in the past, to the diagnosis of illnesses such as chronic fatigue syndrome and fibromyalgia as being psychosomatic in origin, with stress as the underlying cause. There are many people that will test positive for these types of infections but present no symptoms until a trigger event takes place.

 **Cytokines** are chemical messengers that cause inflammation, swelling, abnormal cell communication, and a chemical cascade of events that can lead to the generation of free radicals. All of these result in tissue damage, but free radicals inflict the most damage by binding DNA and RNA, which causes them to produce abnormal proteins; indeed, many of these proteins have been implicated in cancer as well as neurodegenerative disease.

Since mycoplasmas are capable of causing a wide variety of symptoms common to fibromyalgia, chronic fatigue, and many other disorders, a blood test was developed to assess the prevalence of these organisms. Dr. Garth Nicolson of the Institute for Molecular Medicine in Huntington Beach, California, developed a specialized forensic DNA test for detection of multiple types of mycoplasma organisms. In a study employing this test with 93 CFS and fibromyalgia patients, multiple mycoplasma infections were detected in over 50% of the patients. The severity of the infection correlated with the severity of the signs and symptoms reported by the patients. The tests also revealed that patients with multiple infections had a longer history of their illness, indicating that additional infections may have developed over time.

### Autoimmunity as a Cause of CFS/Fibromyalgia

Since cells infected with mycoplasma organisms bear a close resemblance to normal cells, the immune system will target them as well as healthy cells, thereby initiating an autoimmune response or no response at all. These bacterial infections have been associated with several acute illnesses such as asthma, pneumonia, inflammatory bowel disease, chronic fatigue syndrome, fibromyalgia, rheumatoid arthritis, and Gulf War illnesses. Mycoplasmas have also been detected in the lining of blood vessels, causing the release of prostaglandins and thromboxanes, which are chemical mediators of inflammation.

Like rheumatoid arthritis, fibromyalgia is classified as a rheumatoid disorder. In a similar study done with rheumatoid arthritis patients, multiple mycoplasma organisms were detected in the joint tissue. Since rheumatoid diseases are thought to be autoimmune in origin, blood leukocytes—a type of white blood cell—were tested for the presence of these organisms. The results indicated that 50% of the patients were infected with multiple mycoplasma organisms. A specific form of mycoplasma occurring in animals is known to trigger and worsen arthritis by increasing the production of free radicals and cytokines by damaging the membrane of the healthy cell. An autoimmune reaction occurs in response to the transformed cell surface. This particular organism is also known to suppress the action of specific white blood cells while promoting the production of inflammatory mediators by others.

### Multiple Chemical Sensitivity (MCS) and Fibromyalgia/CFS

There is increasing evidence to support the theory of multiple chemical sensitivity as a promoter of chronic fatigue and fibromyalgia syndromes. Multiple chemical sensitivity is associated with a low tolerance to environmental chemicals such as chlorinated hydrocarbons, hydrocarbons, and pesticides and has been reported in 20% to 47% of those diagnosed with CFS/fibromyalgia, compared with 4% to 6% of the general population. These chemicals are normally considered nontoxic, but they elicit varying symptom responses in the bodies of individuals possessing different levels of susceptibilities.

This increased sensitivity is believed to arise from the inhibition of acetylcholinesterase by these chemicals. This enzyme functions to break down acetylcholine. Increased levels of acetylcholine result in repeated chemical stimulation of brain receptors, which in turn creates increased levels of nitric oxide. It is thought that MCS is a result of cell membrane damage and subsequent free-radical–induced production of cytokines. These mediators of inflammation can cause increased sensitivity to organic compounds in all organ systems of the body.

It is important to remember that fatigue is still the overwhelming complaint of these patients. In patients diagnosed with MCS, CFS, and/or fibromyalgia, low-level carbon monoxide poisoning has been detected. Carbon monoxide is present as a result of the breakdown of chemicals we are exposed to in the environment. It is an odorless, colorless, tasteless gas that can be produced by the body from chemicals such as formaldehyde and dichloromethane. The most common carbon monoxide sources include tobacco smoke, automobile exhaust, and wood and coal stoves.

Seventy-five percent of the body's carbon monoxide is produced only as a result of the breakdown of old red blood cells by an enzyme called hemeoxygenase. The remainder of carbon monoxide can be generated through oxidation of lipid membranes (fats) and organic compounds. Hemeoxygenase, also known as heat shock protein 32 (HSP-32), is induced or stimulated by stressors such as cytokines, heavy metals, free radicals, infections, physical and psychological stress, sound, and heat. Therefore, exposure to these stressors can cause a chronic low level of carbon monoxide to exist. While a majority of carbon monoxide is exhaled through the lungs, some of it remains bound to hemoglobin. The hemeoxygenase enzyme can be detected in different organs by testing the blood or by measuring the amount of carbon monoxide exhaled from the lungs.

Carbon monoxide binds to the heme in hemoglobin—the oxygen-carrying protein in blood—more tightly than oxygen, especially in cardiac muscle tissue. This interferes with the tissue's ability to bind oxygen, thereby causing tissue hypoxia or fatigue. Carbon monoxide will also bind to cytochrome oxidase, an enzyme found in the electron transport chain of the mitochondria, which will decrease the activity of the metabolic cycle. Carbon monoxide can interfere with the binding of oxygen in any tissue, thereby affecting all organs of the body.

The difference between acute and chronic carbon monoxide poisoning is that symptoms will vary in severity over a period of time and will not always be present. This is a result of the body's direct response to the environment. The most common symptoms reported are headache, muscle pain and cramps, nausea and vomiting, memory loss, dizziness, chest pain and rapid heartbeat, shallow breathing, and changes in sensitivity of the senses. Treatment cannot be initiated until the environmental triggers have been determined.

## Nitric Oxide Synthase (NOS)

As stated earlier, we know that the trigger events for both chronic fatigue syndrome and fibromyalgia include viral and bacterial infections, which stimulate the production of inflammatory cytokines. The result is the stimulation of an enzyme known as nitric oxide synthase (NOS), which exists in two forms.

As part of many different types of cells, NOS acts to convert arginine to nitric oxide, which is an important signaling chemical involved in smooth muscle relaxation, neurotransmission, and immune system regulation. It is the second form of NOS, known as inducible nitric oxide synthase, which is elevated by the inflammatory cytokines mentioned earlier.

The mitochondrial electron transport chain, as well as the bacterial killing processes of the immune system cells known as macrophages, produce a free radical known as superoxide, which readily reacts with nitric oxide to form peroxynitrite. This is a highly reactive oxidant that will damage cell membrane lipids and proteins. Blood tests can detect the severity of damage by measuring chemical products produced by these reactions. Of particular importance here are the vital membrane lipids that house the electron transport chain, which is in close proximity to the mitochondrial DNA.

With oxidative damage to the lipids, membrane function is seriously impaired; this can be measured by the amount of the by-product produced, known as malondialdehyde. Once the proteins of this energy-producing complex are damaged, cellular production of energy is significantly reduced and is coupled with an increase in superoxide production. This free radical will cause significant damage to the mitochondrial DNA; the damage can be measured by the resulting mutations and deletions.

## Immunology 101—Related Causes Point to Cellular Dysfunction

Before discussing the innovative treatment known as lipid replacement therapy, it is important to understand exactly how the body defends itself under normal circumstances. You now have a good idea of the theoretical causes for fibromyalgia and CFS. Lipid replacement therapy suggests that an advanced nutritional program can indeed bring the body's cells back into balance, creating the protection and communication the cell needs to create energy. Before we can share how a single compound can create such a profound change in fatigue, we must explain how the body fights pathogens as well as inflammation.

The immune system produces cells called phagocytes to engulf and destroy bacteria. The main types of phagocytes are leukocytes (neutrophils) and macrophages. Neutrophils are produced by the bone marrow and released into the blood, making up between one half and two thirds of all leukocytes. Macrophages are also produced by the bone marrow and circulate in the blood as monocytes. They increase in numbers when infections are present to engulf foreign particles. They also exist in different tissues such as brain, liver, lung, and connective tissue. The engulfing of foreign particles is done by actual fusion with the particle by the macrophages, which then release enzymes to digest the particle.

The process of killing bacteria, etc., is accomplished through the generation of reactive oxygen molecules such as superoxide; this is called the "respiratory burst" due to the increased consumption of oxygen by the cell. The process also requires glucose and lactate for the cell's increased energy needs.

The oxygen molecules are then converted to hydrogen peroxide, which is stable enough to enter different tissues of the body and thus exert a strong antimicrobial effect. Hydrogen peroxide can also be further converted into the highly reactive hydroxyl radical, which is noted for tissue damage. Protection of normal, healthy cells from this process is provided by antioxidants such as glutathione and superoxide dismutase, normally present in all cells but markedly decreased in people diagnosed with chronic fatigue and/or fibromyalgia.

As mentioned earlier, nitric oxide is also a highly reactive free radical that is toxic to bacteria and abnormal cells, such as tumors. However, this free radical has been known to result in the breakdown of the iron-sulphur molecules located in the mitochondrial electron transport chain, which in turn generates the hydroxyl radical. The end result is severe and debilitating bouts of fatigue and further depletion of cellular antioxidants.

Acute phase proteins produced in response to tissue damage also kill microbes. These proteins continue to circulate to prevent any further tissue damage. During this response by the body to bacteria and the like, plasma proteins, such as albumin, actually decrease in concentration. Transferrin, a circulating protein for iron transport, also decreases during times of infection to limit the availability of iron to microbes.

## Inflammation Is the Body's Whistle-Blower

The body creates inflammation in order to begin healing and repair of tissue damage. This begins with the release of chemical mediators from nearby tissue mast cells and vascular cells. They begin the healing process by constriction, followed by dilation of blood vessels at the site of injury. The redness of the area is due to the increased blood flow to the area. These chemical mediators also cause an increased permeability of nearby capillaries, which results in leakage of plasma to the site of injury. We see this as swelling and edema. White blood cells such as macrophages and neutrophils also accumulate at the site and produce the noticeable warmth of the skin at the injury site. Other cells involved in this process include platelets and endothelial cells. Platelets can provide several functions in times of inflammation, such as coagulation and the production of proinflammatory cytokines. These include prostaglandins, leukotrienes, and thromboxanes, which promote inflammation, pain, and changes in the cardiovascular system. Endothelial cells will produce nitric oxide, a potent vasodilator. This chemical cascade is important in states of chronic inflammation like fibromyalgia, because the system continues to produce mediators, which perpetuate tissue damage. Chronic injury to tissues depletes the cell of its natural defense systems while also increasing free-radical production.

The immune system contains a negative feedback system whereby antibodies produced in response to an abnormal cell can actually limit or depress the immune system by effective elimination of the foreign material. However, in the case of fibromyalgia, these antibodies do not distinguish between normal and abnormal cells and will attack even healthy cells, resulting in an autoimmune response. A study was done to assess the presence of antinuclear antibodies in a group of patients with chronic fatigue, a group with fibromyalgia, and a healthy control group. Autoantibodies to a connective-tissue protein were present in 15.6% of the patients with fibromyalgia and 13.2% of patients with chronic fatigue, compared with the healthy control group, in which no antinuclear antibodies were present at all. What was most notable about this study was the more frequent reports of sleep disorders and difficulty in concentration among the patients with chronic fatigue and fibromyalgia. The presence of the antinuclear antibodies in these patients suggests it might be a useful clinical marker.

In another study involving chronic fatigue patients, 30 of whom also suffered from fibromyalgia, the researchers were able to isolate the actual protein that the antinuclear antibodies were reacting to. Out of a sample of 60 patients, 52% tested positive for these autoantibodies. These antinuclear antibodies are only present in patients with rheumatic disease, connective tissue disease, and hepatitis.

These and similar studies provide direct evidence for an autoimmune response where there is a chronic, low-level activation of the immune system in chronic fatigue and fibromyalgia patients.

### The Role of Cytokines

Cytokines are proteins produced by all cells in the body that contain a nucleus, in response to infection, chronic disease, and other agents causing physiological stress to the body. Their activity is regulated by their ability to bind to a specific receptor. They can also stimulate the production of other cytokines important for immune system activity, cell growth, and differentiation. Cytokines such as interleukin-6 are produced by T helper cells of the thymus gland and act on white blood cells to stimulate the production of antibodies. Once the antibodies effectively neutralize the foreign particle, they send a negative feedback signal to the immune system to limit any further response by the immune system. Interleukin-6 also induces the production of acute phase proteins during inflammatory states.

Depletion of magnesium during periods of inflammation elevates plasma levels of interleukin-6. Magnesium deficiency has also been reported frequently in cases of fibromyalgia. Immune system cells require energy in the form of ATP in order to effectively rid the body of foreign particles, and magnesium is a critical cofactor for this process. Therefore, in the case of fibromyalgia, an overactive immune system would deplete magnesium stores over time.

As I stated earlier, there is often a triggering event that precedes the development of fibromyalgia. The event is usually an infection that, when coupled with a weak genetic profile, creates an overactive immune system response. It may be an abnormal immune system, which impedes recovery from infections and disease and predisposes the individual to this syndrome. The immune system response by the thymus gland involves two sets of cells, T helper 1 cells (Th1) and T helper 2 cells (Th2). The Th2 cells are responsible for a response to bacteria and chronic viral conditions. These two classes of helper cells, also known as CD4+ T cells, produce different classes of cytokines.

The Th1 cell line promotes the transformation of CD8 cells into natural killer cells for the killing of viruses. The Th2 cell line produces proinflammatory cytokines such as interleukin-6, interleukin-10, and tumor necrosis factor and activates B cells for the production of antibodies in response to infection. It is the overabundance of B cells and autoantibodies that can trigger autoimmune disease and severe allergic reactions. This particular immune response is overly active when there is a high level of cortisol (stress hormone) present.

The body normally exists in equilibrium between both lines of defense. In those affected with fibromyalgia, however, the body does not return to equilibrium after a response to infection by the Th2 cell line; instead, it remains in a pattern that perpetuates the inflammatory process. This pattern is usually seen in patients with allergies, asthma, rheumatoid arthritis, and chronic viral conditions. When this state of immune defense prevails, CD8 killer cells normally produced by the Th1 cell line are very depressed.

## *Mitochondrial Abnormalities and Dysfunction*

Now we return to the energy-producing cellular engine, the mitochondria. When any of the causes mentioned above compromise the phospholipid communication and preservation functions, mitochondrial function is compromised. Mitochondrial dysfunction is an important factor when looking at the development of chronic, degenerative disease. Age-related changes to the cellular process of energy generation by the electron transport chain enzymes within the mitochondria have been documented by the presence of mitochondrial DNA damage and deletions.

Genetic damage of this type causes defects in these enzymes, which results in less efficient energy output by the cell and a corresponding increase in the generation of superoxide and hydrogen peroxide free radicals. The decline of mitochondrial function with age due to the accumulation of mitochondrial DNA mutations is most often present in skeletal muscle and brain tissue and could be responsible for the progression of degenerative disease.

As previously stated, fibromyalgia is classified as a rheumatic disorder due to the presence of specific tender points on the body. The main symptoms reported are muscle pain, stiffness, and muscle fatigue. While inflammatory cytokines can cause sensitization of pain receptors in the muscle, muscle fatigue has been thought to be due to a defect in the electron transport chain enzymes, resulting in a lower respiration rate. The tender areas are actually hardened areas of muscle known as myogelosis, which are easily found by physical palpation. When samples of muscle tissue from patients with a diagnosis of chronic pain were examined by microscopic analysis, distinct changes were found. Muscle tissue from healthy patients showed normal, considerable space between the actual muscle fibers, in contrast to tissue of myogelotic areas, which showed a considerable narrowing between the fibers, as well as a considerable increase in thickness. Tissue from these samples also showed a moth-eaten appearance, with split fibers and ragged red fibers.

Studies have documented the age-related damage to mitochondrial DNA, resulting in mutations and deletions, as the underlying cause of muscle-fiber defects. These deletions and/or mutations to mitochondrial DNA cause the synthesis of defective electron transport chain enzymes. Changes to the respiratory enzymes concentrate in certain muscle fibers with age, causing the above-mentioned changes. Research has proven a direct correlation between age-related electron transport chain abnormalities and mitochondrial DNA deletions and mutations. These abnor-

> To help the body balance its pain centers and to enhance the energy production of the cells, a nutritional protocol should be considered. It is also important to consider the basic components of cell health, as that is truly where energy begins. Many nutritional programs are considered for fibromyalgia and CFS, but the "missing link" of cell health, the lipids, may hold the key to better energy.

malities are not present in muscle fibers containing spontaneous mutations, thus indicating that they arise from age-related damage to mitochondrial DNA by free radicals.

### Reduced ATP Energy in Patients with Fibromyalgia

Abnormal mitochondria produce even more reactive oxygen species, which cause further damage and disrupt the cellular process of muscle protein synthesis. Respiratory chain deficiencies are also common in the patients exhibiting these mutations and deletions; these are clinically evident by the presence of significant muscular fatigue. The abnormalities in the respiratory chain ultimately result in a decreased ATP or energy output by the cell. This genetic profile, coupled with a trigger event, can lead to increased levels of calcium and phosphate through osteoporosis, decreased excretion of phosphate by the kidneys, and increased phosphate absorption. Constant high output of insulin during chronic stress also increases phosphate retention by increasing levels of phosphate within cells. The triggering event, which places a higher demand on the body for ATP, coupled with the genetic abnormalities in the respiratory chain, lead to the progression of fibromyalgia symptoms. In addition, when compared with healthy controls, the levels of ATP are found to be significantly lower in fibromyalgia patients.

## Restoring Cellular Energy through Lipid Replacement Therapy

To help the body balance its pain centers and to enhance the energy production of the cells, a nutritional protocol should be considered. It is also important to consider the basic components of cell health, as that is truly where energy begins. Many nutritional programs are considered for fibromyalgia and CFS, but the "missing link" of cell health, the lipids, may hold the key to better energy. This section will consider what has been termed lipid replacement therapy. The components of this therapy are phospholipids, essential fatty acids, antioxidants, other nutrients, and targeted biochemical constituents for the production of ATP energy. Clinical evidence supports this therapeutic approach, and indicates that a targeted combination of these nutritional and biochemical ingredients that directly support the production of cellular energy, aided by the use of phospholipids, can improve ATP production; this can, in turn, help to relieve feelings of fatigue and enhance the antioxidant capability of the cell.

### Phospholipids in Cellular Energy

The phospholipids used in lipid replacement therapy are produced from soy and derived from an extraction process that enhances their energy-production capability beyond that of lecithin, which is considered the perfect nutritional phospholipid. This extraction process produces a "supercharged" phospholipid that the body recognizes and immediately uses. This is important for several reasons: (1) the body of the CFS or fibromyalgia patient (which is already tired) does not have to use energy to convert the soy phospholipid to the form the body needs, and (2) the effects of the phospholipids can immediately start helping the cell in its energy production.

Cell and mitochondrial membranes are made up of varying ratios of phospholipids and proteins. The phospholipids are organized in soldier-like fashion, with two lines facing each other on their fatty-acid ends. Enmeshed within the membrane fabric are proteins that can move laterally in any direction, sort of like checkers on a checkerboard. The proteins perform many functions, from serving as channels through which minerals can pass, to processing electrons and oxygen to produce energy, to producing more protein-like enzymes. What all proteins have in common is that all of their functions are driven by an electrical "push and pull" process.

For example, for a mineral that is a positively charged unit to be able to pass through a protein channel, the interior of the cell or mitochondria must have a substantial negative charge. Then, like the opposite ends of a magnet, they will pull together. The phospholipid fabric maintains and builds the electrical charges. Phospholipids are unique molecules, fundamental in nature, and they have the dual ability to function in both watery regions and fatty regions. This is important, because we need both water-soluble and fat-soluble nutrients. Phospholipids also have both a positive charge and a negative charge, exactly like a car battery. When they line up in soldier-like fashion, these direct-current batteries increase their electrical charges exponentially, dramatically increasing energy and nutrient utilization, including oxygen. Since oxygen accounts for 80% to 90% of our energy, that is no small consideration.

Cell and mitochondria membrane fabric is weakened when individual phospholipids go rancid and, as a result, interrupt the flow of electricity and energy. When enough lipids go bad, the membrane begins to stiffen; it loses electrical potential and the integral proteins cannot move as freely. This compounds the problem, since the proteins cannot do what they are supposed to do and end up producing free radicals, specifically reactive oxygen species (ROS). The premise of antioxidant use is to try to protect these individual phospholipids and membranes from going bad.

Due to technological breakthroughs, we can now deliver phospholipids directly to the cells of the gastrointestinal tract, where they will diffuse throughout the body. The most successful method that has been used to reverse damage to tissue mitochondria is to replace damaged mitochondrial membrane phospholipids and other lipids by lipid replacement therapy. This has been accomplished by replacing damaged lipids with polyunsaturated phosphatidylcholine (PPC), other phospholipids, and fatty acids that are essential structural and functional components of all biological membranes.

Lipid replacement therapy requires several key nutritional elements to succeed, however. The lipid delivery system would mean little if it did not deliver these essential nutrients, which include vitamins, minerals, amino acids, essential fats, antioxidants, and digestive constituents. Lipid replacement therapy works with the digestive tract to ensure that the absorption of nutrients is fulfilled, through the use of essential fatty acids and probiotic or "friendly" bacteria. As a result, from digestion to absorption of key micronutrients, to breakdown of proteins allowing for amino acids, to mitochondrial delivery and protection through the lipids, lipid replacement therapy is sustained. This means that the cellular fuel is more readily available for the energy-producing function and, in essence, the delivery of raw materials from the phospholipid "train" is on track and the factory is back operating at full capacity.

By providing targeted nutrients for brain function, for instance, these phospholipids will break down to produce polyunsaturated phosphatidylcholine (PPC), thereby enhancing cellular energy and cognitive thought and providing more mental energy. The benefits to the body are not just related to the cells, however. From the delivery system's support of the digestive tract, the absorption of nutrients and the transportation of such are greatly improved, aiding in immune support and organ strength. In essence, the delivery system not only makes sure the raw materials (nutrients) are on the train and delivered to the cells, it also repairs the train tracks all along the way.

In preclinical experiments with lipid replacement therapy, controlled studies were conducted and published in peer-reviewed medical literature under the supervision and authorship of Michael Seidman, M.D., of the Department of Otolaryngology at Henry Ford Hospitals in Bloomfield, Michigan. These studies proved that the nutrient delivery system, a phospholipid-rich supplement known as NT Factor™, demonstrated improved mitochondrial function and nerve function by 20% over controls.[1] Another double-blind, placebo-controlled, randomized crossover clinical trial, performed in a multisite study approved by the Harbor-UCLA institutional review board, involved subjects who were chemotherapy patients. The purpose of the study was to determine the effect of NT Factor when combined with the nutrient groups mentioned above. Because one of chemotherapy's side effects is a significant reduction in energy, the aim of the study was to test the subjects for energy sustained through the chemotherapy regimen. The results, published in the *Journal of the American Nutriceutical Association*, showed a marked improvement through the use of NT Factor, compared with the control group.[2] Another multisite open label trial, conducted simultaneously and reported in the same journal, found nearly identical results, eliminating any possibility that the fatigue reduction and improved quality of life results were a placebo effect. The authors of the studies stated that since patients are expected to become sick and tired during chemotherapy, the overwhelming success of the formulation in alleviating fatigue and improving the quality of life for patients while undergoing chemotherapy was important. Overall, 81% of patients reported a quality of life equal to or better than when they started chemotherapy.[3]

The combination of these trials and my own clinical experiences with patients has convinced me that lipid replacement therapy is one of the key elements in combating fatigue. My practice focuses on cancer treatments; for years I would watch with concern while many of my patients suffered the effects of fatigue and other quality-of-life issues. Through the use of lipid replacement therapy, I have been able to help them regain their energy and stamina and feel better both during the initial healing process and afterward, when they need all their energy to recover fully.

I have seen many products that claim to increase energy, but few, if any, would I endorse. As a practitioner, I require clinical proof for the efficacy of any supplements I consider for my patients and I must be assured that they are both safe and offer measurable results. NT Factor meets both those tests. In addition, due to the multiple causative factors of fibromyalgia and chronic fatigue, it is extremely difficult to find a comprehensive approach to treatment using nutritional supplements alone. Sufferers of both conditions who have used nutritional supplements as part of their treatment can attest to this. This is so because issues of cell health, free-radical proliferation, suppressed immunity, and mycoplasmic deviations can all force a negative response to cellular energy. Lipid replacement therapy addresses these issues by working directly at the cellular level to boost the immune system, enhance the neurocognitive aspect of energy function, and improve nutrient absorption and utilization. In addition, lipid replacement aids in the body's response to pain, through prostaglandin modulation. Therefore, I recommend its use as an integral part of any CFS or fibromyalgia treatment program.

Now it's time to look at how lipid replacement can be used as part of a complete integrative approach for treating CFS, fibromyalgia, and related conditions.

## Putting It All Together: Dr. Jimenez's Comprehensive Treatment Protocol for Treating Fibromyalgia Pain and Chronic Fatigue

As valuable as I have found lipid replacement therapy to be in relieving and eliminating CFS and fibromyalgia, for best results it is essential to combine it with other natural therapeutic approaches in order to most effectively address all of the causative factors related to these conditions.

### Digestion: The Genesis of Lipid Replacement Therapy

It may surprise you to know that we use 25% of our calories during the process of digestion. As we age or undergo health problems and treatments using conventional medications, our digestion suffers. Further, the immune system, 60% of which encircles the digestive tract, suffers from poor absorption. The body's natural defenses would suggest that the immune system is fed first, and this could account for the proximity of the immune system to the digestive tract.

Many sufferers of fibromyalgia and CFS report problems with digestion and elimination, both of which can contribute to a breakdown in immune function. When digestion is impaired, there will invariably be nutritional deficiencies. It is therefore important to nourish the digestive system itself and eliminate any form of dysbiosis (also referred to as "leaky gut syndrome"). The effectiveness of nutritional supplementation depends on the effectiveness of our body's absorption function. I find that the use of NT Factor in combination with proper nutrient supplementation results in a marked improvement in digestion, which is of value for those with fibromyalgia and CFS, as it helps them to counter problems of diarrhea, constipation, and acidity. But support for the immune system must also come from elements other than nutrients within the intestinal tract, such as the friendly bacteria that support the immune system in its efforts to neutralize harmful viral and bacterial invasion. Friendly bacteria create white blood cells called leukocytes to serve as "signal" cells for pathogenic invasion, alerting the immune system to take protective action. In the digestive ecosystem, fiber, essential fatty acids, and bacteria all work in harmony to break down food, eliminate toxins, and supply routes for absorption. The body utilizes some 300 species of friendly bacteria for its digestive purposes.

Friendly, or probiotic (meaning "pro-life"), bacteria are created under normal situations by the fermentation of fibrous particles in the gastrointestinal tract. Though they have a short but active life, these bacteria create vitamins, protect the channels of supply for nutrients, maintain a balance between intestinal yeast, and protect the gastrointestinal system as they are eliminated.

Although normally there are literally trillions of these friendly organisms in and on the body, one strong course of antibiotics can destroy the body's stores, creating a number of problems. Once the body's population of friendly bacteria is diminished, the immune system becomes impaired, due to reduced absorption and leukocyte signaling. The digestion function will be impaired as well, potentially causing elimination problems. Further, the body will suffer from vitamin deficiency, both from diminished absorption and the reduced production of vitamins from the bacteria. In essence, use of antibiotics, as well as other conventional medications, is like turning loose a weapon of mass destruction within the body—and the fallout from the "bomb" is as bad as the "explosion" itself. This cascade of dysbiosis affects the body's cells and structures (muscles, organs, and so on), and is compounded by the fact that reversing dysbiosis is often a slow process or does not happen at all, thus potentially resulting in serious health problems.

As part of lipid replacement therapy, this element of health is essential. Probiotic bacterial organisms coupled with essential fatty acids help to repair the digestive tract and return balance to the ecosystem. This allows the digestive tract to return to its primary function: absorbing nutrients for energy and immune health. By creating rich absorption channels through the intestinal tract, the body begins the delivery of essential materials to the energy-producing plants within the cells.

It can now be shown that the phospholipids play an important role in this process, but without the intestinal involvement, the efficacy of the lipids would also be minimized. Thus, for lipid replacement therapy to be most effective requires the additional support of the probiotic activity. This is very important for fibromyalgia and CFS sufferers, as it provides for a better absorption of nutrients and fats, which are important in both immune system support and regulation of prostaglandins, which balance the body's inflammatory processes.

## Essential Fatty Acids: Regulators of Pain

Essential fatty acids (EFAs) regulate the body's prostaglandin response. Deficiencies of these important nutrients can create a state of prostaglandin stimulation that, left unchecked, will lead to added pain influence. EFAs are also quite important for the reduction of muscle fatigue, a common symptom of fibromyalgia and CFS sufferers.

Though EFAs are found in certain foods—such as cold-water fish, avocados, nuts, and some grain plants—for purposes of lipid replacement therapy, I recommend a rich infusion of EFAs through supplementation.

As with nutrients, the essential fatty acids depend on a sound digestive function for widespread use throughout the body. Impairment of essential fatty acids—and, therefore, impairment of prostaglandin regulation—occurs if there is a digestive malady, which is a common symptom among sufferers of both fibromyalgia and CFS. The body uses all available essential fats to help heal digestion problems; theoretically, this could reduce the available supply of EFAs to the pain centers. Supplementing with essential fatty acids is, therefore, a valuable complement to lipid replacement therapy.

## Antioxidants: Defenders of All Life

Much study has been devoted to antioxidants, beginning with the work of Dr. Denham Harman, who formulated the free-radical theory of aging. All antioxidant nutrients have similar properties of defense against free-radical damage, as previously described. Among the most common and effective vitamins and minerals antioxidants are vitamins

C and E, beta-carotene (pro-vitamin A) and other carotenoids (such as lutein and lycopene), retinol (Vitamin A), several of the B vitamins, manganese, zinc, and selenium. The nutrient coenzyme Q10 (coQ10) is also well known for its role in protecting the cells against free-radical damage, as is alpha lipoic acid, a key antioxidant in the protection of the cell mitochondria, due to its ability to sustain the antioxidant capacity of vitamins C and E.

Several amino acids also act as potent antioxidants, including N-acetyl-cysteine (NAC), L-glutathione, and L-lysine and L-proline, both of which work in tandem with vitamin C to retard cellular degradation. One of the body's major enzyme systems, known as glutathione peroxidase, is specific to antioxidant protection; it utilizes fat-soluble nutrients, amino acids, and enzymes to serve the body's defensive needs. With the help of antioxidants, fibromyalgia and CFS sufferers may gain added support for their immune system and guard against cellular breakdown. Within the understanding of lipid replacement therapy, phospholipids also play an antioxidant role by replacing the electron transport chain and sustaining it against degradation. This action helps keep the basic cellular program intact and prevents the oxidation of the mitochondrial membrane.

Antioxidants work in concert, much like the members of a symphony orchestra, to either directly address antioxidant needs or serve as precursors to the defense. For this reason, it is important to eat foods rich in all the antioxidants and to supplement with a full array as well.

### ATP Nutrition: Creating the Heat for the Energy Furnace

Consideration must also be given to nutrients that are targeted toward the creation of ATP energy. Although not specifically used in the general creation of ATP, the nutrients noted above serve as precursors for this action. The body also requires special nutritional synergy to produce energy, relying on nutrients such as creatine, alpha-ketoglutaric acid, coQ10, and others for this purpose. These are the essential raw materials necessary for the fundamental source of cellular energy. In order to be most effective, these and other nutrients must be combined with phospholipids, which serve as the "delivery train" that initiates the process of stoking the cells' energy-producing furnace. The action of these basic nutritional elements, coupled with the heavy influence of the phospholipids, ensures that the basic materials are being delivered and used to influence cellular energy, while at the same time supporting the biological functions that are the recipients of the cellular energy process.

> Though it is possible to obtain temporary relief of the symp-
> toms experienced by CFS and fibromyalgia patients through
> conventional drug therapies, complete relief from these types
> of chronic illnesses only comes about through a multitiered
> program that includes detoxification, nutrition, immune system
> support, and physical and relaxation exercises.
>
> *—Tony Jimenez, M.D.*

### Malic Acid and Magnesium: Contributing to the Greater Good

I have found that the addition of malic acid and extra magnesium, when coupled with lipid replacement therapy, provides fibromyalgia sufferers with a fundamental nutritional supplement approach for dealing with their symptoms. Malic acid converts sugar and fat into ATP-ready elements. Magnesium is an extremely important mineral, as it performs many functions in the body, and people suffering from fibromyalgia are known to be deficient in it. It plays a role in cellular health and is particularly important to muscle and nerve function. It is also considered one of the body's natural sleep aids. I have found that the use of malic acid, in combination with magnesium, strengthens the body's ability to recover from and reduce fatigue.

All the above elements should be considered as part of a comprehensive approach to fibromyalgia and CFS healing. I have found the nutritional product Propax™ to be so effective for patients with CFS and fibromyalgia that I recommend it for this purpose. Propax contains a synergistic combination of vitamins, minerals, amino acids, EFS, and other nutrients, along with NT Factor, to ensure that the nutrients are most effectively absorbed and utilized at the cellular level.

### Other Components of Dr. Jimenez's Integrative Approach for Treating CFS and Fibromyalgia

Though it is possible to obtain temporary relief of the symptoms experienced by CFS and fibromyalgia patients through conventional drug therapies, complete relief from these types of chronic illnesses comes about only through a multitiered program that includes detoxification, nutrition, immune system support, and physical and relaxation exercises. Therefore, my treatment plan also includes the following:

***Detoxification:*** Eliminate toxins at a slow, consistent pace so that you don't overwhelm an already overtaxed body. First, eliminate or significantly reduce potentially harmful foods such as coffee, soda, alcohol, sugar, and processed foods. Then begin to incorporate more raw and steamed fresh vegetables into your diet, along with whole grains and fresh fish. The oils from the fish are especially important in modulating prostaglandins, the body's response mechanism for inflammation. Once these goals have been accomplished, your body will be ready for more aggressive detoxification programs, such as fasting, colonic therapy, chelation, or herbal detoxification.

***Nutrition:*** Feed your body the nutrients it needs to fight your illness and reduce accompanying pain. Certain foods are good for reducing inflammation, while others may actually stimulate pain. For example, one of the key enzymes in the body that heightens the inflammatory response is solanine, which is found in the nightshade family of vegetables, which includes certain peppers, tomatoes, eggplant, and tobacco. It is important to avoid these foods or to check whether they are affecting your pain threshold.

As we have already discussed, patients who suffer from fibromyalgia and CFS usually have common nutritional deficiencies, including lack of magnesium, malic acid, friendly bacteria, and B vitamins. Find a practitioner who can analyze these deficiencies and develop a nutritional protocol that is specific to your needs.

 For more about **detoxification therapies**, see chapter 5.

For more about **nutritional therapies**, see chapters 8 and 10.

For more information about **restoring immune vitality**, see chapter 4.

***Immune System Support:*** It is essential that individuals who suffer from fibromyalgia bolster their immune system. A variety of natural immune therapies can be employed to help create a stronger immune system.

***Exercise and Physical Therapy:*** Stress exacerbates the pain and suffering of fibromyalgia and CFS patients. To help relieve the effects of stress, I recommend a gentle, circulatory (not deep-tissue) massage. A daily workout routine is also essential. Light exercise that begins gently and is gradually increased so that muscle fibers are not aggravated is perhaps the best approach. Just as for patients suffering from rheumatic conditions, hydrotherapy (exercising in water) is preferred, as it helps to cushion the muscle action and is less jarring than other forms of exercise.

*Relaxation Therapies:* Mental and emotional well-being is extremely important to the success of any treatment strategy. Relaxation techniques involving psychospiritual counseling, mediation, prayer, and guided imagery and visualization can all be effective as a means of enhancing mental and emotional health.

*Biological Dentistry:* In my clinic, I have a biological dentist on staff to determine whether cavitations, root canals, and metal (mercury) amalgam fillings are contributing to my patients' chronic health conditions. Through careful assessment, a treatment program can be developed whereby hidden oral infections and other long-term oral problems can be detected and eliminated.

If necessary, all components of this treatment plan can be used in conjunction with conventional care. Over time, I have found that this comprehensive and integrative approach can dramatically reduce CFS and fibromyalgia flare-ups, and in most cases resolve and eliminate them altogether.

For more information on **healing psychological and emotional factors**, see chapter 11.

For more information about **biological dentistry**, see chapter 7.

**Tony Jimenez, M.D.:** Rapha Clinic. United States mailing address: 482 San Ysidro Blourevard, Suite 1589, San Ysidro, CA 92173; tel: (800) 670-9124. Website: www .hope4cancer.com. For further information about **NT Factor and Propax**: Nutritional Therapeutics, Inc., P.O. Box 5963, Happauge, NY 11788; tel: (800) 982-9158. Website: www.propax.com.

# fourteen

# Additional Alternative Therapies for Treating Chronic Fatigue and Related Disorders

In addition to the therapies covered in previous chapters of this book, in recent years a number of other alternative healing approaches have shown benefit in treating chronic fatigue syndrome (CFS), fibromyalgia, and related conditions. Among the most promising and effective of these are Jaffe-Mellor Technique (JMT™), electro-therapeutic point stimulation (ETPS^SM), Bowen therapy, prolotherapy, Qigong, and aromatherapy.

## Jaffe-Mellor Technique (JMT)

Jaffe-Mellor Technique (JMT) is one of the fastest-growing and most revolutionary therapeutic methods for treating so-called "autoimmune diseases" among alternative medicine practitioners today. It was code-veloped by Carolyn Jaffe, D.Ac., Dipl. NCCA, Ph.D.(c), and Judy M. Mellor, R.N., Ph.D.(c), founding directors of Jaffe-Mellor Associates, Ltd. in Wyomissing, Pennsylvania. Drs. Jaffe and Mellor originally developed JMT as a treatment for rheumatoid and osteoarthritis, but today it is being used successfully by increasing numbers of alternative practitioners to treat a host of disease conditions, including chronic fatigue syndrome and fibromyalgia.

"Throughout the many years of our combined medical practice our goal has always been the same," Dr. Jaffe says, explaining the origins of JMT. "To provide our patients with the best possible care, with the least amount of intervention, in the most expedient way. We strongly believe that the magnificent human body is programmed to self-correct, with a little prodding from caring and knowledgeable health-care providers."

Guided by their holistic philosophy, Drs. Jaffe and Mellor have explored numerous noninvasive techniques to ease their patients' pain. "We tried nutrition, acupuncture and herbs, vitamin therapy, lymphatic drainage and detoxification, enzyme therapy, homeopathy, naturopathy, allergy elimination, magnet therapy—you name it, we tried it," Dr. Jaffe says. "Yet even with our most dedicated patients—the ones who met the cost and commitment of ingesting large volumes of vitamins, herbs, and other supplements; the ones who kept up with exhausting routines of moderating their food intake, doing cleanses, and applying topical analgesics—there was only minimal change at best. We were very frustrated, but we remained convinced that there had to be a solution that would help people, and we were determined to find out what it was."

## Some Conditions Treated by JMT

osteoarthritis
rheumatoid arthritis
psoriatic arthritis
chronic fatigue syndrome
fibromyalgia
allergies
asthma
emotional disharmony
Crohn's disease
colitis
irritable bowel syndrome (IBS)
interstitial cystitis
lupus erythematosus
multiple sclerosis
myasthenia gravis
Guillain-Barré syndrome
Lyme disease
scleroderma
immune mediated thyroid disease
trauma related pain disorders

Continuing their research, Drs. Jaffe and Mellor began to keep a record of all similarities among their arthritic patients, including comparisons of medical histories and lifestyle choices, hoping to find common causal factors involved in their patients' illness. Instead, their records revealed a wide range of differences, and led them to examine an exhaustive number of potential causes, including allergens, parasites, different strains of bacteria, fungi, molds, and viruses. Eventually, their persistence paid off, as they discovered several common denominators that tested positive in every one of their arthritis patients. "Finding the causative agents allowed us to begin developing JMT, which eventually enabled us to stop our patients' pain without their needing to make any lifestyle changes whatsoever," Dr. Jaffe says. "We believe we have found a technique to halt the progression of so-called autoimmune disease itself.

> Throughout the many years of our combined medical practice
> our goal has always been the same. To provide our patients
> with the best possible care, with the least amount of inter-
> vention, in the most expedient way. We strongly believe that
> the magnificent human body is programmed to self-correct, with
> a little prodding from caring and knowledgeable health-care
> providers. —*Carolyn Jaffe, D.Ac., Dipl. NCCA, Ph.D.(c)*

"To discover the causative agents, we theorized that a disease such as arthritis might be the result of the presence of a highly adaptive microorganism residing in the host [body]. Interestingly, pathogenic microorganisms are able to transform and adapt to their changing environments very quickly when necessary—often avoiding detection as a result. For the longest time, however, Western science has assumed that the relationship between the pathogen and its host naturally migrates toward peaceful coexistence, and the pathogen itself toward less aggressive behavior in an effort to keep the host alive. Unfortunately, this is not always true."

As Drs. Jaffe and Mellor continued their investigations, they increasingly came to realize that diseases caused by pathogenic organisms are far more prevalent in contemporary life than commonly believed. They concluded that the presence of organisms they call External Pathogenic Factors (EPFs) is at the heart of many chronic disease conditions, including CFS and fibromyalgia. Further, they discovered that the immune system of every single one of their patients who exhibited symptoms of such conditions had been either temporarily or chronically stressed, opening the way for an EPF to take hold.

"When an EPF sets up housekeeping in the body, the brain alerts the nervous system to continuously send out attacks on all areas on or around the part of the body that the EPF has colonized," Dr. Jaffe explains. "This includes muscles, joints, cartilage, and bone tissue itself. The pattern of attacks becomes increasingly more intense, going ever deeper and wider, and eventually destroying the healthy tissue as the immune system wages its war against the EPF." Dr. Jaffe likens the process to a group of fighter pilots who have been commissioned to continuously drop bombs on whole villages of innocent people in an attempt to exterminate an enemy in hiding. "Add to this the land patrols with torches setting fire to every

## Is the Term "Autoimmune Disease" a Misnomer?

The basic definition of an autoimmune disease, which is how many diseases are commonly classified today, is a degenerative condition caused by an immune system that has simply lost its ability to distinguish between "self" and "nonself" and has begun using its immunological defenses to attack "self," the body's own tissues or organs. This type of response is sometimes called "hyperactive," but is more often known as an "autoimmune response." Among conditions that are so classified are lupus, Crohn's disease, fibromyalgia, multiple sclerosis, myasthenia gravis, and others.

The problem with this definition, say Drs. Carolyn Jaffe and Judy Mellor, is that in the context of such conditions "autoimmunity" does not exist. In other words, the immune system of a patient with such conditions is not attacking body tissues without reason; it is doing exactly what it should be doing, what it is programmed to do to save the host: attempting to eliminate a pathogen.

"Pathogens are the actual triggers of what appears to be an immune system attacking the body's own tissue for no reason," says Dr. Jaffe. "When we isolated External Pathogenic Factors, which are the causes of many diseases typically labeled autoimmune or autoimmune-related, in a sense we turned the theory of autoimmune response inside out. We demonstrated that these factors instigate the immune system's so-called hyperactive response, and we can therefore dismiss the notion that the immune system acts somehow irrationally.

"This 'autoimmune' response is actually a normal, pathogen-induced immune defense reaction. Fortunately, we have been able to reverse many of these diseases by using JMT. Yet, if we had not seen these patients before and after treatment with our own eyes, we would have found it hard to believe how quickly they reversed. These successes contradict the popular notion of intractable 'autoimmune' disease."

hut and shelter to snuff out the hidden enemy, and you have the metaphor of what is happening in the body of a person invaded by an EPF," she says.

### How JMT Works

According to Dr. Jaffe, JMT's effectiveness lies in its ability to restore the normal control systems that the body uses to maintain health, especially the symbiotic relationship between the nervous system and the immune system. "Since the nervous system has the ability to communicate with all parts of the body, and because the immune system is on patrol throughout the entirety of the body, it is reasonable to assume the nervous system plays a major role in governing the activity of the immune system," Dr. Jaffe explains. "This is further confirmed by research in the field of psychoneuroimmunology, which has proven the interaction that exists between the immune system and the nervous system. For instance, we now know that certain cells have neurotransmitter receptors. This discovery has provided the proof that the nervous system acts as a primary player in the regulation of immune system activity."

According to Dr. Jaffe, the nervous system is unique among all body systems in that it has been designed to adapt to change in response to signals from the external environment. "Incredibly, the nervous system actually transforms itself structurally in response to the inflow of data fragments along nerve pathways," she says. "It then modifies the synaptic connections in response to these data fragments, thereby changing both its own structure and its function based on its experience. In this way it is very much like a computer. And, because the nervous system has the ability to change, its function can be modified to return the body to normal function without using harmful drugs or dangerous invasive techniques. This is exactly what JMT does."

During the initial session, the patient first completes an intake form that informs the practitioner about the symptoms they have, the treatments they have been exposed to, and the results of those treatments. The patient is then interviewed and examined to determine whether their condition involves the presence of EPFs or if there are other underlying causes related to the disorder.

Using muscle response testing (MRT)—a unique form of Applied Kinesiology that was first introduced by George Goodheart, D.C., back in the early 1960s as a diagnostic tool—the JMT practitioner observes changes in the strength of an isolated muscle against an established baseline. Typically, the anterior deltoid muscle of the patient's dominant arm is used as an indicator; however, any muscle can be used. "MRT testing is particularly helpful because it accesses the autonomic nervous system (ANS)—which operates on a subconscious level and is involved in controlling every bodily function," Dr. Jaffe says. "Unlike the conscious mind, the ANS subconsciously influences the heart rate, digestion, dilation and contraction of the pupils of the eyes, and so forth. MRT is unique in that it can circumvent the conscious mind and disclose what is happening in the internal environment. We investigate the various pathways of the autonomic nervous system, then fine-tune it for clear reception by dictating certain queries that allow us to investigate internal functioning. The isolated testing muscle acts as a reception device in much the same way a television screen does, receiving bits of information to form a clear picture. So, MRT should not be thought of as some sort of mysterious magic trick, but simply as a type of conversation and exchange of information that takes place on a nonverbal level between the practitioner and the patient's subconscious. Ultimately, the practitioner is inputting information to the patient, which travels along the sensory pathways of the patient's nervous system. The patient's ANS evaluates the input data and responds over its motor pathways with a reflex response in the selected muscle that will either exhibit no change and remain strong, or exhibit a clear temporary weakening that relays a yes/no, positive/negative response to the testing. The test has nothing to do with dexterity, but simply informs the practitioner about functional neurology."

Patients are instructed in how to be the subject of an MRT examination at their first JMT treatment. They are directed to lie face up and relax. In an attempt to access the subconscious part of the nervous system, the practitioner advises the patient to refrain from asking questions or talking once the session has begun. This is done to avoid stimulating the conscious mind. When the examiner begins the MRT examination, the dominant arm is chosen. The examiner will apply gently increasing force against the arm while the patient resists. The patient is told to use only their shoulder muscles to meet the examiner's resistance. One of two responses is possible in the patient during MRT examination— either they will be able to meet the examiner's resistance, or they will see the arm test weak.

Originally, JMT practitioners used small glass vials filled with distilled water and the energetic signature of some chosen test substance to evaluate the reflex response. The ampule was placed somewhere on the patient's body—commonly in the hand—and the patient was asked to resist the practitioner's stress against the arm. The vial could contain the energetic signature of EPFs or, if testing for allergic sensitivities, various foods, inhalants, or contactants. The test vials were manufactured by a method that electronically imprinted the water with a binary energetic signature that caused it to appear to the body as the "real thing." This method of replicating any substance in its energy form is similar to creating homeopathic remedies in which a water-alcohol solution is imprinted with the energetic signature of the component medicinals that are to be a part of the homeopathic preparation. When the patient demonstrated a positive (weak) MRT reaction to a vial containing the energetic signature of a certain pathogen (EPF), this informed the practitioner that the contents of the vial had prodded the ANS to recognize the underlying cause of the patient's problem to be the presence of microorganisms that had incited unregulated immune system activity. The same assumption existed when the patient demonstrated a weak

MRT in response to vials containing the energy of allergens. Again, the reflexive "weak" response indicated a malfunction in the autonomic nervous system, showing that the cells of the immune system were agitated and overreacting without regulation. In either case, the weak muscle response indicated that the patient was a good candidate for being treated with the JMT protocol.

More recently, however, Drs. Jaffe and Mellor have made new advancements that now enable practitioners to investigate the ANS for glitches without using vials. "While the energized vials were a means to an end, the process of resolving allergies and complex degenerative disorders was slow and tedious," Dr. Jaffe says. "The vials that were placed in the patient's hand were only as good as the speculation on the part of the practitioner as to why the patient was demonstrating symptoms in the first place. Each time the practitioner placed a vial in the patient's hand, s/he looked for a clear indication from the testing arm that would put the practitioner on some course. The problem, however, was that the vials in and of themselves never really revealed anything. The key to uncovering the true cause of the disorder lay with the practitioner's ability to access the ANS—and this is done with the MRT. While the ANS is perfectly capable of communicating on a subconscious level with its internal environment, it has no way of communicating to the conscious level verbally. Its only communication to the external environment is by subtle changes, like the ones observed in a muscle test."

According to Dr. Jaffe, since the ANS depends on all stimuli flowing in via its sensory pathways to moderate the necessary changes, the energy of the spoken word from the JMT practitioner provokes the internal evaluation for function. So any corrections that would be made hinge on the practitioner's ability to interrogate the ANS appropriately and then make the necessary changes, using specific verbal commands. "Pathway after neurological pathway, the JMT practitioner combs for bits of negative information that might be embedded and impairing the patient's ability to recover optimum health," she explains. "Like a bad flashback, these perverse data patterns, left unresolved, continue to hold the negative energy of bodily insults—pathogens, trauma, allergies, emotional upheaval, etc.—and they are played out in the body over and over again. But once this negative information that has been embedded for so long in a specific pathway is removed using JMT, proper functioning is rapidly restored."

The method for accomplishing this involves gentle tapping at the paraspinal muscles located laterally along the spine, using either an Activator® Adjusting Instrument (used in the Activator Methods Chiropractic Technique [AMCT]) or an ArthroStim Instrument—a device that provides mild percussion in rapid succession. The technique produces specially selected sensory input to initiate more correct control of body function by the nervous system.

"The JMT protocol allows for as many as ten corrections during any one visit, but this too is guided by the responses from the patient's autonomic nervous system," Dr. Jaffe says. "On subsequent office visits, evaluation continues: the ANS, its many neurological pathways, and other systems within the body are tested to ensure that the patient is moving in a positive direction. Further steps in treatment involve using MRT to determine which tissue sites are under attack by the immune system and using specific approaches to trigger the immune system to stop its attack on those body tissues. Once the destructive behavior of the immune system has been checked, subsequent treatments are performed to prompt the body to optimize repair of damaged tissues. In a very real sense, what we are describing here is a sort of informational medicine— quite functional, quite effective, quite fast, and quite observable."

Not only is JMT treatment exceedingly safe, it does not require dietary modifications or lifestyle changes, although nontoxic homeopathic medicines and nutritional supplements may be recommended temporarily to help the body eliminate toxic materials that have built up in the tissues as a result of the disease process and to thus hasten the return to health. In addition, unlike other treatment approaches for chronic degenerative diseases that may span many months and even years, JMT treatments commonly take from 3 to 24 visits to achieve lasting results, depending upon the complexity of the disorder. "The more acute the onset of the problem, the more likely the recovery will be swift," Dr. Jaffe says. "Commonly, trauma-related pain syndromes can resolve within two to four treatments."

During the course of successive treatments, the immune system "eventually has nothing left to lash out against," according to Dr. Jaffe. "At that point, the flare-ups of pain and other symptoms usually terminate altogether."

## Success Story:
## Using JMT to Reverse Fibromyalgia

For many patients suffering from the chronic degenerative diseases for which JMT has been found to be effective, the painful muscle aches and joint pain begin to disappear after four to five treatments, sometimes even sooner. But in the case of Grace S., a 68-year-old patient with a medical diagnosis of osteoarthritis and a ten-year history of severe fibromyalgia, 16 JMT sessions were required before Grace reported that her pain was down to "zero to one" on a scale of one to ten. Dr. Jaffe says, "What's amazing is that, when Grace first came to us, she described her pain as a twelve on the scale, with ten being unbearable. She said she spent 'many a sleepless night' crying because of the pain. And she had reached the point where she found no relief despite the many prescription drugs—Elavil, Voltaren, prednisone, and others—she had available in her medicine chest.

"We did a complete intake on Grace, and when we performed muscle testing, we discovered several of the EPFs often found in patients presenting with symptoms associated with osteoarthritis, fibromyalgia, and digestive disorders such as irritable bowel syndrome, colitis, and Crohn's. After Grace's seventh treatment, about 65% of her pain and discomfort was gone." Dr. Jaffe reports that this relief was achieved without prescribing any herbs, topical or internal remedies, cleanses, or dietary restrictions. By the time they finished her treatments, Grace was so excited she went on a hometown radio show to share her good news. A year later, Grace reported that she was "living a fairly active life."

By the end of a patient's last treatment, Dr. Jaffe reports that there is usually a 100% resolution of all symptoms. Resolution appears to be permanent, based on follow-up evaluations conducted 3, 6, 9, 12, and 18 months later. According to Dr. Jaffe, persons with rheumatoid arthritis, as well as those with Crohn's disease or fibromyalgia, and a high percentage of lupus and MS patients, usually demonstrate between a 75% and 100% decrease in symptoms, with no further relapse shown during the same follow-up period. "JMT does not require patients to change their diet or lifestyle for its benefits to occur," Dr. Jaffe points out, "nor do they need to take any drugs, herbs, or other special ingestants or other substances. We do encourage healthy nutrition and lifestyle choices to further assist the immune system, but even when patients continue to eat a 'junk food' diet, it does not appear to reduce the efficacy of JMT in any way and patients are free to resume a normal, active lifestyle."

While Drs. Jaffe and Mellor both hesitate to use the word "cure" to describe JMT's ability to resolve symptoms of many degenerative diseases, they do believe they have developed a simple, risk-free, and expedient method for relieving the suffering from such conditions. And their view is shared by the many physicians, nurses, chiropractors, and other health-care practitioners whom they have trained in the use of JMT.

"Our goal at this point," Dr. Jaffe says, "is to train and certify as many qualified health-care practitioners as possible, so that people around the world may benefit from JMT. We would like to see all so-called autoimmune disorders become a thing of the past during our lifetimes."

**For more information or to locate a practitioner of JMT,** contact: Jaffe-Mellor Associates, Ltd., 928 Penn Ave., Wyomissing, PA 19610; tel: (610) 685-1800. Website: www.jmttechnique.com.

## Electro-Therapeutic Point Stimulation (ETPS)

Developed by Bruce Hocking, D.Ac., who was named Practitioner of the Year by the World Congress of Acupuncture in 2000, Electro-Therapeutic Point Stimulation (ETPS) is rapidly gaining acceptance among physicians and therapists as an innovative and effective method for treating and relieving chronic pain. According to Dr. Hocking, among the conditions for which ETPS has proven effective are chronic back and neck pain, headache and migraine, carpal tunnel, menstrual cramps, whiplash, temporomandibular joint syndrome (TMJ), tennis elbow, frozen shoulder and shoulder pain, plantar fasciitis, most neuromyofascial pain syndromes, and fibromyalgia. Dr. Hocking reports that "dramatic results" can be achieved using ETPS in as little as one or two sessions lasting only ten minutes. Since its inception, he has trained over 10,000 practitioners in its use, and that number continues to grow.

### How ETPS Works

ETPS combines the principles of acupuncture, massage therapy, electrotherapy, and physical therapy and is based on four basic therapeutic concepts: (1) increasing or decreasing circulation, as necessary, through the use of electrical impulses; (2) stimulating "gateways" in the nervous system to calm the body; (3) relaxing contracted muscles to relieve pressured nerves; and (4) releasing endorphins, the body's natural painkillers.

According to Dr. Hocking, ETPS is a form of transcutaneous electrode nerve stimulation (TENS), a therapy that is commonly used to treat pain conditions. TENS practitioners use electrode patches to stimulate nerve fibers that compete with those in the body's pain-producing areas, thus tricking the nervous system into not feeling the pain. In place of the bulky electrodes, ETPS employs the Stim Pro, an electrode wand developed by Dr. Hocking that is similar in appearance to a large digital thermometer and available for $350 to $600. In addition, ETPS extends the

> When the legs differ in length, the pelvis is out of line, or the patient's gait is asymmetrical, the spine is compressed and stressed and the muscles contract unevenly, causing nerve impingement that directly affects pain.

use of mild electrical currents to acupuncture points—to treat specific regions of the body and to relieve certain conditions—and trigger points, the areas in tight bands of muscles that massage therapists and physical therapists manipulate to help patients relax. Patients choosing to purchase a Stim Pro can also be taught basic ETPS techniques and use them at home on themselves to achieve additional benefit.

While ETPS therapy varies according to each patient's specific needs, it usually follows a five-step process. The therapist begins by evaluating the patient's gait, to determine whether the legs are equal in length and whether the pelvis is parallel to the floor, then assesses the range of motion or injury, the degree of the patient's disability, and the level of pain.

When the legs differ in length, the pelvis is out of line, or the patient's gait is asymmetrical, the spine is compressed and stressed and the muscles contract unevenly, causing nerve impingement, according to Dr. Hocking. "The flow of impulses through the nerves will directly affect pain," he says.

In the second step of ETPS, the therapist manipulates the patient's leg to give a simple manual stretch of the piriformis muscle, located between the femur and the pelvis. This helps to align the hip to the pelvis.

In the last three steps, the therapist uses the Stim Pro to deliver a mild electric current to the various acupuncture points, dermatomes (the nerve pathways to specific tissues), and muscular trigger points that correspond to the part of the body that is in pain. Each stage treats a specific pathway, group of muscles, spinal segment, acupuncture point, or scar tissue.

Although ETPS draws upon a number of different therapies to address chronic pain, Dr. Hocking claims it goes several steps further. "The strength of our therapy is that we incorporate anything that works," he says. "I didn't make up acupuncture. I took acupuncture and trigger points and integrated them into other therapies. The hip positioning was original; I corrected it through a very simple stretch. That was the missing link."

Another core concept behind ETPS is electrotherapy. Physicians have long been able to measure the electrical impulses at acupuncture pressure points. Dr. Hocking's Stim Pro device measures these impulses and emits a beep when it detects that impulse points are blocked. The device then applies a low-level electrical current to open the blockage and relax the muscle.

Because it uses no needles and the signal helps the patient to quickly find the acupoints and indicates when the block has opened up, the Stim Pro is an easy device to use at home, allowing patients to address chronic pain whenever it strikes. That's a key advantage of ETPS, according to Jay Shah, M.D., a physiatrist in the Clinical Center of the National Institutes of Health, who uses the Stim Pro to relieve his own pain, as well as to treat patients with a variety of pain conditions. Dr. Shah has studied acupuncture and finds that ETPS offers many of the same benefits in terms of relaxing muscles to ease pain. "It's a wonderful tool patients can use to treat themselves," he says, "and it causes them to rely less on medications. You can give pain medication, but are you really getting to the underlying cause of the problem?" While Dr. Shah urges anyone with acute pain to get a complete physical exam to determine the cause, he says that ETPS offers a simple way to find out whether the problem is muscular. If it is, ETPS may very well be an effective therapy for people who might otherwise think their only recourse is pain medication.

While medications only address symptoms, ETPS enables patients to both treat the symptom and address its source if it is muscular in nature, which is often the case with fibromyalgia. Additionally, ETPS has several healing effects. It stimulates the pituitary gland to release endorphins that help ease pain, and it causes the release of adrenocorticotropic hormone and hydrocortisols to repair soft-tissue damage.

## ETPS As an Aid to Conventional Therapies

The most important advantage to ETPS may be that it offers an effective alternative to pain medication or surgery. Cindy Cornell uses ETPS at the Cigna Pain Clinic outside Phoenix, Arizona, where she is both a nurse educator and a pain treatment specialist. Though her initial training was in conventional medicine, she realized there had to be a solution for pain beyond medication alone.

Cornell knows the benefits of ETPS firsthand, finding that it worked for her when no other treatment did, after an in-line skating accident left her suffering with headaches and neck pain for three years. As a result, she now offers ETPS to her patients at the pain clinic, noting that it is a covered benefit. She says that many physicians now send their patients with soft-tissue pain to see her first, to determine whether they can avoid surgery. Since incorporating ETPS in her practice, she has used it to treat chronic pain, whiplash, fibromyalgia, migraine, high blood pressure, and even pain and nausea from breast cancer treatment. She reports that the treatment works for about 85% of her patients—for some, in a single session; for others, after two or three; and for those with recurrent pain, as an ongoing home therapy.

According to Majid Ali, M.D., author of numerous books on health and anti-aging and president of Capital University of Integrative Medicine in Washington, D.C. (where Dr. Hocking is a faculty member), "Pain and fear feed the fires of suffering in many chronic disorders. Every safe and effective therapy that alleviates pain and frees the person from fear markedly improves long-term clinical outcomes in these disorders. The energetic-molecular basis of pain relief obtained with ETPS has been extensively documented. For other symptoms—such as poor sleep, anxiety, and depression—the only thing we clearly understand about ETPS is that it is safe and it works. This empiricism—

**Dr. Bruce Hocking** teaches ETPS seminars nationwide and at Capital University in Washington, D.C. He can be reached at Acumed Medical Ltd., 44 Royal York Road, Toronto, Ontario, Canada M8V 2T4; tel: (800) 567-7246. Website: www.acumedmedical.com.

what works and is safe in real-life circumstances—is the guiding principle in integrative medicine. Most practitioners in the university community who employ ETPS speak enthusiastically about the results obtained with this noninvasive methodology. I have personally observed impressive results with it. The practitioners, however, must recognize that they need to vigorously identify and address nutritional, ecologic, and immune disorders that set the stage for the development of the chronic disorders they treat with ETPS."

## Bowen Therapy

According to Jo Anne Whitaker, M.D., F.A.A.P., director of the Bowen Research and Training Institute in Palm Harbor, Florida, Bowen therapy is a unique, gentle, hands-on therapy that has minimal side effects and works on mind, body, and spirit. "It involves specific moves that defy explanation, but our research indicates that the technique stimulates the body to balance the autonomic nervous system or ANS," Dr. Whitaker says.

Bowen therapy was developed in the 1950s by an Australian healer named Thomas Bowen, who successfully demonstrated the effectiveness of his method to relieve the pain of many acute and chronic conditions by personally treating tens of thousands of patients, many of whom were regarded as "hopeless cases" before coming to him. Over time, Bowen developed a reputation for being able to "cure the incurable," and at one point in his career he was treating over 13,000 patients per year, most of whom required only two or three sessions with him in order to become well. Today, Bowen therapy is well known in Australia, New Zealand, and parts of Europe, but is still little known in the United States. "Anyone is eligible to take the courses, but practicing Bowen depends on local licensing laws," Dr. Whitaker says.

### How Bowen Therapy Works

Dr. Whitaker's research indicates that Bowen therapy's ability to relieve the pain of a wide range of acute and chronic disease conditions—including chronic fatigue and fibromyalgia—is due to its effectiveness in stimulating the body to balance the autonomic nervous system. "For any peak performance, all body systems—including the autonomic nervous system, the central nervous system, and the motor nerves—must be in concert with the personality of each individual," she explains. "The ANS regulates 80% to 90% of our physiological and emotional functions and governs such things as digestion, respiration, heart and circulatory function, blood pressure, muscles, glands, immune function, and gross and fine motor skills."

The ANS is divided into two parts: the sympathetic and the parasympathetic. "The sympathetic nervous system readies us to achieve the task before us or can escalate into fear, acute anxiety, and panic," Dr. Whitaker says, "whereas the parasympathetic nervous system comes into play to maintain the balance needed for peak performance, providing an inner calmness to go along with the readiness. Bowen therapy, because of its ability to positively affect the ANS, allows the body to adjust physiologically and psychologically to bring itself into a balanced state, and provides an efficient and extremely gentle and noninvasive way to support inner calmness without harmful effects."

A typical Bowen session involves an interview to assess the person's history and problems. The technique is performed on a padded table or bed, beginning in the prone position with the person fully clothed, preferably in loose-fitting clothes. The desired effect is enhanced by a quiet environment, one in which the client can relax and be as comfortable as possible.

"The treatment involves a series of moves consisting of pulling the skin away from the underlying muscle or tendon, applying gentle pressure against the side of a muscle or tendon, and holding and releasing it, allowing the underlying structure to spring back to its normal position," says Dr. Whitaker. The moves are performed in a specific pattern. The basic treatments involve three sets of moves on the lower back, upper back, and neck. Other moves, specific to the client's problem, can also be added.

"The moves are so subtle people often wonder how this technique can be of benefit," Dr. Whitaker continues. "Bowen is like homeopathy in the sense that less is best." Between moves, the therapist steps out of the client's energy field to allow the full energetic effect of the treatment. There are also waiting periods between sets of moves. Sessions typically last from 20 to 45 minutes.

At the end of the session, the client is assisted to a sitting position and then to stand, putting weight equally on both feet, before walking briefly around the room, to help the body absorb the full effect of the changes that have been made. Posttreatment instructions include drinking plenty of water, not sitting for longer than 30 minutes without walking around for a short time on the day of treatment, and avoiding other therapies for five to seven days.

The effects of the treatment may be immediate, or may take place over the next few days. "Occasionally clients experience a residual soreness or flu-like symptoms on the day following treatment," Dr. Whitaker reports, "but that will subside with more water intake and walking. Emotional release may also occur during treatment or afterward, often resulting in the resolution of long-term emotional conflicts. In the majority of cases, the client's physical symptoms are completely relieved in one to three treatments, although chronic conditions may involve more long-term therapy."

Bowen therapy can be performed on healthy or ill individuals and on any age group, from newborns to the elderly. Among the conditions for which Bowen therapy can provide noticeable benefit are acute and chronic pain; arm, shoulder, neck, and cranial problems; digestive and gastrointestinal disorders; frozen shoulder; fibromyalgia; headache and migraine; leg problems, including hamstrings, knees, and ankles; respiratory conditions; sports and work-related injuries; stress; and TMJ. In addition, clients typically report greater energy, enhanced positive moods, and reduced feelings of tension, fatigue, anger, depression, and confusion with Bowen therapy.

## Bowen Therapy for Fibromyalgia

Dr. Whitaker conducted research into the effectiveness of Bowen therapy as a treatment for fibromyalgia using a test called Heart Rate Variability (HRV— SEE QUICK DEFINITION), which is recognized by alternative medicine physicians as a dependable, noninvasive indicator of how the nervous system responds to any type of medical treatment. HRV evaluates both cardiac and ANS function and serves as a prognostic indicator of risk associated with a variety of chronic diseases, behavioral disorders, and aging and mortality. Measurements made using time intervals from a single-lead EKG are converted into data representing the sympathetic and parasympathetic components of the ANS.

Twenty fibromyalgia patients participated in Dr. Whitaker's study. Prior to receiving Bowen therapy, all 20 patients were found by HRV to have very low power and little or no parasympathetic activity. "This corresponds with the sleep disturbances many fibromyalgia patients have," Dr. Whitaker says. "Sleep disturbances result from low parasympathetic activity." After a series of Bowen treatments, HRV

 **Heart Rate Variability (HRV)** is a form of biofeedback that provides a computerized graph of the shape of the pulse wave of the heart's left and right carotid arteries. The approach is called "noncognitive" biofeedback, because it works without the patient's conscious participation or awareness. Instead, the HRV device "talks" directly with the patient's autonomic nervous system (ANS). When the heart rate shifts, the change is routed by computer into audiovisual signals (light flashes and intermittent sounds) that the patient becomes aware of through the use of headphones and a TV screen. Frequency information obtained by HRV is then returned to the patient through light and sound waves generated in accordance with the specific rhythm of the heart, which in turn help to rebalance the ANS.

HRV testing can also reveal imbalances in the patient's ANS even when he or she reports feeling well. This is valuable because an imbalance in the ANS will eventually produce physical symptoms. If imbalances are caught early, steps can be taken to prevent the onset of symptoms.

 **To learn more about Bowen therapy,** contact: Bowen Research and Training Institute, Inc., Connell Square, 38541 U.S. Highway 19 N., Palm Harbor, FL 34684; tel: (727) 937-9077. Website: www.bowen.org.

clearly showed that the parasympathetic response had dramatically improved and that each patient's power had doubled or tripled. Moreover, all of the test subjects reported that their sleep problems had dissipated and that their overall sense of well-being had greatly improved.

# Prolotherapy

Prolotherapy (also known as reconstructive therapy, sclerotherapy, or proliferative therapy) is a nonsurgical method that stimulates the body's natural healing abilities to repair injured tissues and joints. Its name is derived from the root word *prolo*, which is short for *proliferation*, and it is so named because it causes new collagen (SEE QUICK DEFINITION) to grow, or proliferate, in areas of the body where it has been weakened or injured.

A simple, cost-effective alternative to drugs and surgery, prolotherapy is most commonly known as a proven solution for a variety of pain conditions, including degenerative arthritis, back and neck pain, joint pain, carpal tunnel, migraine headaches, and torn ligaments and cartilage. More recently, it has also been shown to provide benefit for patients suffering from fibromyalgia.

**Collagen** is a component of ligaments, tendons, cartilage, muscle, and the outer covering of muscle called fascia. All soft tissue in the body is composed of collagen.

**Ligaments** are sheets or bands of connective tissues that provide stability to the joints of the body by connecting two or more bones together. When ligaments become weak or damaged, healing is often slow and the injury may not fully heal, primarily because the blood supply to ligaments is limited. Ligaments also contain many nerve endings that can exacerbate the pain a person feels when ligaments are injured or loosened.

**Tendons** are fibrous connective tissues made out of collagen, which connect muscles to bones. Like ligaments, when tendons are damaged they can cause pain.

## How Prolotherapy Works

Prolotherapy facilitates healing and eliminates or reduces pain by stimulating the body to produce more connective tissue, which helps to strengthen weak or damaged areas. "As a result, the patient will often experience less pain and greater strength and endurance," says William Faber, D.O., director of the Milwaukee Pain Clinic in Wisconsin and a leading authority on prolotherapy. Greater mobility and range of motion are other benefits of prolotherapy treatment.

During a prolotherapy session, a local anesthetic and a natural irritant, sodium morrhuate (a purified derivative of cod-liver oil), or dextrose, phenol, minerals, or other natural substances are injected into areas of the body that are weak or torn (tendons, ligaments, or cartilage). The injections are completely safe and trigger the same natural healing response that normally occurs after an injury. When used to repair ligament or tendon damage, in many cases treatment produces ligaments or tendons that are stronger and more stable than they were prior to injury. Prolotherapy is most effective when used in conjunction with

> Stimulating growth with prolotherapy, thereby strengthening the ligaments and tendons, can relieve most chronic painful conditions.
> —*Ross Hauser, M.D.*

proper diet, treatment for bacterial and fungal infections, and proper balancing of omega-3 fatty acids.

"Prolotherapy is based on the concept that the cause of most chronic musculoskeletal pain is ligament and/or tendon weakness or laxity," explains Ross Hauser, M.D., founding medical director of Caring Medical and Rehabilitation Services in Oak Park, Illinois, and author of *Prolo Your Fibromyalgia Pain Away!* "Ligaments connect the bones together to provide stability for the joints, whereas tendons connect muscles to the bone, providing movement of the joints. When ligaments become weakened, the overlying muscles contract to stabilize the particular joints because the ligaments can no longer do their job. The results are muscle spasms and 'knots.' Movement is painful because the tendons are weakened and the muscles are in spasm. Stimulating the growth with prolotherapy, thereby strengthening the ligaments and tendons, can relieve most chronic painful conditions."

Researchers have studied and validated prolotherapy's effectiveness for over 50 years. One such study, conducted over a 16-year period by Harold Wilkinson, M.D., former Chair of Neurosurgery at Massachusetts Medical Center, found that "a sizeable portion of people with unresolved chronic pain had more than a year's pain relief with only one [prolotherapy] injection."[1]

During the same 50-year period, over one million patients have been successfully treated with prolotherapy in the United States, including former U.S. Surgeon General C. Everett Koop, M.D., who for more than two decades suffered from chronic back pain before prolotherapy entirely cured it.

The benefits of prolotherapy over other methods of treatment include:

- Eliminating the need for drugs or surgery
- Stimulating the body's natural healing mechanism, causing natural regrowth of structural tissue
- A low risk of side effects
- Permanent results when a full treatment course is completed

## Conditions Benefited by Prolotherapy

Common symptoms and conditions that respond well to prolotherapy include the following:

degenerative arthritis

back and neck pain

degenerated discs

bursitis

carpal tunnel syndrome

Achilles tendon tears

heel spurs

tennis elbow

rotator cuff tears

bunions

herniated discs

fibromyalgia

headache and migraine

hip degeneration

knee injuries

polio

sacroiliac sprain

sciatica

scoliosis and other spinal defects

whiplash

temporomandibular joint dysfunction (TMJ)

Prolotherapy is also recommended for weak joints; joints requiring a brace; joints that continually pop, snap, or grind; and joints that cannot maintain alignment, even after chiropractic or osteopathic treatments. It is also effective as a treatment for a wide range of musculoskeletal problems caused by failed surgery, compression fractures, degenerated discs, and muscular dystrophy.

According to Marc Darrow, M.D., codirector of the Joint Rehabilitation and Sports Medical Center in Los Angeles, California, patients generally make dramatic improvements after the first four to six prolotherapy injections. "Often, two to four treatments are all that is necessary to bring joints back to full strength and function," he says. However, response time varies from patient to patient, depending on each person's healing ability, and some patients may require as many as 12 to 30 treatments. Once treatment begins, the physician can gauge individual response and provide a more accurate estimate of how many sessions will be required.

### Success Story: Fibromyalgia Disappears after Prolotherapy Treatment

Pamela came to see Dr. Hauser after having received a diagnosis of fibromyalgia. She had also suffered from painful migraine headaches for eight years, as well as chronic sinus infections. In addition, she had trouble sleeping, was chronically exhausted, and experienced persistent muscle aches. Prior to receiving treatment from Dr. Hauser, she had tried various medications and antibiotics and consulted with chiropractors, physical therapists, orthopedists, neurologists, and internists, all to little avail.

Commenting on Pamela's case, Dr. Hauser says, "My advice to anyone with the diagnosis of fibromyalgia is to immediately find a physician who practices natural medicine, for such

> My advice to anyone with the diagnosis of fibromyalgia is to immediately find a physician who practices natural medicine, for such doctors know that the constellation of symptoms known as fibromyalgia can be cured. —*Ross Hauser, M.D.*

doctors know that the constellation of symptoms known as fibromyalgia can be cured."

Dr. Hauser notes that in Pamela's case, the key to her condition started in her neck. "She said that her neck was constantly sore," he says. "This was an indication of ligament laxity and was found on palpatory examination to elicit a positive 'jump sign.' The same chronic ligament laxity that led to her neck pain and migraine headaches was also the main cause of her chronic insomnia. People with chronic pain typically do not get much deep sleep. That is why they wake up feeling unrested even after ten hours of sleep. Fortunately, when chronic insomnia is related to a pain complaint in a particular part of the body, there is an excellent chance that prolotherapy can cure the problem."

That proved to be the case with Pamela. After Dr. Hauser performed prolotherapy on her neck, her pain soon abated, enabling her to achieve restful sleep. But Dr. Hauser's treatment did not end there. "Given the fact that Pamela had been on several antibiotics before she came to see me, I tested her for yeast antibodies in her blood and found high levels present," he says. "Antibiotics destroy the normal and necessary bacteria in the intestines and cause *Candida* (yeast) overgrowth. Pamela's intestinal wall was too permeable, meaning she had a 'leaky gut.'" Dr. Hauser prescribed herbs known to have antiyeast properties and acidophilus to replenish the normal intestinal bacteria. He also advised her to follow a high-protein, low-carbohydrate diet. "Such a diet is necessary for someone with her condition," he explains.

To contact **Ross Hauser, M.D.**: Caring Medical and Rehabilitation Services, Medical Arts Building, 715 Lake Street, Suite 600, Oak Park, IL 60301; tel: (708) 848-7789. Website: www.caringmedical.com. To contact **William Faber, D.O.**: Milwaukee Pain Clinic, 6529 West Fond du Lac Avenue, Milwaukee, WI 53218; tel: (414) 464-7246. Website: www.milwaukeepainclinic.com. To contact **Marc Darrow, M.D.**: Joint Rehabilitation and Sports Medical Center, 11645 Wilshire Boulevard, Suite 120, Los Angeles, CA 90025; tel: (310) 231-7000. Website: www.jointrehab.com.

Dr. Hauser's multifaceted approach resulted in a complete resolution of Pamela's fibromyalgia symptoms, as well as an end to her sinus problems. "Prolotherapy is not an isolated treatment," he points out. "The physician must investigate all possible factors that may be involved with a person experiencing diffuse body pain, because chronic pain always has a cause. For fibromyalgia pain, besides ligament laxity, other causes include multiple chemical sensitivities, hypoglycemia, yeast infection, viral infection, chronic insomnia, increased intestinal permeability, nutrient deficiencies, and poor tissue oxygenation. To cure the pain, people diagnosed with fibromyalgia will be much better served by a physician or health-care professional who utilizes natural treatments that address all of those causes."

## Qigong

Among the more systematized programs of exercise and movement therapy that can be applied to treating serious illness is qigong ("CHEE-gung"), developed centuries ago in China. In China, it is estimated that nearly 100 million people, from the healthy to the severely ill, practice qigong every day. Qigong is used in almost all hospitals in China today, and thousands of qigong institutes provide qigong instruction, while major research centers in Beijing, Shanghai, and Guangzho train qigong teachers and carry out government-sponsored research.

Qigong movements are gentle and unhurried; the slow rate tends to synchronize with the rate of breathing. People engaged in these activities experience a sense of deep relaxation and heightened alertness. In fact, many derive an immediate positive sensation from the practice, and this gives them an incentive to continue practicing on a regular basis.

Qigong literally means "to work with or cultivate the *qi*"—the vital life-force energy that flows through the body like a river. The Chinese consider the existence of *qi* to be a fundamental truth. In one laboratory demonstration performed by a qigong master upon a group of patients, researchers measured the following results: a 30% reduction in cervical cancer cells; a 50% reduction in flu viruses; and a 60% to 80% reduction in bacteria. In addition, test subjects showed measurable changes in brain states during qigong practice.[2]

*Qi* is a naturally occurring, internally produced, self-healing resource, according to Roger Jahnke, O.M.D.—author of *The Healing Promise of Qi*, and a practitioner of traditional Chinese medicine in Santa Barbara, California—who uses qigong as part of his support treatment for

> Qigong can facilitate the free flow of energy throughout the body, which supports and promotes blood and lymph flow and even the flow of neurological impulses necessary for good health. The primary benefit is to activate the bioelectrical currents that flow along the energy channels through breathing regulation, deep relaxation, and gentle movement.
>
> — *Roger Jahnke, O.M.D.*

patients with serious illness. "Qigong can facilitate the free flow of energy throughout the body, which supports and promotes blood and lymph flow and even the flow of neurological impulses necessary for good health," says Dr. Jahnke. "The primary benefit is to activate the bioelectrical currents that flow along the energy channels through breathing regulation, deep relaxation, and gentle movement."

One advantage of this kind of exercise is the lack of strain on the body's joints and organ systems, a problem associated with high-impact aerobic activities. "Qigong is simple and easy to learn," says Dr. Jahnke. "My goal as a physician is to teach and inspire my patients to learn these techniques for themselves, so they can play an active role in their recovery."

### The Health Benefits of Qigong

From Dr. Jahnke's perspective, the regular practice of qigong has three primary health benefits.

*Improved Oxygen Supply.* Under healthy conditions, body cells and tissues receive oxygen as needed; this helps repel invading pathogens, including those associated with chronic fatigue syndrome and fibromyalgia, since bacteria, viruses, and fungi cannot thrive in a high-oxygen environment. During qigong practice, the body becomes deeply relaxed and oxygen is absorbed from the blood by the tissues. But unlike more vigorous physical activities in which this oxygen is utilized by the muscles, during qigong, oxygen is distributed throughout the body.

"Qigong accelerates oxygen distribution in the body at a time when your muscles are not rapidly using it as they would be in running and other high-stress forms of exercise," Dr. Jahnke says. "The higher the oxygen supply, the more readily your body can reverse a disease condition." At the same time, there is an increased efficiency of cell metabolism and tissue regeneration through increased circulation of oxygen and nutrient-rich blood to the brain, organs, and tissues.

*Improved Balance of Autonomic Nervous System.* The second major health benefit of qigong involves the person's psyche and its effect on the autonomic nervous system (ANS). As mentioned earlier, the ANS, which controls most of our basic body functions, contains two branches: the sympathetic and parasympathetic systems. The sympathetic nervous system is associated with arousal and stress; this system prepares us physically when we perceive a threat or challenge, by increasing our heart rate, blood pressure, and muscle tension. The hormones released in this process tend to suppress the immune system, however, which is why a calm or centered way of responding to potentially difficult situations is more desirable.

During qigong practice, says Dr. Jahnke, the individual can achieve a state of deep relaxation, enabling the parasympathetic nervous system to neutralize the stress response. Qigong tends to reduce the sympathetic system's functioning to ensure that a balance exists between the two branches of the autonomic nervous system. This, in turn, decreases heart rate and blood pressure, dilates the blood vessels (enhancing the oxygen supply further), and supports optimal immune function.

"When the two parts of the autonomic nervous system are in balance, the immune system is more highly activated," says Dr. Jahnke. "There's a tremendous benefit to this deep relaxation state, and qigong is one of the most effective methods among the body-centered practices under investigation." A related benefit, Dr. Jahnke adds, is a reduction in depression and anxiety. "One of the most striking features of qigong is the optimism and cheerfulness of the practitioners."

*Improved Lymphatic Function.* Qigong also exerts a powerful positive influence on the lymphatic system, which Dr. Jahnke regards as the "garbage disposal system" of the body. "People who are not well are generally not mobilizing their lymphatic systems. This system is moved by a kind of 'composite heart,' including all the body's muscles, the breath, the cells' production of water, gravity, and an automatic contraction of the ends of the lymph vessels. Qigong practice stimulates circulation of the lymph fluid through the system, carrying the immune cells to key areas and eliminating toxins from the tissue spaces." The impact of this qigong-induced detoxification is evidenced by the improved skin condition of people who have practiced regularly for one to two months.

The combined effects of improving the oxygen supply, balancing the nervous system, enhancing mood and relaxation, and strengthening the lymphatic system make up qigong's main therapeutic benefits for persons with chronic fatigue and fibromyalgia. "The beauty of qigong is that you can literally feel the sensation of the activation of the natural healing response internally," says Dr. Jahnke. "The Chinese call this '*qi* sensation.' We might call it the sensation of naturally occurring self-healing resources."

## A How-to Introduction to Qigong Practices

This section contains detailed instructions from Dr. Jahnke on a specific set of therapeutic qigong practices that can easily be practiced by anyone with CFS, fibromyalgia, or related disorders as a means of improving health and well-being. Since the act of reading can interfere with the fluidity of the practice, you may find it useful to tape record this entire section as you read it aloud so that you will be able to listen as you practice qigong movements in subsequent sessions.

### *Tracing Acupuncture Meridians to Circulate Vital Life Energy*

The goal of this practice is to move the *qi* along the acupuncture meridians (SEE QUICK DEFINITION). Rub your hands together to build up heat and increase *qi*. They will become warmer if you are relaxed and your environment is comfortable. As if washing your face, stroke your palms upward across the cheeks, eyes, and forehead; continue over the top and side of your head, down the back of the neck, and along the shoulders to the shoulder joint (see figure 1).

Continue under the arm and down the sides to the rib cage. At the lower edge of the rib cage, move the palms around to the back, across the buttocks, down the back and sides of the legs, and out the sides of the feet. Trace up inside the feet and the inner surface of the legs, up the front side of the torso and onto the face again, begin-

**Acupuncture meridians** are specific pathways in the human body for the flow of life force or subtle energy, known as *qi* ("chee"). Typically, meridians run up and down both sides of the body and correspond to individual organs or organ systems, designated as Lung, Small Intestine, Heart, and so on. There are twelve principal meridians and eight secondary channels. More than a thousand points of heightened *qi*, called acupoints, exist on the body's surface along the meridians. Each is potentially a place for acupuncture treatment.

Fig. 1. Tracing acupuncture meridians to circulate vital life energy.

ning the second round. You may rub the palms together before each round. Imagine that you are standing in a pool of healing water and that you are bathing your whole body in a profound medicine.

### Directing Vital Life Energy to Internal Organs.

Again, rub your hands together to build up heat. Apply the right hand to the area over the liver at the lower right edge of your rib cage. Visualize the liver—the largest, most complex organ in the body—receiving the *qi* and its benefits (see figure 2).

Apply the left hand to the area over the spleen and pancreas at the lower left side of the ribs. The spleen—a blood-storing and lymphatic organ—is the producer of white blood cells; the pancreas produces digestive enzymes as well as insulin and glucagon (the hormone that regulates blood sugar level and energy metabolism). Move your hands in a circular way, continuing to create heat, breathe restful breaths, and

Fig. 2. Directing vital life energy to internal organs.

relax. Feel the heat, or *qi*, moving through the surface of the skin and penetrating the organs as the entire metabolic process becomes more efficient.

Still holding the hands over the organs, continue to feel the heat penetrate. On exhalation, visualize the *qi* circulating from the center of the body out along the arms and into the hands, to finally penetrate into the organs.

Now, move your left palm to cover the navel and your right palm to cover the breastbone. The navel is the human's original connection to life and nourishment, and the Chinese feel that in adulthood it still connects, energetically, to the whole body. The breastbone protects several vital organs: the heart and the thymus. The heart pumps the blood, of course, but the Chinese believe it is also the resting place of one's emotional and spiritual self. The thymus is the original source of T cells, some of the most powerful immune agents. Visualize them benefiting from the warmth, the *qi*, pouring into the navel, heart, and thymus, gathering strength to carry out their essential functions.

Move the palms around to cover the lower back. In traditional Chinese medicine, this area is thought to be directly connected to the kidneys, which not only remove toxins from the blood but also are the storehouse of vital life energies. The adrenal glands rest on top of the kidneys and control much of what the Chinese associate with the regulation of our energy. Rub these areas, penetrating the *qi* deep into the body to improve the ability of the kidneys and adrenals to do their work. Visualize the kidneys and adrenals receiving the *qi* and being empowered to efficiently eliminate waste products, produce energy, and activate healing throughout the whole body.

### Massaging the Acupuncture Microsystems

In modern Chinese medical terminology, the hands, feet, abdomen, and ears are called reflex microsystems. Pressure properly applied to these areas, usually with the thumbs, can stimulate *qi* throughout the body.

With your thumbs, vigorously press all areas of the palms and the soles of the feet. Find sore points and concentrate pressure on them several times. Press out along each segment of the fingers and toes. At the tips of the fingers and toes, press on the lateral sides of the base of the finger or toenails (feel for an indentation). Continuing to press, roll the receiving finger or toe under the pressure of the thumb and forefinger of the working hand. Return to give additional pressure to those hand or foot points that were particularly tender.

Now, using the thumbs and forefingers, massage both ears simultaneously. Begin with moderate pressure and work over the entire ear on both sides, until the ears begin to feel hot. Notice any areas of discomfort and rub the uncomfortable areas vigorously a second or third time.

### Building Up Vital Life Energy with Breathing

Sit or stand, keeping your eyes lightly closed or just slightly open, with your attention focused inward. Try to feel anything you can about your physical body or emotional state. Relax your shoulders and allow your head to rest directly on top of the shoulders and spine. Hold your hands two inches below the navel with palms facing upward, fingertips pointing toward each other.

Slowly inhaling, bring the hands upward to the lower edge of the breastbone. Then, take in three additional short puffs of breath to maximally fill the lungs, raising the hands a bit with each puff to the level of the center of the heart. Hold for a movement. Turn the palms face down and exhale slowly, gradually lowering the hands to the navel. Exhale three additional puffs of breath, to empty the lungs completely. Lower the hands a bit to the beginning level. Hold for a moment. Turn the palms upward and repeat.

On the exhalations you may feel a warm or tingling sensation spreading outward from the center of your body toward your hands. On inhaling, visualize the *qi* accumulating deep inside the pelvic and abdominal cavities (known as "the sea of energy").

## Contracting and Relaxing While Breathing

In this exercise, the body musculature contracts on exhalation and deeply relaxes on each inhalation. The breath and the contraction together help to cleanse the tissues of the body.

While sitting or standing, bring the hands in front of the heart/ breastbone, inhale, and relax. Begin to exhale, pressing the hands forward as if pushing something heavy. Contract as many of the body's muscles as possible. Grip the floor or ground with the toes and, while the hands slowly push forward, contract the perineal muscles (the muscles used to curtail the flow of urine, located on the pelvic floor between the genital and anal areas).

When the hands are extended, all muscles contracted, the breath is completely exhaled. Now relax, release tension from all muscles, and float the hands back toward the heart with a deep inhalation. Release the toes, the perineum, and the abdomen.

Repeat the same cycle, pressing the hands upward as high as possible, as if lifting a great weight off yourself, exhaling and contracting. Then relax completely, inhale slowly, and return the hands to the position before the heart.

Next, repeat, pushing out to the sides, then repeat, pressing downward. Continue for several rounds, pressing forward, then up, then to the sides, and finally downward. Contraction and release of the muscles pumps large volumes of lymphatic fluid away from the tissues, carrying metabolic by-products and pollutants through the lymph to the bloodstream, for elimination through the liver and kidneys.

## Qigong Concentration

This practice can be done standing, sitting, or lying down. In the severely ill, it can mobilize important healing resources; in a healthy person, it can help maintain health and coordinate body, mind, and spirit.

> One factor makes qigong an inevitable innovation in Western culture: the staggering cost of postsymptomatic medical intervention. With qigong, individuals learn to heal themselves and maintain their health—this is a profoundly cost-effective feature.
>
> — *Roger Jahnke, O.M.D.*

In this exercise, natural forces accelerate through breath, relaxation, intention, and visualization. On inhalation, visualize a concentration of *qi* in the abdominal area. On exhalation, visualize these resources circulating out from the center to all the parts of the body: extremities, organs, tissues, and glands. Continue, through thought and visualization, to circulate healing energy with deep breathing and deep relaxation. On the inhalations, powerful healing *qi* gathers; on the exhalations, these healing resources circulate throughout the body.

## Maintaining the Therapeutic Practice of Qigong

If you are able, Dr. Jahnke recommends that you practice qigong for 30 to 60 minutes daily. If you feel you have the resources and energy to carry out qigong practice more aggressively, then you should practice it several times a day. It is important that you apply yourself on a vigilant yet gentle basis, until you begin to experience some benefits. "There is great value in a continuing practice to ensure long-term healing and the increase of vitality," Dr. Jahnke says. Practicing qigong with other people, as is commonly done in China, provides positive reinforcement and makes the practice easier to maintain.

Some physicians recommend qigong to their patients as a "last resort," when other therapies fail. Dr. Jahnke considers this a grave mistake, since qigong aids in the recovery process by enhancing the immune system function. "Qigong should be incorporated into every treatment approach from day one. It is better as a first resort," he says. "It is an excellent way to improve the patient's appetite and sleep, as well as increase their overall immune resistance, energy level, and emotional well-being. Why would anyone want to experience these benefits as a last resort?"

Although qigong exercises are increasingly practiced in the United States, the conventional medical community has been resistant to its use in a medical context. "Yet," says Dr. Jahnke, "one factor makes qigong an inevitable innovation in Western culture: the staggering cost of postsymptomatic medical intervention. With qigong, individuals learn to heal themselves and maintain their health—this is a profoundly cost-effective feature."

For more information about qigong, contact: **Roger Jahnke, O.M.D.**, Institute of Integral Qigong & Tai Chi, 243 Pebble Beach Drive, Goleta, CA 93117; tel: (805) 685-4670. Website: www.FeelTheQi.com.

## Aromatherapy

Aromatherapy is a unique branch of herbal medicine that utilizes the medicinal properties found in the essential oils of various plants. Because of these medicinal properties, certain essential oils can greatly benefit suffers of CFS, fibromyalgia, and related conditions. "The main symptoms that are present with chronic fatigue syndrome, fibromyalgia, and environmental illness are pain, lack of energy, toxicity, depression, stress, viruses, overgrowth of bacteria, digestive imbalances, impaired immune function, and a decrease in circulation of the blood, lymphatic, and nervous system fluids," observes Anne Vermilye, C.C.H.T., C.M.T., C.M.A., a researcher and aromatherapist in Mill Valley, California. "These are all factors that can be effectively cared for by the use of essential oils."

The therapeutic atmosphere created during the use of essential oils is also a powerful adjunct in the healing process, Vermilye adds, pointing out that "deep benefits can be had from some of the application techniques themselves, such as massage, baths, saunas, and diffusing into room air. The healthy attributes of essential oils on the immune system; psyche and emotions; the nervous, circulatory, and digestive systems; pain and stress management; energy levels; and libido are all well documented. Essential oils also work extremely well in conjunction with medical protocols of all types."

### How Essential Oils Work

"The chemical make-up of essential oils gives them a host of desirable pharmacological properties, ranging from antibacterial, antiviral, and antispasmodic, to uses as diuretics, vasodilators, and vasoconstrictors," says Kurt Schnaubelt, Ph.D., director of the Pacific Institute of Aromatherapy in San Rafael, California. "Essential oils also act on the adrenal glands, ovaries, and thyroid, and can energize or pacify, detoxify, and facilitate the digestive process." The oils' therapeutic properties

> Essential oils, unlike pharmaceutical drugs, are in a complete and balanced form that our bodies are designed to absorb and use beneficially.    — *Anne Vermilye, C.C.H.T., C.M.T., C.M.A.*

also make them effective for treating infections, interacting with various branches of the nervous system, modifying immune response, and harmonizing moods and emotions, all of which can be important for people suffering from CFS, fibromyalgia, and related disorders.

Essential oil preparations are generally broad spectrum, meaning that they benefit multiple areas of the body simultaneously. "Essential oils, unlike pharmaceutical drugs, are in a complete and balanced form that our bodies are designed to absorb and use beneficially," Vermilye says. "Hundreds of different molecules assist in the activity of each oil, not just a 'most active ingredient.'"

### The Physiological Effects of Fragrance

Aromatic molecules that interact with the top of the nasal cavity emit signals that are modified by various biological processes before traveling to the limbic system, the "emotional switchboard" of the brain.[3] There, they create impressions associated with previous experiences and emotions. Because the limbic system is directly connected to those parts of the brain that control heart rate, blood pressure, breathing, memory, stress levels, and hormone balance, scientists have learned that inhalation of oil fragrances may be one of the fastest ways to achieve physiological or psychological effects. "Through inhalation, essential oils are absorbed into the bloodstream through the tissues of the lungs while they pass through the olfactory nerves," Vermilye explains. "As these vapors pass through the olfactory nerves, they affect the following areas of the brain: the cortex, which governs all thought processes; the pituitary, which oversees all hormonal activity, including adrenal hormones; and the hypothalamus, which plays a direct role in controlling anger and aggression."

### How to Use Aromatherapy

Aromatherapy uses essential oils to affect the body in several ways. The benefits of essential oils can be obtained through inhalation or external application, or orally by ingestion.

## Inhalation Methods

Essential oils can be inhaled via diffusers, steam tents, a nose cone, or floral waters.

Diffusers disperse microparticles of the essential oil into the air. They can be used to achieve beneficial results in respiratory conditions, or to simply charge the air with the mood-lifting or calming qualities of the fragrance.

Steam tents are an efficient way to deliver concentrated doses of essential oils into the respiratory tract, according to Vermilye. To employ this method, boil water in a stainless steel or glass pot. Remove from the stove and add two or three drops of essential oil. "Rosemary, lavender, tea tree, eucalyptus, *Ravensara aromatica*, palmarosa, and chamomile are ideal oils for steaming," Vermilye says. Quickly tent your face over the pot by covering your head with a towel. Be sure to raise yourself high enough to avoid getting burned. Keep your eyes shut and breathe deeply for five minutes.

The nose cone method involves applying two drops of essential oil to a napkin or tissue folded into a 2 1/2-inch square. Once the oil is applied, the paper can be folded in half and rolled up to fit into the nostril. "Place the dry end, with no oil, into the nostril and keep it there for 20 minutes," Vermilye instructs.

Floral waters are easily made and can be sprayed into the air or directly onto the skin. Combine ten drops of essential oils with purified water and pour into a 4-ounce glass atomizer bottle.

**External Applications.** Essential oils are readily absorbed through the skin. Convenient external applications are baths, massages, hot and cold compresses, floral water sprays, or a simple topical application of diluted oils.

Essential oils added to a hot bath can stimulate the skin, induce relaxation, and energize the body. The heat of the bath helps the oils penetrate the skin faster and enhances circulation, Certain oils, such as rosemary, can also stimulate elimination of toxins from the skin. When you get out of the bath, Vermilye advises, quickly wrap yourself in a flannel sheet and warm blanket and lie

**Kurt Schnaubelt, Ph.D.:** Pacific Institute of Aromatherapy, P.O. Box 6723, San Rafael, CA 94903; tel: (415) 479-9120. Website: www .pacificinstituteofaromatherapy.com. **Anne Vermilye, C.C.H.T., C.M.T., C.M.A.:** Bio Excel, 775 East Blithedale, Suite 337, Mill Valley, CA 94941; tel: (707) 933-0577. Website: www.bioexcel.com.

down to rest. "The sweating this will promote is extremely beneficial. Be sure to drink plenty of water and wash off afterward in a shower so you do not reabsorb the toxins," she says, adding that essential oils can also be used in a foot bath.

Massage works the oils into the skin and, depending on the oil and massage technique, can either be calming or stimulating. "Since massage oil blends are quite potent, they should be kept within a range of 10 to 30 drops of essential oil per ounce of carrier oil," Vermilye says. Good carrier oils include sweet almond, avocado, sesame, hazelnut, safflower, jojoba, and sunflower. Although it is preferable to use a fresh blend for each application, some blends will keep for up to two months. To further enhance the absorption rate, once the massage is finished, cover yourself in a flannel sheet or warm blanket.

 Cancerous tissues or lymph nodes should not be massaged with essential oils.

**Internal Application.** For certain conditions, it can be advantageous to take oils internally, but since certain oils can cause a toxic reaction if ingested, it is important to consult with a medical expert trained in the use of aromatherapy before using this approach.

### Essential Oils for CFS and Fibromyalgia

Vermilye recommends the following essential oils to help ease symptoms associated with—or causative factors related to—CFS, fibromyalgia, and similar conditions:

- **To treat viral, fungal, or bacterial factors:** Clove, *Ravensara aromatica,* tea tree, niaouli, *Eucalyptus radiata,* lavender, rosemary, thyme, palmarosa.

- **To aid in detoxification:** Niaouli, tea tree, *Ravensara aromatica,* Roman chamomile, bay laurel, rosemary cineole, palmarosa, lavender.

- **To relieve stress and manage emotions:** Lavender, neroli, frankincense, jasmine, rose, ylang ylang, Roman chamomile, bergamot.

- **To aid in digestion:** Cardamom, Roman chamomile, peppermint, lemon, tea tree, *Ravensara aromatica,* German chamomile, thyme.

- **To help balance the nervous system:** Lavender, tarragon.

# fifteen

# Treating and Preventing Lyme Disease Using Alternative Medicine

Although Lyme disease is said to have been first discovered in 1977, after a mysterious outbreak of arthritis near the town of Lyme, Connecticut, it was actually first identified in Germany in 1883, in the town of Breslau.[1] It is caused by the spirochete (a slender, spiral microorganism) *Borrelia burgdorferi (Bb)*, first identified in 1982 by Willy Burgdorfer, Ph.D., M.D. (hon).

Conventional wisdom holds that Lyme disease is relatively rare and only transmitted by ticks. In actuality, it is epidemic; and it can be spread by other insects in addition to ticks—including fleas, mosquitoes, mites, and flies—as well as by human-to-human contact, including breast-feeding. Transmission may also occur via blood transfusion, according to Katrina Tang, M.D., H.M.D., of Reno, Nevada.

Although Lyme is typically identified by an initial rash, known as erythema migrans (EM), that affects the skin in a "bull's-eye" pattern, only 30% to 40% of adults with Lyme disease and less than 10% of infected children exhibit the EM rash, meaning that a sizeable number of people suffering with the disease do not know they have it. For this reason, Lyme disease—which, if left untreated, inevitably spreads into the joints and nervous system—is sometimes called "The Great Imposter," because of how often it is un- or misdiagnosed, leading patients, and often their physicians, to mistake it for a variety of other chronic health conditions. These include chronic fatigue syndrome, fibromyalgia, borderline thyroid-gland dysfunction, multiple sclerosis (MS), amyotrophic lateral sclerosis (ALS; also known as Lou Gehrig's disease), and other debilitating conditions, many of which can also mimic environmental illness. Today, many physicians regard Lyme disease not as a simple infection, but rather as a complex illness that often consists of other co-infections. Additionally, since one hallmark of Lyme disease is fatigue unrelieved by rest, growing numbers of health practitioners—especially among those who practice alternative medicine—share the view of Jo Anne Whitaker, M.D., of Palm Harbor, Florida, who believes that Lyme is at the base of most cases of chronic fatigue syndrome. Therefore, if you have symptoms associated with CFS or any of the other illnesses mentioned above, it is prudent to determine whether you may have Lyme disease.

In this chapter, we examine the symptoms and history of Lyme disease; outline preventive measures to avoid contracting it; evaluate conventional and alternative testing methods; and learn how leading alternative medicine physicians employ an integrative approach of conventional and alternative methods to effectively treat and reverse the condition.

> **Important:** If you have symptoms associated with chronic fatigue syndrome or other chronic, debilitating illnesses, it is prudent to determine whether you may have Lyme disease.

## Symptoms of Lyme Disease

According to Karen Vanderhoof-Forschner—cofounder and chair of the Lyme Disease Foundation, and author of *Everything You Need to Know About Lyme Disease and Other Tick-Borne Disorders*—the signs and symptoms of Lyme disease manifest over three stages: localized disease, disseminated early disease, and disseminated later disease.[2] In the first, or localized disease, stage, the only visible manifestation of Lyme disease is the EM rash without other symptoms. The rash will appear at the site of the tick or other insect bite that leads to *Bb* infection.

During the disseminated early disease stage, which is caused as the *Bb* spirochete starts to migrate throughout the body, the primary symptom is widespread inflammation, which can be accompanied by flu-like symptoms. "More severe symptoms at this stage may suggest that more serious and hard-to-treat disease will follow," Vanderhoof-Forschner warns, pointing out that *Bb* can begin spreading through the body even before the EM rash manifests.[3]

The third, or disseminated late disease, stage typically occurs approximately three months after a person first contracts *Bb*; it can result in

> The course of disseminated Lyme disease is far from pre-
> dictable. New signs and symptoms associated with infection
> are still being discovered. Clearly the infection is protean—
> that is, ever changing—and because so many body systems
> are involved, it takes a seemingly infinite array of forms.
>
> *—Karen Vanderhoof-Forschner, cofounder and chair*
> *of the Lyme Disease Foundation*

organ damage and impairment of other body systems. In some cases, however, symptoms of Lyme disease can take much longer (as long as 15 years, according to some estimates) to become visible, which is one more reason why the illness is so difficult to detect, let alone to treat.

"The course of disseminated Lyme disease is far from predictable," Vanderhoof-Forschner says. "New signs and symptoms associated with infection are still being discovered. Clearly the infection is protean— that is, ever changing—and because so many body systems are involved, it takes a seemingly infinite array of forms."[4]

Marylynn S. Barkley, Ph.D., M.D., associate professor of neurobiology, physiology, and behavior at the University of California at Davis, notes that approximately 15% of Lyme patients develop serious problems. For such patients, chronic debilitation and extreme pain can change their lives dramatically and in some cases has even led to suicide, she says.

### Localized Symptom

As mentioned, the primary initial symptom of Lyme disease is the EM rash, which, if it occurs, will do so at the site of the tick or insect bite. Other symptoms, similar to those of the flu—such as minor aches and pains, headache, and/or fever—may also be present. Because of its distinctive "bull's-eye" pattern, the appearance of an EM rash is usually sufficient for a confirmed diagnosis of Lyme disease. But more than half of all adults and 90% of children affected with Lyme disease never exhibit the rash. Moreover, in many cases, particularly among African-Americans and others with dark skin, the rash may not be noticed, due to its lightness, or it may be mistaken for a bruise. Further compounding the problem is the fact that, although the EM rash will typically manifest within a few days of infection, in other cases it may not appear for months, by which time *Bb* can be well-advanced throughout the body.

## The Appearance of the EM Rash Isn't Always a "Bull's-Eye"

Though the EM rash that can accompany early signs of Lyme disease is usually described as having a "bull's-eye" pattern, according to Karen Vanderhoof-Forschner, cofounder and chair of the Lyme Disease Foundation, the rash can also take other, less recognized forms.

"The typical rash begins as a small, reddish bump about one-half inch in diameter that is sometimes raised," she explains. "It soon begins to expand outward, usually clearing in the center and reaching a final size that may be as little as two inches in diameter or it may be large enough to cover your entire back or to wrap around your arm or leg until the two ends meet. The characteristic 'bull's-eye' form of the rash is a series of bright red and paler skin colors resembling the ripples created when a rock is thrown into a pond. However, there are many other well-recognized variations of the Lyme rash. It may be uniformly discolored and may range in color from reddish to purple to bruised-looking. An EM can be shaped like a ring, a triangle, an oval, or a long, thin, ragged line and may be hot to the touch, icy, burning, or painful. Alternately, the skin at the bite may be numb. You may also see blistering, ulceration, or scaling, and very occasionally there will be some bleeding."[a]

Another distinctive characteristic of the EM rash, compared to rashes caused by other tick or insect bites, is its duration; it typically lasts from one week to several months before disappearing, compared to other rashes or localized skin inflammation or discolorations, which start to fade within a day or two.[b]

---

[a] Vanderhoof-Forschner, Karen. *Everything You Need To Know About Lyme Disease and Other Tick-Borne Disorders*, 2nd ed. (Hoboken, NJ: John Wiley & Sons, Inc., 2003): 51–52.
[b] Ibid.

### Disseminated Disease Symptoms

Symptoms of Lyme disease in both the early and late stages of dissemination are variable and include unrelieved fatigue, headache, weakness, muscles aches and pain, back pain, joint pain and swelling (similar to arthritis), chills, fever, sore throat, nausea, vomiting, facial paralysis, swollen lymph glands, enlarged spleen, profuse perspiration, irregular heartbeat, seizures, blurry vision, memory loss, cranial and Bell's palsy, impaired muscle coordination, gait problems, stabbing pains along the extremities, diminished reflexes, brain and spinal cord infection, bladder and kidney problems, infertility, liver problems (including, in some cases, hepatitis), and skin disorders.

Vanderhoof-Forschner notes that Lyme disease may also lead to psychiatric disorders. The most commonly observed disorder in this category is depression, which affects as many as one-third of all Lyme disease patients. Other disorders in this category include mood swings, dementia, personality changes, hallucinations, panic attacks, impulsive violence and verbal aggression, paranoia, schizophrenia, eating disorders, and suicide.[5]

> Lyme disease eludes many doctors because it can mimic many other diseases. This poses a health risk, because doctors may treat the wrong disease or not find the true cause, thus delaying treatment. — *Katrina Tang, M.D.*

Lyme disease can also be a cause of or contributing cofactor in a variety of other degenerative diseases, including ALS, Alzheimer's, fibromyalgia, and multiple sclerosis. It can also cause or play a role in bipolar disorder (manic depression), neurological disease, and even heart disease (Lyme carditis). Many people who are thought to have such conditions are misdiagnosed and actually have Lyme disease, according to Charles Ray Jones, M.D., of New Haven, Connecticut. Dr. Tang adds, "Lyme disease eludes many doctors because it can mimic many other diseases. This poses a health risk, because doctors may treat the wrong disease or not find the true cause, thus delaying treatment."

Despite all of its mimicking effects, conventional wisdom still considers the incidence of Lyme disease to be rather limited. The U.S. Centers for Disease Control and Prevention (CDC), for instance, reports that there have been fewer than 200,000 confirmed cases of Lyme disease since 1980, but others strongly dispute such figures. "If it weren't for AIDS," states Nick Harris, Ph.D., director of the International Lyme and Associated Disease Society (ILADS), "Lyme would be the number-one infectious disease in the U.S. and Western Europe. Lyme is grossly underreported. In the U.S., we probably have 200,000 cases per year." W. Lee Cowden, a world-renowned expert in the field of integrative medicine, puts the number even higher. "There are very few symptoms where you shouldn't consider Lyme, especially given that a quarter of the U.S. population may be affected," he says. "More than 50% of ill people may have Lyme contributing to their condition."

What is the reason for the discrepancy between the CDC's statistics and the experience of front-line alternative medicine physicians who treat Lyme disease? Dr. Jones explains, "The CDC criteria was developed only for surveillance; it was never meant for diagnosis. Lyme is a clinical diagnosis. The test evidence may be used to support a clinical diagnosis, but it doesn't prove one has Lyme. About 50% of patients I've seen have been seronegative [blood test negative] for Lyme but meet all the clinical criteria."

> If it weren't for AIDS, Lyme would be the number-one infectious disease in the U.S. and Western Europe. Lyme is grossly underreported. In the U.S., we probably have 200,000 cases per year. —*Nick Harris, Ph.D., director of the International Lyme and Associated Disease Society (ILADS)*

Making matters worse, researchers now know that Lyme disease is transmittable from one human to another. "Of the more than 5,000 children I've treated, 240 have been born with the disease," states Dr. Jones, who specializes in pediatric and adolescent medicine. "Twelve children who've been breast-fed have subsequently developed Lyme. *Bb* can be transmitted transplacentally, even with *in vitro* fertilization. I've seen eight children infected this way." A study presented by Gregory Bach, D.O., P.C., of Colmar, Pennsylvania, to the American Psychiatric Association in November 2000 revealed that Lyme can also be transmitted during sex via semen. Dr. Bach confirmed the presence of *Bb* in semen using the polymerase chain reaction (PCR) test. He calls *Bb* a "brother" to the syphilis spirochete because of their genetic similarities. (Syphilis, like Lyme disease, can manifest as a wide variety of symptoms; in fact, it preceded Lyme as the original "Great Imposter" in medical circles.) For this reason, when he treats a Lyme patient in a relationship, Dr. Bach often treats the spouse or partner as well. Otherwise, he points out, both partners can continue to pass *Bb* back and forth, reinfecting each other.

Dr. Tang adds that there are other avenues of infection. "Transmission may also occur via blood transfusion and through the bites of mosquitoes or other insects." Dr. Jones says, "People from Asia who came to me with the classic Lyme rash have been infected by fleas and gnats." Dr. Cowden contends that unpasteurized goat or cow milk can also transmit *Bb* infection.

Nor is Lyme disease a simple infection; it is a complex illness that can consist of other infectious cofactors, especially the parasitic pathogens *Babesia* and *Ehrlichia*. When diagnosed at a very early stage, Lyme disease can be cured by a course of oral antibiotics, such as doxycycline. When treatment is delayed, however, the results can be disastrous, since in its later stages, "Lyme also includes collateral conditions that result from being ill with multiple pathogens, each of which has a

## The History of Lyme Disease

Conventional wisdom has it that Lyme disease was first observed in 1977 in Lyme, Connecticut, hence its name. The truth, however, is that Lyme disease is not new, nor did it originate in the United States. As Karen Vanderhoof-Forschner, cofounder of the Lyme Disease Foundation, documents in her book *Everything You Need to Know About Lyme Disease and Other Tick-Borne Disorders*, Lyme disease has been written about in medical journals for over a century, primarily in Europe, where the disease was first described by German physician Alfred Buchwald in 1883.[a] In 1909, Swedish physician Arvid Afzelius first presented research about the expanding ring-like lesion that is now known as the erythema migrans (EM), a characteristic of Lyme disease, and in 1921 the first report concerning the severe joint pain and swelling that can also accompany Lyme disease was published, followed a year later by published reports denoting a link between the EM rash and the neurological disorders that can be associated with it.[b] "By 1945, researchers had already described much about what we now call Lyme disease," Vanderhoof-Forschner writes, "includ-ing the variety of skin problems, the common arthritic conditions, and many of the neurological, cardiac, and ophthalmologic problems that suggest the involvement of multiple body systems."[c] Yet, despite the large body of published research dating back 120 years, to this day most people still believe that Lyme is a fairly new disease and limited in occurrence to only certain geographical regions in the United States, when in actuality it is also common in Canada and Europe, and cases have been documented as far away as Australia and New Zealand.[d]

---

[a] Buchwald, A. (1883). "Ein Fall von diffuser idiopathischer Haut-Atrophie." *Arch Dermatol Syph* 10: 553–56. Referenced in: Vanderhoof-Forschner, Karen. *Everything You Need To Know About Lyme Disease and Other Tick-Borne Disorders*, 2nd ed. (Hoboken, NJ: John Wiley & Sons, Inc., 2003): 37, 187.
[b] Vanderhoof-Forschner, Karen. *Everything You Need To Know About Lyme Disease and Other Tick-Borne Disorders*, 2nd ed. (Hoboken, NJ: John Wiley & Sons, Inc., 2003): 39.
[c] Ibid, 37.
[d] Ibid, 46.

profound impact on the person's overall health," states Joseph J. Burrascano, Jr., M.D., of East Hampton, New York. "Together, damage to virtually all bodily systems can result."

## Making a Definitive Diagnosis

"Despite the breadth of symptoms that characterize Lyme disease, it remains an extremely difficult disease to diagnose," observes Vanderhoof-Forschner. "Although multiple laboratory tests are available, it is impossible to be entirely sure what the results mean." She adds that negative findings are no guarantee that a person is free of Lyme disease, nor is a positive test result proof that Lyme is present; it indicates only that at some point in the past a person was infected with *Bb* and created antibodies to fight it.[6]

### Conventional Testing Methods

The most common conventional testing methods used to diagnose Lyme disease fall into two categories: antibody and direct detection.

Antibody tests include the enzyme-linked immunosorbent assay (ELISA) test, an automated and standardized procedure that uses enzymes to detect *Bb* antibodies. Some laboratories employ an ELISA "capture test," which uses two different methods to detect *Bb* antibodies and is considered more sensitive than the more commonly available version of the ELISA test.

The indirect fluorescent antibody (IFA) test was the original test used to diagnose Lyme disease, and it is still used by some labs despite its high risk of error. In this test, fluorescent dye is added to a slide containing a blood sample mixed with a dead *Bb* specimen. The slide is then placed under a microscope under fluorescent or ultraviolet light. If a green color appears, it is considered a positive reading.

With both the ELISA and IFA tests, a positive reading usually results in a follow-up Western Blot test. In this test, a strand of *Bb* is fragmented by the use of detergent, then the mixture is applied to a side of a gelatinous strip and receives a charge of electrical current, which causes the *Bb* specimen to further fragment and separate according to weight. A reagent (a substance used to detect the presence of another substance) is then applied to check for the presence of *Bb* antibodies.

Other antibody tests include the Borreliacidal antibody test (BAT), the immune complex test, the prevue test, and the C6 Lyme peptide test.

Direct detection testing methods include culturing, staining, antigen tests, and the PCR test already mentioned.

### Unreliable Testing

Most standard conventional tests used to detect Lyme are notoriously unreliable, according to Dr. Harris. "The initial thing patients usually get is a Western Blot antibody test," he points out. "This test is not positive immediately after *Bb* exposure, and only 60% or 70% of people ever show antibodies to *Bb*. Unfortunately, the CDC five-band criteria [checking for a limited number of antibody types] became the standard for the Western Blot. We go beyond this criteria, as do some other labs."

Dr. Cowden favors two tests developed, respectively, by Dr. Whitaker and Lida Mattman, Ph.D., director of the Nelson Medical Research Institute in Warren, Michigan. However, neither of these tests has as yet won FDA approval for diagnostic use. "We have developed the Rapid

> When a person is sick, antibodies get tied up in the tissues, in what is called an immune complex, and are not detected in the patient's blood plasma. So it's not that the antibody isn't there or hasn't been produced, it just isn't detectable. Thus, the tests that are based on detecting antibodies give false negatives.
> — *Lida Mattman, Ph.D.*

Identification of Bb (RIBb) test in order to more effectively screen for Lyme disease," Dr. Whitaker says. "During the RIBb test, a highly purified fluorescent antibody stain specific for *Bb* is used to detect the organism. This test provides results in 20 to 30 minutes, a key to getting the right treatment started quickly."

The test developed by Dr. Mattman is a culture test that also uses a fluorescent antibody staining technique, which allows her to study live cultures under a fluorescent microscope. "When a person is sick," says Dr. Mattman, "antibodies get tied up in the tissues, in what is called an immune complex, and are not detected in the patient's blood plasma. So it's not that the antibody isn't there or hasn't been produced, it just isn't detectable. Thus, the tests that are based on detecting antibodies give false negatives." Both tests used and developed by Drs. Whitaker and Mattman do not look for antibodies but rather for the organism, in the same way that tuberculosis is diagnosed.

### A Master of Elusiveness

There are several reasons why Lyme is so difficult to test for and difficult to treat. In addition to the fact that the bull's-eye EM rash that is characteristic of Lyme disease appears in only 30% to 40% of infected adults and in only 10% of children, Lyme can rapidly disseminate throughout the body. In its classic spirochete form, the *Bb* bacteria can contract like a large muscle and twist to propel itself forward. Moreover, because of this spring-like action it can actually swim better in tissue than in blood. It can also travel through blood vessel walls and through connective tissue. Animal studies have shown that in less than a week after the host is infected, the Lyme spirochete can be deeply embedded inside tendons, muscle, the heart, and the brain. It invades tissue, replicating and destroying its host cell as it emerges. Sometimes the cell wall collapses around the bacterium, forming a cloaking device, allowing it to

> No currently available test, no matter the source or type, is definitive in ruling out infection with the pathogens associated with Lyme disease or determining whether these infections are responsible for the patient's symptoms. The entire clinical picture must be taken into account, including a search for concurrent conditions, alternative diagnoses, and other reasons for some of the presenting complaints. Often, much of the diagnostic process in late, disseminated Lyme involves ruling out other illnesses and defining the extent of damage that might require separate evaluation and treatment.
>
> — *Joseph Burrascano, Jr., M.D.*

evade detection by many diagnostic tests, as well as by the body's immune system.

But the main reason that Lyme is so resistant to detection and therapy is that it is pleomorphic, meaning it can radically change form. "We have examined blood samples from over 800 patients whose Lyme disease was clinically diagnosed with the RIBb test and we have rarely seen *Bb* in anything but a cell wall deficient (CWD) form," Dr. Whitaker reports. "In addition, we have found *Bb* in urine, EDTA blood, spinal fluid, eye fluid, finger joint fluid, shoulder fluid, semen, breast milk, extracted teeth, tonsils, and adenoids. The problem is that a CWD organism doesn't have a fixed exterior membrane presenting information—a target—that would allow our immune systems or drugs to attack it, or allow most current tests to detect it." Dr. Mattman points out that *Bb*, as a CWD organism, is extremely diverse in its appearance, its activity, and its vulnerability. Dr. Cowden adds, "Because *Bb* is very pleomorphic, you can't expect any one antibiotic to be effective. Also, bacteria share genetic material with one another, so the offspring of the next bug can have a new genetic sequence that can resist the antibiotic."

### The Clinical Diagnosis: Key to Effective Treatment

Although alternative medicine physicians who treat Lyme disease all have their own testing preferences, they all agree that Lyme disease is a clinical diagnosis for which testing and retesting can add support, but not provide a definitive result one way or the other.

"We look at the patient's history and symptoms, genetic tendencies,

# A Symptom Checklist for Lyme Disease

Because Lyme disease is so often misdiagnosed, it can often be confused with other disease conditions. Or it can go undiagnosed altogether, leaving sufferers in the dark about their symptoms and not knowing how to get relief. The following symptom checklist, created by Joseph Burrascano, Jr., M.D., a specialist in the integrative treatment of Lyme disease, can help patients and their physicians make a more accurate diagnosis. The checklist is not meant to be used as definite diagnostic criteria, but it can be helpful in determining whether Lyme disease is present. The more Yes answers a patient marks on the checklist, the more likely it is that Lyme is indeed involved.

## RISK PROFILE (Check all that apply)

Tick-infested area__ Frequent outdoor activities__ Hiking __ Fishing __
Camping __ Gardening __ Hunting __ Ticks noted on pets __
Do you remember being bitten by a tick? No__ Yes__ When? ____
Do you remember having the "bull's-eye" rash? No__ Yes__
Any other rash? No__ Yes__

Have you had any of the following symptoms? Circle the number for all Yes answers:

1. Unexplained fevers, night or day sweats, chills, or flushing
2. Unexplained weight change (loss or gain)
3. Fatigue, tiredness, poor stamina
4. Unexplained hair loss
5. Swollen glands (list areas_____)
6. Sore throat
7. Testicular pain/pelvic pain
8. Unexplained menstrual irregularity
9. Unexplained milk production; breast pain
10. Irritable bladder or bladder dysfunction
11. Sexual dysfunction or loss of libido
12. Upset stomach
13. Change in bowel function (constipation, diarrhea)
14. Chest pain or rib soreness
15. Shortness of breath, cough
16. Heart palpitations, pulse skips, heart block
17. Any history of a heart murmur or valve prolapse
18. Joint pain or swelling (list joints_____)
19. Stiffness of the joints, neck, or back
20. Muscle pain or cramps
21. Twitching of the face or other muscles
22. Headache

*(continued)*

## A Symptom Checklist for Lyme Disease *(continued)*

23. Neck creaking and cracking, neck stiffness, neck pain
24. Tingling, numbness, burning or stabbing sensations, shooting pains
25. Facial paralysis (Bell's palsy)
26. Eyes/Vision: double, blurry, increased floaters, light sensitivity
27. Ears/Hearing: buzzing, ringing, ear pain, sound sensitivity
28. Increased motion sickness, vertigo, poor balance
29. Lightheadedness, wooziness
30. Tremor
31. Confusion, difficulty in thinking
32. Difficulty with concentration, reading
33. Forgetfulness, poor short-term memory
34. Disorientation: getting lost, going to wrong places
35. Difficulty with speech, vocalization, or writing; word block
36. Mood swings, irritability, depression
37. Disturbed sleep—too much, too little, fractionated, early awakening
38. Exaggerated symptoms or worse hangover from alcohol

*Source:* Burrascano, Joseph. *Advanced Topics in Lyme Disease: Diagnostic Hints and Treatment Guidelines for Lyme and Other Tick Borne Illnesses*, 13th ed. (May 2000). Available from East End Medical Associates, P.C., 139 Springs Fireplace Road, East Hampton, NY 11937; tel: (631) 324–7337.

metabolism, past immune function problems or infection, as well as history and duration of antibiotic treatment, co-infection, nutritional and micronutritional status, and also psychospiritual factors," explains Steven Bock, M.D., who, with his brother Kenneth Bock, M.D., founded the Centers for Progressive Medicine in Albany and Rhinebeck, New York. Dr. Cowden also employs muscle testing and electrodermal screening (EDS), while Dr. Burrascano has developed a weighted list of diagnostic criteria and an exhaustive symptom checklist. (SEE SIDEBAR.) "No currently available test, no matter the source or type, is definitive in ruling out infection with the pathogens associated with Lyme disease, or whether these infections are responsible for the patient's symptoms," Dr. Burrascano says. "The entire clinical picture must be taken into account, including a search for concurrent conditions, alternative diagnoses, and other reasons for some of the presenting complaints. Often, much of the diagnostic process in late,

For more on **electrodermal screening**, see chapter 2.

## Lyme Disease and Heart Problems

One of the less commonly recognized traits of Lyme disease is that it can cause cardiovascular illness, due to the fact that it affects multiple systems in the body. According to Philip W. Paparone, D.O., director of the Lyme Disease Center for South Jersey in Absecon, New Jersey, patients with unexplained cardiac symptoms who live in regions with a high incidence of Lyme disease should be screened to see if they have been infected with the Bb pathogen.

"The potentially fatal cardiac involvement of Lyme disease remains the least-well-documented complication of this complex, multisystem illness, which often presents with nonspecific signs and symptoms," Dr. Paparone notes. "Although significant advances have been made in our understanding and management of the disease, its cardiovascular manifestations have not yet been fully elucidated."[a] Published research indicates that 8% to 10% of reported Lyme disease cases involve symptoms of cardiac illness,[b] but Dr. Paparone believes that the percentage may be higher due to how easily Lyme disease can go undetected.[c]

Heart conditions due to Lyme disease are known as Lyme carditis. Originally, researchers who observed the link between the two conditions believed that Lyme carditis was both mild and self-limiting, but today it is understood that it is far more serious: it can cause permanent heart damage and even death. "Therefore, physicians who care for patients with Lyme disease must carefully consider the possibility of cardiac involvement," Dr. Paparone says. "The necessity of differential diagnosis in all cases of unclear myocarditis and cardiac arrhythmia in patients living in, or exposed to, areas endemic for Lyme disease should be recognized." He also points out that failure to identify Lyme disease as the cause of heart block can lead to the unnecessary use of permanent pacemakers, as well as permanent heart damage.[d]

What follows is a checklist of the full range of cardiovascular symptoms that can be caused by Lyme disease.[e] Patients who suffer from any of these symptoms for undetermined reasons are advised to consider a clinical diagnosis of Lyme disease.

- **Conduction systems symptoms**—1st, 2nd, and 3rd degree atrioventricular block; Wenckebach periodicity; left, right, and/or fluctuating bundle-branch block; sinus node dysfunction; atrial fibrillation; ventricular ectopy.

- **Other cardiac disease**—cardiomyopathy; cardiac failure; myocarditis/pericarditis; pancarditis; atrial and ventricular tachycardias; cardiomegaly.

- **Other symptoms**—palpitations; syncope; chest pain; shortness of breath; exertional dyspnea; dizziness; fatigue.

---

[a] Paparone, P. W. "Cardiovascular manifestations of Lyme disease." JAOA 97:3 (March, 1997), 156–161.
[b] Vlay, S. C. "Cardiac manifestations of Lyme disease." Pract. Cardiol. 16 (1990), 83–88.
[c] Paparone, P. W. "Cardiovascular manifestations of Lyme disease." JAOA 97:3 (March, 1997), 156–161.
[d] Ibid.
[e] Ibid.

disseminated Lyme involves ruling out other illnesses and defining the extent of damage that might require separate evaluation and treatment."

"In pediatric screening, especially," says Dr. Jones, "we ask about sudden, sometimes subtle, changes in behavior or cognitive function—such as losing skills or losing the ability to learn new material; not wanting to play or go outside; running a fever; or being sensitive to light or noise. If one has joint phenomena, we know that an inflammatory or infectious process is present. Another hallmark of Lyme is fatigue unrelieved by rest."

For women, Dr. Barkley has found that testing around the time of menses increases the probability of discovering the presence of *Bb*. "Women with Lyme disease have an exacerbation of their symptoms around menses," she explains. "Estrogen stimulates an inflammatory response, and progesterone opposes this effect of estrogen in addition to stimulating antibody synthesis. It is the decline in both of these hormones at the end of the menstrual cycle that is associated with worsening of Lyme symptoms."

## Preventing Lyme Disease

Given how often it escapes detection, and how difficult it is to treat once it is detected, when it comes to Lyme disease, the maxim "an ounce of prevention is worth a pound of cure" most definitely applies. To improve your ability to avoid Lyme disease, it is important that you heed the following guidelines, released in 1998 by the U.S. Department of Health and Human Services, especially during the months of May through September, the time of year in which most infections occur.

- Avoid tick-infested areas.
- When outdoors, wear light-colored clothing so ticks are clearly visible. Smooth materials such as windbreakers are harder for ticks to latch onto and are therefore preferable to clothing such as knits.
- Wear long-sleeved shirts, pants, and a hat, and closed shoes and socks. Be sure to tuck pant legs into socks or boots, and tuck shirts into pants.
- Apply insect repellent to pants, socks, shoes, and exposed skin.
- Walk in the center of nature trails to avoid overgrown grass and brush.
- After being outdoors in tick-infested areas, remove, wash, and dry clothing.
- Inspect your body thoroughly and carefully remove any attached ticks. Also check pets for ticks.
- If you find a tick, tug gently but firmly with blunt tweezers near the head of the tick until it releases its hold on the skin. Grasp the tick as close to the skin as possible and pull straight out. To

reduce the risk of infection, try not to crush the tick's body or to handle the tick with bare fingers. Don't attempt to dislodge ticks using heat or chemicals, as this can cause them to inject more pathogens into your skin.

- Swab the bite area thoroughly with an antiseptic to prevent bacterial infection.

## Additional Precautionary Measures

Dr. Burrascano offers additional suggestions for protecting yourself from tick bites:[7]

**Property:** Remove wood piles, rock walls, and bird feeders, as these attract tick-carrying small animals and can therefore increase the risk of Lyme infection.

Property should be treated with Damminix, which consists of cardboard tubes containing cotton balls that have been dipped in insecticide. Lace the tubes around wooded areas and below shrubs. "Mice, which are a key link in the propagation of Lyme disease, find the cotton and bring it back to their burrows to be used as nesting material, with the result being a big decrease in the number of ticks in the area," Dr. Burrascano explains.

Unfortunately, after two years the tick population may once again increase, as other small animals that do not gather cotton become tick hosts. Therefore, according to Dr. Burrascano, the use of Damminix alone is not sufficient. He recommends that it be used in conjunction with liquid or granular insecticides—such as Tempo®, permethrin, and sevin—all of which are available in liquid concentrate or granule form. "If liquid insecticides are used, application should be by fogging, not by coarse sprays," Dr. Burrascano says. "Apply these products in a strip a few feet wide at the perimeter of the lawn at any areas adjacent to woods and underbrush. Also treat any ornamental shrubs near the house that may serve as a habitat for small animals. The best time to apply these products is in late spring and early fall."

**Clothing:** Tick repellents that contain permethrin, such as Permanone® and Permakill, can be sprayed directly onto clothing. "Spray your clothes before you put them on, and let them dry first," Dr. Burrascano instructs. "But do not apply permethrin products to the skin."

Since ticks have a low tolerance for being dried out, after being outdoors in a tick-infested area, Dr. Burrascano recommends placing your clothes in a dryer for a few minutes to kill any ticks that may still be present.

*Skin:* "Insect repellents that contain DEET are somewhat effective when applied to the arms, legs, and around the neck," Dr. Burrascano says. "But do not use any type of repellent over wide areas of the body, since it can be absorbed into the skin, causing toxicity. Also, it is inadvisable to use a product that contains more than 50% DEET, and 25% concentrations are preferred. Use repellents cautiously on small children, as they are more susceptible to their toxic effects, and be aware that these repellents evaporate quickly and must be reapplied frequently. Finally, check carefully for ticks not only when you get home, but frequently while you are still outside."

## Treating Lyme Disease

Treating Lyme disease effectively, especially cases in which the *Bb* pathogen has disseminated throughout the body, involves a comprehensive, knowledgeable approach that integrates the best of both conventional and alternative medicine. Alternative medicine physicians agree that the primary treatment for Lyme disease is antibiotics. They caution, however, that the accepted "standard" antibiotic therapies (of a duration and type acceptable to insurance carriers, HMOs, mainstream physicians, and so on) are insufficient.

"The initial common treatment for people with Lyme disease is two to four weeks of antibiotics therapy," Dr. Whitaker points out. "Unfortunately, that is often not enough. Treatment should be holistic. There should be proper diagnosis to identify the form of *Bb* and to determine whether co-infections are present and, if so, what type. Because we rarely find spirochetes, but we do find cell wall deficient (CWD) forms that hide in immune complexes." In cases where CWDs are involved, Dr. Whitaker adds that the antibiotic of choice must be specific to the cell wall deficient organisms, and it must be able to penetrate through the blood brain barrier or whatever area of the body is affected.

Lyme is sometimes classified as having different stages—early versus chronic, or localized versus disseminated. "The biggest distinction is between early-stage and chronic," Dr. Whitaker says. "In the beginning, many organ systems are invaded while the patient may experience no symptoms. As time goes on we see multiple system symptoms involving the whole body, especially the central and peripheral nervous systems, and the musculoskeletal, skin, and circulatory systems. Many Lyme cases are diagnosed by psychiatrists, a number of whom are studying cognitive and other neuropsychiatric manifestations."

The problem with conventional treatment approaches, according to Dr. Barkley, is that "There isn't an adequate treatment model. So if the physician says you have Lyme and gives you the standard antibiotic therapy, and you aren't better, the thinking is that you must have something else wrong, such as an autoimmune problem, or else you didn't have Lyme disease in the first place. Short-term oral antibiotics are effective in treating localized Lyme, but with disseminated Lyme, the requirement for either intravenously administered antibiotics or long-term oral antibiotics becomes common."

According to Dr. Bock, proper treatment depends on the stage of the disease, and on how the patient responds to it. "The patient's response to each step of treatment determines how I proceed in each subsequent step," he says. "For instance, if a patient has a Herxheimer reaction [caused by rapid die-off of pathogens and/or toxins in the body] three weeks into treatment, it's my experience that he or she requires additional antibiotic treatment for five or six more weeks." Dr. Bock waits until his patients go five to six weeks without symptoms, or at least achieve an acceptable level of symptoms, before he ends antibiotic treatment, in order to minimize the chances of a relapse. In some cases, however, even after three months of antibiotic treatment, symptoms can recur despite no evidence of further tick bites or other new *Bb* exposure.

In his regular practice treating non-Lyme cases, Dr. Bock tries to avoid using antibiotics. But, he says, "If you go back to syphilis, the history of spirochetes is one of being able to hide out and then reappear, causing severe, devastating neurological illness. This isn't a risk I would recommend taking with *Bb*."

Most physicians recommend an immediate short course of antibiotics for anyone bitten by a deer tick, or who exhibits certain symptoms. "It takes a while for the immune system to produce antibodies," says Dr. Barkley. "So Lyme testing—other than by a skin biopsy from an active rash within 14 days following the bite—may yield inconclusive results. Symptoms of Lyme include fever, night sweats, fatigue, or a flu-like illness that does not improve within three to five days." Other symptoms reported by physicians include stiff neck, prolonged joint and muscle pain, heart palpitations, brain fog, or severe headaches.

"I make a tally of all the initial symptoms and signs and try to weed them out one by one," says Dr. Jones. However, he cautions, "Treatment duration varies with each individual. If one stops antibiotics prematurely, a more resilient *Bb* infection will develop that will cause more brain and body injury."

## Types of Antibiotic Treatments and the Challenges They Present

A wide range of antibiotic drugs are now used to treat Lyme disease, with the medications being chosen according to patients' specific symptoms. The more complete a patient's clinical diagnosis is, the more effective the medication is likely to be, although treatment failure is not uncommon even in cases of thorough diagnosis if *Bb* infection is in the later stages of dissemination—especially if conventional medications are used exclusively, without addressing other cofactors that may be involved in the patient's illness.

Antibiotics can be administered orally, intramuscularly, or intravenously, depending on the severity of the disease. When Lyme disease is detected early, prior to dissemination, oral antibiotics are usually employed, typically for up to four weeks, and in the majority of these types of cases this is enough to achieve remission. Success or failure depends on a number of factors, including when treatment begins, the strength and amount of *Bb* that has been disseminated in the body, the areas of the body in which infestation occurs, and the potency of the antibiotic in comparison to the sensitivity of the strain of *Bb* that it is treating. Cell wall deficient strains of *Bb*, for example, cannot be killed by cell wall–activated antibiotics. In addition, according to Vanderhoof-Forschner, "Researchers in Slovenia and Italy have proven *Bb* can revert to a cyst form, in order to survive a hostile environment, only to reemerge later as viable spirochetes."[8]

The antibiotics most commonly used to treat Lyme disease are tetracyclines, penicillins, cephalosporins, and macrolides.

The tetracycline class of antibiotics include doxycycline and minocycline, both of which are absorbed to a high degree by an empty stomach and able to penetrate into the cells and be distributed through the body. Tetracyclines work by inhibiting bacteria's ability to reproduce and, in higher dosages, by killing bacteria. They are not recommended for children under the age of eight, or for pregnant or breast-feeding women, and should also be avoided by people who spend a great deal of time outside, because they can greatly increase the risk of severe sunburn. Other potential side effects, according to Vanderhoof-Forschner, include yeast infections, rash, gastrointestinal disorders, nausea, and vomiting. Certain individuals may also develop liver or kidney disorders, and tetracyclines can also cause burning sensations in the eyes. Vanderhoof-Forschner also cautions that patients taking tetracyclines should avoid

# Managing Yeast Infections

According to Joseph Burrascano, Jr., M.D., "Many patients with Lyme disease develop an overgrowth of yeast. Therefore, it is recommended that on a daily basis the patient eat a full container of yogurt that contains active cultures and take acidophilus supplements (two capsules after each meal)."

What follows are further recommendations by Dr. Burrascano for controlling yeast overgrowth.

**Mouth:** Yeast infection manifests in the tongue as thrush, signs of which include bad breath, beige coating of the tongue, and dysgeusia, a condition in which the sense of taste becomes impaired or normal pleasant food tastes become unpleasant or completely different from normal. To manage oral thrush, Dr. Burrascano recommends using antiseptic mouthwashes. "Whenever the patient brushes their teeth, they must brush the tongue, using the antiseptic mouthwash, followed by thorough rinsing," he says. "Because the effectiveness of a mouthwash is related to how long it is in contact with the germs, it should be kept in the mouth while brushing."

Dr. Burrascano also recommends that patients avoid all simple carbohydrates, starches, fruits, and juices for at least two weeks, or until the problem is gone, because yeast germs feed on sugars. Anti-yeast prescription medications may also be necessary. If so, he recommends Nystatin oral powder (not liquid), which can be mixed with water to be swished and swallowed. In some cases, systemic antifungal medications (Diflucan®, Lamisil®, Nizoral®) may also be necessary.

"The most effective and drastic treatment, employed as a last resort, consists of using 'Dakin's Solution' as a mouth rinse," Dr. Burrascano says. "This is a mixture of one teaspoon of household Clorox combined with four ounces of water. A small amount is held in the mouth while brushing, then spit out, and repeated until the mouth has cleared. This is usually a one-time treatment, but it may have to be repeated every few weeks."

After using an antiseptic mouthwash to clean the mouth, Dr. Burrascano says it is necessary to immediately eat yogurt, chew an acidophilus capsule, or take liquid acidophilus, to replenish the beneficial flora in the mouth. "Because the germ count after such a cleaning will be artificially reduced, and because yeasts are opportunists, they would be the first to come back," he explains. "By having yogurt or acidophilus immediately afterwards, a more normal oral flora will result and thrush will be better controlled."

**Intestinal Tract:** Yeast overgrowth in the intestinal tract leads to fermenting of dietary sugars and starches, which causes acids, gases, and alcohols to form. Symptoms include flatulence, heartburn, stomach pain, and, because of the alcohol, headaches, dizziness, lightheadedness, and/or wooziness. "To clear intestinal yeast, first the tongue and mouth must be cleared so yeast does not reenter the system with every swallow," Dr. Burrascano says. "Avoid sweets, starches, fruits, and juices for two weeks or longer to starve the germs, and eat plain yogurt or acidophilus supplements daily. Usually systemic antifungals are also needed."

**Vaginal Yeast Infection:** "Occasional vaginal yeast infections can be controlled with products such as Monistat® cream or suppositories," Dr. Burrascano says. "If it is a recurrent or ongoing problem, then it often reflects a simultaneous intestinal infection that reinfects the genital area with every bowel movement. Therefore, follow the measures for treating intestinal yeast infection, and apply topical preparations such as Monistat concurrently for two weeks."

---

Source: Burrascano, Joseph. *Advanced Topics in Lyme Disease: Diagnostic Hints and Treatment Guidelines for Lyme and Other Tick Borne Illnesses*, 13th ed. (May 2000). Available from East End Medical Associates, P.C., 139 Springs Fireplace Road, East Hampton, NY 11937; tel: (631) 324-7337.

dairy products, antacids, and iron supplements, as these interfere with the drugs' absorption.[9]

The forms of penicillin most commonly used to treat Lyme disease are amoxicillin, penicillin G (administered intravenously), and benzathine penicillin G (Bicillin), which is typically used intramuscularly. Common side effects, according to Vanderhoof-Forschner, include yeast overgrowth, rash, nausea, fever, and joint swelling. In some individuals, lowered white blood cell count can also result, and on rare occasions penicillin use can be fatal, due to allergy.[10]

The cephalosporin class of antibiotics consists of cefuroxime axetil (administered orally), cefotaxime, and ceftriaxone (both administered intravenously). Cefuroxime axetil was the first drug ever to be approved by the Food and Drug Administration (FDA) for the treatment of Lyme disease, and it is proven to be effective against early *Bb* infection. Side effects associated with these drugs include yeast overgrowth, rash, and diarrhea, and ceftriaxone can also cause gallstones. Like penicillin, cephalosporins can also be life-threatening to people who are allergic to them.[11]

The class of antibiotics known as macrolides include azythromycin and clarithromycin, both of which are administered orally. Common side effects caused by both drugs include rash, cramps, nausea, diarrhea, and vomiting. In some instances, they can also cause liver damage, elevated white cell counts, and temporary hearing loss.[12]

### Supportive Alternative Therapies

While alternative medicine physicians agree that antibiotic therapy should be the first line of defense in treating Lyme disease, they do not rely on antibiotics alone; they also focus on immune system–strengthening protocols, as well as lifestyle changes, and educating their patients about how to more effectively cope with the stress associated with their condition. Therapies employed by alternative medicine physicians to support antibiotic therapy for Lyme disease include the following:

*Diet:* Avoid alcohol and all sugars, because they feed the bacteria associated with Lyme disease and can also contribute to yeast overgrowth.

For more on **food allergies**, see chapter 9.

For more on **enyzme deficiencies**, see chapter 8.

As previously mentioned, Dr. Burrascano also recommends avoiding excessive caffeine intake and advises that plain yogurt containing active cultures should be eaten every day, along with two acidophilus capsules after each meal, to replenish the gastrointestinal tract with healthy intestinal flora, which are killed by antibiotics. Dr. Cowden adds that identifying your metabolic type and eating accordingly can also help, as can increasing your intake of alkaline foods (most green vegetables, complex grains, almonds, yams, lentils, squash), which helps to maintain proper pH balance. Identifying food allergies is also important, as is supplementation with digestive enzymes.

*Nutritional Therapy:* Proper nutritional supplementation can help bolster immune function, which Lyme disease impairs and which can be further compromised by the use of antibiotics. "Studies on patients with chronic Lyme disease have demonstrated that some of the late symptoms are related to cellular damage and deficiencies in certain essential nutrients," Dr. Burrascano says. Among those nutrients proven by double-blinded, placebo-controlled studies to be of value to patients with Lyme disease are essential fatty acids (EFAs), B complex vitamins, magnesium, and coenzyme Q10, as well as a daily multivitamin supplement.[13]

"Studies show that when EFAs are taken regularly, statistically significant improvements in fatigue, aches, weakness, vertigo, dizziness, memory, concentration, and depression are likely," Dr. Burrascano says.[14] Sources of EFAs include omega-3 and omega-6 oils, fish oil, black currant seed oil, and borage oil.

According to Dr. Burrascano, supplementing with B complex vitamins is useful for dealing with the neurological symptoms of Lyme disease. He recommends taking one 50-mg capsule of B complex vitamins daily.

Coenzyme Q10 (coQ10) helps improve stamina, energy levels, resistance to infection, and heart function. Dr. Burrascano recommends taking 200 to 300 mg of standard brand coQ10 daily, in two or three equal doses. "The body will manufacture its own coQ10 when the original infection is controlled, but only if stimulated by aggressive exercise," he says. "Therefore, use this supplement until you are feeling well and exercising regularly." He cautions, however, that patients taking the medication atovaquone (Mepron®) should not take coQ10.[15]

Magnesium is helpful for relieving the headaches, tremors, twitches, cramps, muscle soreness, general weakness, and heart strain caused by Lyme disease, and it can also aid in improving energy levels and cognition. Dr. Burrascano recommends magnesium supplements be taken every 12 hours in the form of magnesium L-lactate dihydrate. "Do not rely on calcium plus magnesium combination supplements, as they are not well absorbed," he says, adding that in some cases intramuscular or intravenous doses of magnesium may be necessary.[16]

Dr. Bock also recommends vitamin C, calcium pantothenate, vitamin B1, biotin, inositol, and the amono acid L-carnitine (for cognitive enhancement). To further boost immunity, Dr. Cowden suggests Thymic Protein A (to enhance thymus gland function), glyconutrients, and the immune-enhancing polysaccharide arabinogalactan (Larix™). He also cautions that vitamin C and grape seed extract can interfere with the tissue uptake of antibiotics, making them less effective.

When using nutritional supplements, "the quality, potency, purity, and bioavailability are often more important than the dose," Dr. Burrascano says. "Megadoses are not recommended. Instead, seek out pharmaceutical-grade supplements wherever possible."[17]

*Herbal Medicine:* Although herbal medicine is best administered under the guidance of a professional trained in their use, the following herbs can be used safely as part of a self-care protocol. For general immune support, Dr. Bock recommends astragalus, ginseng, and maitake and reishi mushrooms, along with milk thistle to support liver function. *Ginkgo biloba* and other herbs can also be used to improve cognitive ability.

Dr. Burrascano also recommends cordyceps, an herb famed in Tibet for its ability to improve stamina and energy levels, reduce fatigue, and enhance lung and antioxidant function. In addition, according to Dr. Burrascano, "It is the only compound known to raise superoxide dismutase (SOD) activity. Although the use of cordyceps is optional, the effects can be so dramatic that I strongly urge all people with fatigue to use it long-term."[18]

*Stress Reduction:* Because stress diminishes immunity and energy levels, it is essential that people with Lyme disease learn how to effectively manage stress levels. Dr. Whitaker advises regular periods of rest, and Dr. Bock advises patients to use relaxation techniques, guided imagery and visualization, and biofeedback. He also recommends joining a support group. Breath work, flower essence therapy, meditation, prayer, and counseling can also be effective in helping to minimize stress.

For more on **herbal medicine**, see chapter 12.

For more about **stress relief**, see chapter 11.

*Lifestyle Changes:* "It is most important to balance saliva pH between 6.7 and 7.0," advises Dr. Cowden. "Sufficient dietary minerals bring pH up if it is low. Reducing stress will help balance pH, as will identifying and removing food, nutrient, and inhalant allergies."

Dr. Bock adds, "It's also important to support the endocrine system. In some cases, cognitive abilities improved when subclinical hypothyroid problems were treated. Chronic stress can cause suppression of the immune system. To better manage the effects of stress on the body, use relaxation techniques and biofeedback, and find a group for emotional support."

In his practice, Dr. Jones has found that Lyme disease patients tend to need to develop a healthier standard of living and get plenty of rest. "We've found that a parent who has a child with Lyme is often feeling guilty," he adds. "One has to work with these difficult feelings. I try to emphasize that it's not a parent's fault; you can't protect your child from Lyme exposure."

*Acupuncture:* Acupuncture combined with physical therapy can reduce the pain associated with Lyme disease, help detoxify the body, and bolster immune function.

*Bowen Therapy:* Bowen therapy, due to its ability to balance and restore proper functioning of the autonomic nervous system, can be very effective in relieving the symptoms of Lyme disease, according to Dr. Whitaker.

*Oxygen Therapy:* Oxidative therapy (ozone) and intravenous hydrogen peroxide therapy, two aspects of oxygen therapy, can both be extremely useful in dealing with chronic Lyme disease cases, according to Dr. Bock. When treating such cases, he also employs photo-ox therapy, a combination of IV hydrogen peroxide or ozone and ultraviolet blood irradiation (UVB); he finds that UVB is very effective in treating persistent microbial infections.

*Transfer Factor:* Both Drs. Whitaker and Cowden recommend antigen-specific transfer factor when dealing with chronic Lyme disease cases.

 For more on **Bowen therapy**, see chapter 14.

For more on **transfer factors**, see chapter 3.

## Lyme Disease Rehabilitation

As Dr. Burrascano points out, "Even with successful treatment, chronic Lyme disease patients will not return to normal unless they pursue a formal program of therapeutic exercise." In the late stages of the disease, he adds, patients experience muscle atrophy, increases in fat content as a percentage of overall body weight, elevated cholesterol levels, and a less favorable balance between HDL ("good') and LDL ("bad") cholesterol. Weakening of the heart muscle also occurs, as does joint, tendon, and nerve pain. A high percentage of patients also experience significant weight gain.

"Because of the extreme fatigue and body pain, many Lyme sufferers end up spending inordinate amounts of time in bed and get far less exercise than they did before they became ill," Dr. Burrascano adds. "This begins a debilitating downward spiral that can be very difficult to reverse. As a result, Lyme patients are stiff, weak, and tired, have poor stamina, and are at increased risk for cardiovascular disease and diabetes. Antibiotic treatment alone cannot correct these effects. Therefore, it is necessary to prescribe physical therapy, the extent of which depends on an individual's condition, followed by a graded exercise program."

In the initial phase of rehabilitation, Dr. Burrascano recommends multiple physical therapies, including massage, heat, TENS, and ultrasound treatments, to relieve pain and muscle spasms, and aggressive range-of-motion exercises, supervised by a physical therapist, to relieve stiffness. "The goal of physical therapy is to prepare the patient for the required gym-based exercise program," he says. "This starts with stretching and mild muscular toning—light calisthenics and weight lifting. Then, the program must expand to include muscular conditioning and strengthening, ideally under the supervision of a credentialed exercise physiologist. Aerobic exercises are not recommended, not even the low-impact variety, until the patient has fully recovered. Patients should exercise no more than every other day, for one hour each session. If the patient is unable to continue for the whole hour, then the program can be modified to decrease its intensity so that he or she can continue for the entire 60 minutes."[19]

## Success Story: Overcoming Lyme Disease Using Integrative Medicine

According to the American Lyme Disease Foundation, Lyme disease is "almost always readily curable," usually with a four-week course of an oral antibiotic, provided the treatment is begun early in the disease process. The problem with Lyme disease, however, is how diversely it can manifest symptoms, compounded by the fact that the laboratory tests for identifying the presence of the *Bb* pathogen associated with Lyme are largely unreliable, so that doctors often miss the diagnosis. Dr. Bock, who has treated Lyme disease for over a decade using an integrative approach that combines both conventional and alternative methods, agrees that antibiotics are needed.

"Although in our practice we don't particularly like antibiotics, I've never seen anyone who didn't need them to kill the *Bb* pathogen," Dr. Bock says. "But there are so many variations of Lyme and you often get a mixture of problems. Sometimes it's hard to sort out whether you need antibiotics or immune support, or a combination." Knowing how to make that determination can make all the difference, as is illustrated in the following case history involving one of Dr. Bock's patients.

Ada, 35, came to Dr. Bock "devastated" by her Lyme disease symptoms, which included fatigue and joint pain. Due to a tick bite seven years earlier, which produced vertigo, fatigue, headaches, joint pain, and mental confusion, Ada had been treated with antibiotics and initially achieved a remission. But then stress brought on by job pressures caused her symptoms to recur. She was placed on a heavy antibiotic regimen, which again subdued her symptoms, but two years later she had another recurrence, requiring yet a third round of antibiotic treatment. This time, however, Ada did not respond. In addition, the antibiotics started to damage her immune system. Her red blood cell count dropped, and when she developed heart palpitations, her doctor put her on beta-blockers, to no avail. Ada's condition continued to deteriorate. She developed mood disturbances, insomnia, and anxiety, leading her doctor to prescribe Depakote®, an anticonvulsive medication for depression, Klonopin® for her anxiety, and Restoril®, a sedative.

Before running Lyme disease tests on Ada, Dr. Bock found that she was suffering from headaches, joint aches, anxiety, depression, sleep disorders, and food and environmental sensitivities. He also determined that she had food allergies, yeast infection, and low adrenal function.

### An Illness of Cycles

According to Dr. Bock, it is difficult to determine the sequence of causes and effects in a case like Ada's. Dr. Bock could not say whether she had the allergies, yeast infections, and stress before contracting Lyme disease and these triggered it, or whether the repeated rounds of antibiotics made her vulnerable to yeast infections and then caused her diminished immune function—especially since the *Bb* pathogen has been known to lie dormant within the nervous system for up to 15 years before becoming active.

Dr. Bock points out that antibiotics are unlikely to kill off all vestiges of the *Bb* pathogen, and while they are employed they weaken the immune system at precisely the same time that it is working harder by attacking the pathogen. "This invites Lyme disease to keep coming back in cycles," he says.

Before he devised Ada's treatment, Dr. Bock ordered a series of tests, beginning with a stool sample, which confirmed her yeast infection by showing high levels of anti-*Candida* antibodies. Next, he ordered an intestinal permeability test to measure nutrient absorption or leakage from the intestines. As he explains, in cases of "leaky gut" syndrome, candidiasis (yeast infection), or intestinal inflammation, immune reactive molecules can be present in the intestinal wall, continuously activating the immune system. Ada tested positive for "leaky gut" syndrome and dysbiosis (an unfavorable ratio of disease-causing to beneficial intestinal microorganisms). A liver test revealed that Ada also had decreased glutathione (a key liver detoxifier), elevated lipid peroxides (a form of free radicals), and oxidative stress, since her liver was overwhelmed by toxins. In addition, testing to determine Ada's vitamin and mineral status revealed that she was deficient in B complex vitamins, and further allergy testing showed that she was allergic to wheat, chocolate, and citrus. Based on this information, Dr. Bock began to develop a treatment plan.

In Ada's case, Dr. Bock's plan featured an integrative blend of antibiotics, probiotics, acupuncture, Chinese herbs, nutritional medicine, bioxidative and light therapies, and psychological counseling in stress reduction.

Dr. Bock had Ada begin a course of probiotics involving supplementation with the "friendly" bacteria *Lactobacillus acidophilus* and *Bifidobacterium bifidus* to help repopulate her intestines with these much-needed microorganisms, since the rounds of antibiotic treatment she had received previously had destroyed them along with a broad spectrum of other bacteria, "good" and "bad."

Then Dr. Bock employed acupuncture to reduce Ada's anxiety levels, help her relax, and rebalance her immune system, and to first reduce, then eliminate, her need for psychiatric medications. The acupuncture treatments also helped to relieve Ada's neck and shoulder pain and headaches. Dr. Bock treated Ada with acupuncture once a week for eight weeks, addressing first her sleep problems, then her anxiety, then her immune status, and finally her pain. As progress occurred, he reduced her treatments to twice a month.

To enhance the benefits of the acupuncture treatments, Dr. Bock prescribed a blend of Chinese herbs in liquid extract form known as Comfort Shen. In Chinese medicine, *shen* refers to subtle energy attributed to the heart, both as an organ and as a meridian (energetic pathway in the body) system. "If a patient has neurological problems, is agitated, or is not sleeping well, this is regarded as a disturbance of the heart energy," Dr. Bock explains. For Ada, he also prescribed melatonin, a hormone that produces well-documented sleep-inducing effects.

In addition, Dr. Bock prescribed a diet that was yeast-free and eliminated sugars and the foods to which Ada was allergic. He also placed her on a multivitamin/multimineral supplement for general fortification; additional vitamin B1, biotin, and inositol to calm her nervous system; borage and fish oils to ensure adequate fatty acid intake; coenzyme Q10 to improve her cellular energy levels; milk thistle, an herb used to protect her liver against the liver-related side effects of antibiotics; and calcium pantothenate, along with adrenal gland extract, to tonify and support her adrenal glands. Ada also underwent vitamin C drip infusions to deal with recurrent infections and bring her immune system back into balance.

## Using Oxygen and Light to Heal

A key element of Dr. Bock's approach to reversing Ada's Lyme disease involved the use of oxidative therapy (SEE QUICK DEFINITION) and photo-ox therapy, which make use of oxygen and light, respectively. The combination of the two therapies is especially useful for chronically ill patients, according to Dr. Bock.

Oxidative therapies deliver measured amounts of powerful oxidants (highly reactive molecules involved in energy production) in the form of medical ozone or hydrogen peroxide, which stimulate healing. For example, Dr. Bock says, white blood cells will use intravenously infused hydrogen peroxide to destroy undesirable microorganisms; he adds that oxidative therapies are controversial not because they are harmful, but because they are not well understood by conventional doctors.

Photo-ox therapy refers to a process in which intravenous hydrogen peroxide or ozone is combined with ultra-

**QUICK DEFINITION**

**Oxygen therapies** involve the use of oxygen; they can be used in various forms to promote healing and to destroy pathogens in the body. Such therapies can be used to treat a variety of conditions, including cancer, infections, circulatory problems, chronic fatigue syndrome, arthritis, allergies, and multiple sclerosis.

There are two principal types of oxygen therapy, classified according to the chemical process involved. **Oxygenation** is the process of enriching the oxygen content of the blood or tissues. Employed under strictly controlled conditions, oxygenation can be highly therapeutic. **Oxidation** is a chemical reaction in which electrons (negatively charged particles) are transferred from one molecule to another. Although uncontrolled oxidation can be destructive, as in the case of free radical damage, it can also provide significant health benefits when used carefully on weak and devitalized cells.

violet blood irradiation (UVB). Together, these produce a synergistic therapeutic effect. In Ada's case, photo-ox therapy was employed as a complement to her antibiotic regimen to aid in killing the *Bb* pathogen and other harmful microorganisms. UVB appears to be highly effective in treating persistent viruses and antibiotic-resistant bacteria, according to Dr. Bock. Not only does it kill unwanted microbes, it also adds oxygen to the body, improves energy-producing activity (oxidative metabolism) at a cellular level, and elevates levels of antioxidants capable of fighting free radicals.

During photo-ox therapy, a small amount of a patient's blood (100 cc or one-half cup) is drawn from the body and exposed to ultraviolet light, which changes the molecular structure of the oxygen in the blood sample to one that is therapeutically more potent. When the irradiated blood is reintroduced into the body, the altered form of oxygen circulates throughout the body.

Ada received photo-ox treatments three times a week for five weeks, during which time Dr. Bock reduced her antibiotic intake. "When you treat Lyme disease with antibiotics in a patient with yeast infections, the *Candida* infestation worsens," he explains. "But when you use oxidative therapies, you can subdue and eliminate both the Lyme bacteria and the *Candida*."

### Stress Relief: The Final Element of Ada's Treatment Program

To help Ada deal with stress, Dr. Bock referred her to his staff psychologist, Peter Kaplan, Ph.D. Dr. Kaplan taught her stress-reduction techniques, biofeedback, and visual imagery. "These are ways you can use the mind's healing power to help with the body's deficiencies," Dr. Kaplan says.

Ada was a perfectionist who operated under a high level of stress at work. The stress, in turn, affected her breathing, so that it became shallow, limited to inhalation high in her chest. Dr. Kaplan taught her how to shift the seat of her breathing to her abdomen, which both served to help keep her calm and improved her oxygen intake. He also instructed her in self-hypnosis with wellness suggestions. "I induced a trance state in Ada, then suggested she imagine a split movie screen and project an image of herself onto both sides," Dr. Kaplan recounts. "One side of the screen was Ada's sick, tired, old self; the other side displayed her as well, vital, strong, and free of Lyme disease. Then she slowly covered up and dissolved the image of her sick self with the well one." The purpose of this exercise was to plant a positive thought in Ada's subconscious mind;

> It's sad where we are with this disease. You're supposed to go through the "standard" treatment first, before turning to alternative treatments. We need to turn this around, into a logical, integrated approach. —*W. Lee Cowden, M.D.*

this would favorably influence the immune system, which, research has proven, is highly sensitive to one's state of mind.

Within her first month on this comprehensive treatment plan, Ada was completely off all psychiatric medications, and within three months she was also off all antibiotics and well on her way to a full recovery. Soon thereafter, she went through the stress and pressure of buying a house and handling all the business transactions, an activity she admits she could not have dreamed of conducting before Dr. Bock's treatments. Today, not only is Ada recovered from Lyme disease, she also reports that she now has the tools—the alternative medicine therapies Dr. Bock introduced her to—to rely on when the pressures of life and work temporarily impact her well-being.

## The Future of Treating Lyme Disease

No health expert claims to completely understand Lyme disease, nor has any physician—conventional or alternative—been able to completely cure it in every case. By its very nature, Lyme disease remains a mysterious illness. Some people infected with the *Bb* pathogen may never manifest the symptoms of Lyme, while others become seriously ill soon after they are infected. This is why alternative medicine physicians stress that treatment must be customized from patient to patient and can vary widely.

"Certain people may clear Lyme without antibiotic therapy," says Dr. Barkley. "However, the other extreme is that even with antibiotics, some people with Lyme have died from this disease." Dr. Jones adds, "We have seen children from one day old to eighteen years of age who have required from three months to six years of antibiotic therapy. We have also had some patients on antibiotic therapy for very long periods, and we've done follow-ups for as long as 15 years post-treatment. The criterion for stopping therapy is that one must be totally Lyme disease–symptom free for two months, with no Lyme flare-up induced by another infection or menses and no Herxheimer reaction caused by the body manifesting symptoms in response to dying *Bb*."

**Marylynn S. Barkley, M.D., Ph.D.**, Division of Biological Sciences, 211 Briggs Hall, University of California at Davis, Davis, CA 95616; tel: (530) 752-0203. **Steven Bock, M.D.**, Rhinebeck Health Center, 108 Montgomery Street, Rhinebeck, NY 12572; tel: (845) 876-7082. Website: www.rhinebeck-health.com. **Joseph J. Burrascano, Jr., M.D.**, 139 Springs Fireplace Road, East Hampton, NY 11937; tel: (631) 324-7337. **W. Lee Cowden, M.D.**, 1333 West Campbell, #113, Richardson, TX 75080. **Nick Harris, Ph.D.**, IgeneX, Inc., 797 San Antonio Road, Palo Alto, CA 94303; tel: (800) 832-3200. Website: www.igenex.com. **Charles Ray Jones, M.D.**, Pediatric and Adolescent Medicine and Lyme Disease, 111 Park Street, Suite F, New Haven, CT 06511; tel: (203) 772-1123. **Lida Mattman, Ph.D.**, Nelson Medical Research Institute, 11664 Martin Road, Warren, MI 48093; tel: (810) 755-6430. **Katrina Tang, M.D.**, Century Wellness Clinic, 380 Brinkby Avenue, Reno, NV 89509; tel: (775) 828-5388. Website: www.centurywellness.com. **Jo Anne Whitaker, M.D.**, Bowen Research and Training Institute, Inc., Connell Square, 38541 U.S. Highway 19 N., Palm Harbor, FL 34684; tel: (727) 937-9077. Website: www.bowen.org.

The following organizations provide further resources and information about Lyme disease: **Lyme Disease Foundation, Inc.**, One Financial Plaza, Hartford, CT 06103; tel: (860) 525-2000. 24-hour hotline tel: (800) 866-LYME. Websites: www.lyme.org, www.jstd.org. **The Lyme Disease Network**, 43 Winton Road, East Brunswick, NJ 08816. Website: www.lymenet.org. **International Lyme and Associated Diseases Society**, P.O. Box 341461, Bethesda, MD 20827; tel: (301) 263-1080. Website: www.ilads.org.

Dr. Cowden says, "It's sad where we are with this disease. You're supposed to go through the 'standard' treatment first, before turning to alternative treatments. We need to turn this around, into a logical, integrated approach."

The impetus for this change must come not only from the patients who have been classically infected by a tick bite, but by those who suffer from "unexplained" muscle and joint pain, unrelieved fatigue, and cognitive impairment—and by those who are afflicted with degenerative diseases that can be caused or aggravated by Lyme disease. Presently, such patients will find few doctors experienced in the comprehensive treatment of Lyme disease, because of the newness and lack of understanding of the disease—and because those doctors who take such a comprehensive approach to diagnosing and treating it are commonly harassed by state medical boards, insurance companies, and HMOs. Therefore, it is up to the patients to actually educate their conventional doctors about the inadequacy of standard testing and the necessity for integrating viable alternative therapies with standard antibiotic care. And it is up to the patients to become politically involved with Lyme advocacy groups, such as those listed in the sidebar, to fight for their right to proper medical care.

The earlier Lyme disease is diagnosed, the easier it is to cure, but for people with chronic Lyme symptoms, the road to recovery can be long. With a combination of the best of conventional and alternative medicine protocols, however, their health can be continually and dramatically improved.

# Endnotes

## Chapter 1. Related Epidemics

1. U.S. Centers for Disease Control. "The Facts About Chronic Fatigue Syndrome." (August 1994). Internet: http://www.cdc.gov/ncidod/diseases/cfs/info.htm#Demo.

2. Stoff, Jesse A., M.D., and Charles R. Pellegrino, Ph.D. *Chronic Fatigue Syndome: The Hidden Epidemic* (New York: HarperCollins, 1992).

3. U.S. Centers for Disease Control. "The Facts About Chronic Fatigue Syndrome." (August 1994). Internet: http://www.cdc.gov/ncidod/diseases/cfs/info.htm#Demo.

4. Ibid.

5. Krieger, Lisa M. "Alarming S.F. Study of Chronic Fatigue." *San Francisco Examiner* (October 14, 1996).

6. Fukuda, Keiji, et al. "The Chronic Fatigue Syndrome: A Comprehensive Approach to Its Definition and Study." *Annals of Internal Medicine* 121 (December 15, 1994), 953–959.

7. Teitelbaum, Jacob, M.D. *From Fatigued to Fantastic!* (Garden City Park, NY: Avery Publishing Group, 1996).

8. Goldenberg, Don, M.D. American College of Rheumatology meeting (1994). Dr. Goldenberg is chief of rheumatology at Newton-Wellesley Hospital in Newton, MA, and professor of medicine at Tufts University School of Medicine in Medford, MA.

9. Van Why, Richard P. *Fibromyalgia Syndrome and Massage Therapy: Issues and Opportunities* (self-published, 1994). Available from: Richard P. van Why, 123 East 8th Street, Frederick, MD 21701. Starlanyl, Devin, M.D., and Mary

Ellen Copeland, M.S., M.A. *Fibromyalgia and Chronic Myofascial Pain Syndrome: A Survival Manual* (Oakland, CA: New Harbinger Publications, 1996), 8.

10. National Institutes of Health. Internet: www.niaid.nih.gov/fact-sheets/cfs.htm.

## Chapter 2. Testing

1. U.S. Department of Health and Human Services. *CFS: A Pamphlet for Physicians* NIH Publication 90-484 (Washington: U.S. Department of Health and Human Services, 1990).

2. Rosenbaum, M., M.D., and M. Susser, M.D. *Solving the Puzzle of Chronic Fatigue Syndrome* (Tacoma, WA: Life Sciences Press, 1992), 44.

3. Chaitow, L. *Post Viral Fatigue Syndrome* (London: Dents, 1989).

4. Gittleman, Ann Louise. *Guess What Came to Dinner: Parasites and Your Health* (Garden City, NY: Avery Publishing Group, 1993).

5. Galland, L., M.D. *Super-Immunity for Kids* (New York: Dell Publishing, 1989).

6. Casemore, D., M.D. "Foodborne Protozoal Infection." *The Lancet* 336 (December 1990), 1427–1432.

7. Bendig, D. W., M.D. "Diagnosis of Giardiasis in Infants and Children by Endoscopic Brush Cytology." *Journal of Pediatric Gastroenterology and Nutrition* 8:2 (1989), 204–206.

8. Lapp, Charles W., M.D. "Chronic Fatigue Is a Real Disease." *North Carolina Family Physician* 43:1 (Winter 1992). Dr. Lapp collaborates with Paul Cheney, M.D., the physician who treated the first cases of CFS in Incline Village, Nevada, and has since become an international authority on the disorder.

## Chapter 3. Eliminating Viruses, Infections, Candidiasis, and Parasites

1. Rosenbaum, M., M.D., and M. Susser, M.D. *Solving the Puzzle of Chronic Fatigue Syndrome* (Tacoma, WA: Life Sciences Press, 1992).

2. Ibid.

3. Editorial. "Depression, Stress and Immunity." *The Lancet* 1:8548 (June 1987), 1467–1488.

4. Galland, L., M.D., et al. *Journal of Nutritional Medicine* 1 (1990), 27–31.

5. Ostrum, Neenyah. "LEM: Exciting News for Good Health." *The New York Native* (July 31, 1989).

6. *HealthWatch* 4:3 (Summer/Fall 1994), 6. *HealthWatch* is available from: CFIDS Buyers Club, 1187 Coast Village Road, #1-280, Santa Barbara, CA 93108; tel: (800) 366–6056.

7. Lawrence, H. S. "The cellular transfer of cutaneous hypersensitivity to tuberculin in man." *Proc. Soc. Exp. Biol. Med*, 71 (1949), 516.

8. Lawrence, H.S., and Borkowsky, W. "A new basis for the immunoregulatory activities of transfer factor—an arcane dialect in the language of cells." *Cell Immunol*, 82 (1983), 102–116.

9. Lawrence, H. S. "The cellular transfer of cutaneous hypersensitivity to tuberculin in man." *Proc. Soc. Exp. Biol. Med*, 71 (1949), 516; Kirpatrick, C. H. "Activities and characteristics of Transfer Factors." *Biotherapy* 9 (1-3) (1996), 13.

10. Harthoorn, A. M., and Lynda M. Martin. "The Homeopathic Treatment of Myalgic Encephalomyelitis (ME) Based on 219 Case Histories." *Biomedical Therapy* 15:2 (1997), 60–63.

11. Juven, B., et al. "Studies on the Mechanism of the Antimicrobial Action of Oleuropein." *Journal of Applied Bacteriology* 35 (1972), 559–567.

12. Walker, Morton, D.P.M. "Antimicrobial Attributes of Olive Leaf Extract." *Townsend Letter for Doctors & Patients* ( July 1996), 80–85.

13. Rosenbaum, M., M.D., and M. Susser, M.D. *Solving the Puzzle of Chronic Fatigue Syndrome* (Tacoma, WA: Life Sciences Press, 1992), 131.

14. Trowbridge, J., and M. Walker. *The Yeast Syndrome* (New York: Bantam Books, 1986).

15. Pizzorno, J. E., and M. T. Murray, eds. *A Textbook of Natural Medicine* (Seattle, WA: John Bastyr College Publications, 1988–1989).

16. Chaitow, L. *Post Viral Fatigue Syndrome* (London: Dents, 1989).

17. Crinnion, W. J. *Clinical Trial Results on Neesby's Capricin* (unpublished manuscript, September 10, 1985). Available from: Probiologic, Inc., 1803 132nd Avenue NE, Bellevue, WA 98005.

18. Pizzorno, J. E., and M. T. Murray, eds. *A Textbook of Natural Medicine* (Seattle, WA: John Bastyr College Publications, 1988–1989).

## Chapter 4. Restoring Immune Vitality

1. Carrow, Donald J., M.D. "Beta-1,3-Glucan as a Primary Immune Activator." *Townsend Letter for Doctors & Patients* ( June 1996), 86–91.

2. Meira, D. A., et al. "The Use of Glucan as Immunostimulant in the Treatment of Paracoccidioidomycosis." *American Journal of Tropical Medicine and Hygiene* 55:5 (November 1996), 496–503.

3. Browder, W., et al. "Synergistic Effect of Nonspecific Immunostimulation and Antibiotics in Experimental Peritonitis." *Surgery* 102:2 (August 1987), 206–214.

4. Whitaker, Julian, M.D. "Give Your Immune Cells a Natural 'Shot in the Arm.'" *Health & Healing* 7:3 (March 1997), 1–3. Beardsley, Terry R., et al. "Induction of T-cell Maturation by a Cloned Line of Thymic Epithelium (TEPI)." *Proceedings of the National Academy of Sciences* 80 (1983), 6005–6009.

Hays, Esther F., and Terry R. Beardsley. "Immunologic Effects of Human Thymic Stromal Grafts and Cell Lines." *Clinical Immunology and Immunopathology* 33 (1984), 381–390. Hale, Peter. "The FIV Connection." *Searchlight* (Summer 1996), 21–23. O'Brien, C. J. "In Vitro Effect of TP-1 (a Calf Thymic Extract) on Suppressor T-cell Function of Patients with Autoimmune Chronic Active Hepatitis." *International Journal of Immunopharmacology* 10:6 (1988), 651–666. Podwysocka, M., et al., "Correction of the Abnormal Ratio of OKT4+ to OKT8+ Peripheral Blood Lymphocytes in Patients Suffering Arthritis (JCA) by the Extract from Calf Thymuses." *Archivum Immunolgiae et Therapiae Experimentalis* 37:1-2 (1989), 127–132. Pontiggia, P., et al. "Effect of Treatment with Thymustimulin (TP-1) on T and B Cells in Lymphoproliferative Disorders." *Blut* 47:3 (1983), 153–156.

5. Papenburg, R., et al. "Dietary Milk Proteins Inhibit the Development of Dimethylhydrazine-induced Malignancy." *Tumour Biology* 11:3 (1990), 129–136. Bounous, Gustavo, M.D., et al. "Whey Proteins as a Food Supplement in HIV-seropositive Individuals." *Clinical and Investigative Medicine* 16:3 (1993), 204–209. Lang, C. A., et al. "Low Blood Glutathione Levels in Healthy Aging Adults." *Journal of Laboratory and Clinical Medicine* 120:5 (1992), 720–725. Julius, M., et al. "Glutathione and Morbidity in a Community-based Sample of Elderly." *Journal of Clinical Epidemiology* 47:9 (1994), 1021–1026.

## Chapter 5.  Detoxifying the Body

1. Burton Goldberg Group. *Alternative Medicine: The Definitive Guide* (Tiburon, CA: Future Medicine Publishing, 1995), 3.

2. Ibid., 4.

3. Elmer, Gary W., Ph.D., et al. "Biotherapeutic Agents: A Neglected Modality for the Treatment and Prevention of Selected Intestinal and Vaginal Infections." *Journal of the American Medical Association* 275:11 (March 20, 1996), 870–876.

4. Crayhon, Robert. *Health Benefits of FOS* (New Canaan, CT: Keats Publishing, 1995).

## Chapter 6.  Reversing Hidden Thyroid Problems

1. *Natural Medicine Newsletter* 1:2 (March 1997).

2. Ibid.

## Chapter 7.  Eliminating Heavy Metal Toxicity

1. "Dental Mercury Hygiene: Summary of Recommendations in 1990." *Journal of the American Dental Association* 122 (August 1991), 112.

2. Patient records of David J. Nickel, O.M.D., L.Ac.

3. van Benschoten, M. M. "Acupoint Energetics of Mercury Toxicity and Amalgam Removal with Case Studies." *American Journal of Acupuncture* 22:3 (1994), 251–262.

4. "Dental Amalgam: A Scientific Review and Recommended Public Health Service Strategy for Research, Education and Regulation." *Final Report of the Subcommittee on Risk Management of the Committee to Coordinate Environmental Health and Related Programs.* (Washington: U.S. Public Health Service, 1993).

5. Melillo, W. "How Safe Is Mercury in Dentistry?" *The Washington Post Weekly Journal of Medicine, Science and Society* (September 1991), 4.

6. Hahn, L. J., et al. "Dental 'Silver' Tooth Fillings: A Source of Mercury Exposure Revealed by Whole-Body Image Scan and Tissue Analysis." *FASEB Journal* 3 (1989), 2641–2646. Hahn, L. J., et al. "Whole-Body Imaging of the Distribution of Mercury Released from Dental Fillings into Monkey Tissues." *FASEB Journal* 4 (1990), 3256–3260.

7. Vimy, M. J., Y. Takahashi, and F. L. Lorscheider. "Maternal-Fetal Distribution of Mercury Released from Dental Amalgam Fillings." *American Physiological Society* 258 (1990), R939–R945.

8. For an excellent article on the subject of mercury fillings, see Lorscheider, Fritz, et al. "Mercury Exposure from 'Silver' Tooth Fillings: Emerging Evidence Questions a Traditional Dental Paradigm." *FASEB* Journal 9 (1995), 504–508.

## Chapter 8. Replenishing Enzyme Deficiencies

1. Howell, E., M.D. *Food Enzymes for Health and Longevity* (Woodstock Valley, CT: Omangod Press, 1980).

2. Morley, J. E., M. B. Sterman, and J. H. Walsh, eds. *Nutritional Modulation of Neural Function.* UCLA Forum in Medical Sciences 28 (San Diego, CA: Academica Press, 1988).

3. Jaeger, C. B., et al. "Polymer Encapsulated Dopaminergic Cell Lines as 'Alternative Neural Grafts.'" *Progress in Brain Research* 82 (1990), 41–46.

## Chapter 9. Addressing the Allergy Connection

1. Prince, T., et al. "Chronic Fatigue in a 43-year-old Woman." *Annals of Allergy* 74 (June 1995), 474–478.

2. Patient records of Helen Thomas, D.C., of Santa Rosa, California.

3. "Quercetin: The Anti-Allergy Bioflavonoid." *Let's Live* (September 1992).

## Chapter 10. Ending Nutritional Deficiencies with Supplements

1. Patient records of Guillermo Asis, M.D.

2. *Natural Medicine Newsletter* 1 (September 1996).

3. Murray, Michael, N.D. *Encyclopedia of Nutritional Supplements* (Rocklin, CA: Prima Publishing, 1996).

4. Murray, Michael, N.D. *Chronic Fatigue Syndrome* (Rocklin, CA: Prima Publishing, 1994), 55.

5. Ibid., 56.

6. Pao, E. M., and S. Mickle. "Problem Nutrients in the United States." *Food Technology* (September 1981), 58–79.

7. U.S. Department of Health and Human Services. *Dietary Intake Source Data: U.S. 1976–1980* DHHS Publication (PHS) 8361. (Washington: U.S. Department of Health and Human Services, 1983). Data from the National Health Survey 11:231.

8. Machlin, L. J., and M. Brin. "Vitamin E." In: *Human Nutrition—A Comprehensive Treatise*, Vol. 3, edited by R. Alfin-Slater and D. Kritchevsky (New York: Plenum Press, 1980).

9. Werbach, M. R., M.D. *Nutritional Influences on Illness* (Tarzana, CA: Third Line Press, 1993).

10. The CFIDS Information Line of the CFIDS Association of America, Inc. (P.O. Box 220398, Charlotte, NC 28222-0398; tel: [800] 442-3437; fax: [704] 365-9755).

11. U.S. Department of Agriculture. *Nutritive Value of American Foods in Common Units* Agriculture Handbook No. 456 (Washington: U.S. Department of Agriculture).

12. Lark, Susan M., M.D. *Chronic Fatigue Self Help Book* (Berkeley, CA: Celestial Arts, 1995).

13. Machlin, L. J., and A. Bendich. "Free Radical Tissue Damage: Protective Role of Antioxidant Nutrient." *FASEB Journal* 1:6 (1987), 441–445.

14. Cunha, Burke A., M.D. "Beta Carotene Stimulation of Natural Killer Cell Activity in Adult Patients with Chronic Fatigue Syndrome." *The CFIDS Chronicle* (Winter 1993).

15. Murray, Michael, N.D. *Encyclopedia of Nutritional Supplements* (Rocklin, CA: Prima Publishing, 1996), 36.

16. Cameron, E. T., et al. "Ascorbic Acid and Cancer: A Review." *Cancer Research* 39 (1979), 663–681.

17. Yonemoto, R. H. "Vitamin C and Immunological Response in Normal Controls and Cancer Patients." *Medico Dialogo* 5 (1979), 23–30.

18. Lombard, Jay, M.D., and Carl Germano. *The Brain Wellness Plan: Breakthrough Medical, Nutritional, and Immune-Boosting Therapies* (New York: Kensington Books, 1997), 184.

19. Werbach, M. R., M.D. *Nutritional Influences on Illness* (Tarzana, CA: Third Line Press, 1993).

20. Cheraskin, E., et al. "Daily Vitamin C Consumption and Fatigability." *Journal of the American Geriatric Society* 24:3 (1976), 136–137.

21. Cathcart, Robert, M.D. Internet: www.mall-net.com/cathcart/cfids .html.

22. Murray, Michael, N.D. *Encyclopedia of Nutritional Supplements* (Rocklin, CA: Prima Publishing, 1996), 438.

23. U.S. Department of Agriculture. *Nutritive Value of American Foods in Common Units* Agriculture Handbook No. 456 (Washington: U.S. Department of Agriculture).

24. Murray, Frank. "Advanced New Form of Vitamin C: Ester C." *Better Nutrition for Today's Living* (January 1993).

25. Lark, Susan M., M.D. *Chronic Fatigue Self Help Book* (Berkeley, CA: Celestial Arts, 1995).

26. Murray, Michael, N.D. *Encyclopedia of Nutritional Supplements* (Rocklin, CA: Prima Publishing, 1996), 438.

27. Werbach, M. R., M.D. *Nutritional Influences on Illness* (Tarzana, CA: Third Line Press, 1993).

28. Gridley, D. S., et al. "In Vivo and In Vitro Stimulation of Cell-mediated Immunity by Vitamin B6." *Nutrition Research* 8:2 (1988), 201–207.

29. Lark, Susan M., M.D. *Chronic Fatigue Self Help Book* (Berkeley, CA: Celestial Arts, 1995).

30. Simpson, L. "M. E. and B12." *JRS Medicine* (October 1991), 633.

31. Lapp, C. W. "Chronic Fatigue Syndrome Is a Real Disease." *North Carolina Family Physician* 443:1 (1992), 6–11.

32. Ellis, F. R., and S. Nasser. "A Pilot Study of Vitamin B12 in the Treatment of Tiredness." *British Journal of Nutrition* 30:2 (1973), 277–283.

33. Lindenbaum, J., et al. "Neuropsychiatric Disorders Caused by Cobalamin Deficiency in the Absence of Anemia or Macrocytoses." *New England Journal of Medicine* 318 (1988), 1720–1728.

34. Lindenbaum, J., et al. "Prevalence of Cobalamin Deficiency in the Framingham Elderly Population." *American Journal of Clinical Nutrition* 60 (1994), 2–11.

35. Teitelbaum, Jacob, M.D. *From Fatigued to Fantastic!* (Garden City Park, NY: Avery Publishing Group, 1996), 20–21.

36. Werbach, M. R., M.D. *Nutritional Influences on Illness* (Tarzana, CA: Third Line Press, 1993).

37. Botez, M. I., et al. "Neuropsychological Correlates of Folic Acid Deficiency: Facts and Hypotheses." In: *Folic Acid in Neurology, Psychiatry, and Internal Medicine*, edited by M. I. Botez and E. H. Reynolds (New York: Raven Press, 1979).

38. Schroeder, H. *The Poisons Around Us* (Bloomington, IN: Indiana University Press, 1974), 126.

39. Underwood, E. *Trace Elements in Human and Animal Nutrition*, 4th ed. (New York: Academic Press, 1977), 267.

40. Faloona, G. R., and S. A. Levine. "The Use of Organic Germanium in Chronic Epstein-Barr Virus Syndrome (CEBVS): An Example of Interferon Modulation of Herpes Reactivation." *Orthomolecular Medicine* 3:1 (1988), 29–31.

41. Kidd, P. M. "Germanium-132 (Ge-132): Homeostatic Normalizer and Immunostimulant. A Review of Its Preventive and Therapeutic Efficacy." *International Clinical Nutrition Review* 7:1 (1987), 11–20.

42. Werbach, M. R., M.D. *Nutritional Influences on Illness* (Tarzana, CA: Third Line Press, 1993).

43. Buetler, E., et al. "Iron Therapy in Chronically Fatigued Non-Anemic Women: A Double Blind Study." *Annals of Internal Medicine* 52:378 (1960).

44. Cox, I. M., et al. "Red Blood Cell Magnesium and Chronic Fatigue Syndrome." *The Lancet* 337 (March 30, 1991), 757–760.

45. "Top CFIDS Researchers and Physicians Find Nutritional Supplement to Reduce Muscle Pain and Fatigue in Some Cases." *Health Watch* 4:3 (Summer/Fall 1994), 3.

46. Ibid.

47. "Management of Fibromyalgia: Rationale for the Use of Magnesium and Malic Acid." *Journal of Nutritional Medicine* 3 (1992), 49–59. "Alternatives: Fibromyalgia." *What Doctors Don't Tell You* 6:6 (September 1995), 9.

48. Keen, C. L., and S. Zidenberg-Cherr. *Present Knowledge in Nutrition*, 6th ed. (Washington: International Life Sciences Institute, 1990).

49. Gershwin, M. E., et al. "The Potential Impact of Nutritional Factors on Immunological Responsiveness." In: *Nutrition and Immunity* (Orlando, FL: Academic Press, 1985), 201–204.

50. Werbach, M. R., M.D. *Nutritional Influences on Illness* (Tarzana, CA: Third Line Press, 1993).

51. Snively, W. D., and R. L. Westerman. "The Clinician Views Potassium Deficit." *Minnesota Medicine* (June 1965), 713–719.

52. Gaby, A. R. "Aspartic Acid Salts and Fatigue." *Currents in Nutritional Therapeutics* (November 1982).

53. Murray, Michael, N.D. *Encyclopedia of Nutritional Supplements* (Rocklin, CA: Prima Publishing, 1996), 176.

54. Fan, A. M., and K. W. Kizer. "Selenium: Nutritional, Toxicological, and Clinical Aspects." *Western Journal of Medicine* 153 (1990), 160–167. Burk, R. F. "Recent Developments in Trace Element Metabolism and Function: Newer Roles of Selenium in Nutrition." *Journal of Nutrition* 119 (1989), 1051–1054.

55. Kiremidjian-Schumacher, L., et al. "Supplementation with Selenium and Human Immune Cell Functions; II, Effect on Cytotoxic Lymphocytes and Natural Killer Cells." *Biological Trace Element Research* 41 (1994), 115–127.

56. Boik, John. *Cancer and Natural Medicine* (Princeton, MN: Oregon Medical Press, 1995), 147.

57. Werbach, M. R., M.D. *Nutritional Influences on Illness* (Tarzana, CA: Third Line Press, 1993).

58. Krotkiewski, M., et al. "Zinc and Muscle Strength and Endurance." *Acta Physiologica Scandinavica* 116:3 (1982), 309–311.

59. Kuratsune, H., et al. "Acylcarnitine Deficiency in Chronic Fatigue Syndrome." *Clinical Infectious Diseases* 18:Suppl. 1 (January 1994), S62–S67.

60. Eaton, K. K., and A. Hunnisett. "Abnormalities in Essential Amino Acids in Patients with Chronic Fatigue Syndrome." *Journal of Nutritional Medicine* 2 (1991), 369–375.

61. Kuratsune, H., et al. "Acylcarnitine Deficiency in Chronic Fatigue Syndrome." *Clinical Infectious Diseases* 18:Suppl. 1 (January 1994), S62–S67.

62. Plioplys, S., and A. V. Plioplys. "Serum Levels of Carnitine in Chronic Fatigue Syndrome: Clinical Correlates." *Proceedings of the American Association of Chronic Fatigue Syndrome* 1 (1994), 19.

63. Kuratsune, H., et al. "Acylcarnitine Deficiency in Chronic Fatigue Syndrome." *Clinical Infectious Diseases* 18:Suppl. 1 (January 1994), S62–S67.

64. Lombard, Jay, M.D., and Carl Germano. *The Brain Wellness Plan: Breakthrough Medical, Nutritional, and Immune-Boosting Therapies* (New York: Kensington Books, 1997), 188.

65. Murray, Michael, N.D. *Encyclopedia of Nutritional Supplements* (Rocklin, CA: Prima Publishing, 1996), 296.

66. Lapp, C. W. "Chronic Fatigue Syndrome Is a Real Disease." *North Carolina Family Physician* 443:1 (1992), 6–11.

67. Teitelbaum, Jacob, M.D. *From Fatigued to Fantastic!* (Garden City Park, NY: Avery Publishing Group, 1996), 57, 71.

68. Horrobin, D. F. "Post-viral Fatigue Syndrome, Viral Infections in Atopic Eczema, and Essential Fatty Acids." *Medical Hypotheses* 32:3 (1990), 211–217.

69. Behan, P. O., et al. "Effect of High Doses of Essential Fatty Acids on the Post-viral Fatigue Syndrome." *Acta Neurologica Scandinavica* 82:3 (1990), 209–216. Behan, P. O., and W. Behan. "Essential Fatty Acids in the Treatment of Post-viral Fatigue Syndrome." In: *Omega-6 Essential Fatty Acids: Pathophysiology and Roles in Clinical Medicine*, edited by D. F. Horrobin (New York: Alan R. Liss, 1990), 275–282.

70. Murray, Michael, N.D. *Encyclopedia of Nutritional Supplements* (Rocklin, CA: Prima Publishing, 1996), 438.

## Chapter 11. Healing Psychological and Emotional Factors

1. Teitelbaum, Jacob, M.D. *From Fatigued to Fantastic!* (Garden City Park, NY: Avery Publishing Group, 1996), 73.

2. Stoff, Jesse A., M.D., and Charles R. Pellegrino, Ph.D. *Chronic Fatigue Syndrome: The Hidden Epidemic* (New York: HarperCollins, 1992), 89.

3. Ibid., 327.

4. Teitelbaum, Jacob, M.D. *From Fatigued to Fantastic!* (Garden City Park, NY: Avery Publishing Group, 1996), 73.

5. Cass, Hyla, M.D. "Alternative Medical Treatments for Depression." In: *Sacred Sorrows: Embracing and Transforming Depression*, edited by John E. Nelson, M.D., and Andrea Nelson, Ph.D. (New York: Jeremy P. Tarcher/Putnam, 1996), 92–101.

6. Hodgkinson, N. "'Yuppie Flu'—It Is All in the Mind Say Doctors." *The Sunday Times London* (July 17, 1988).

## Chapter 12. Treating Chronic Fatigue with Herbs

1. Lark, Susan M., M.D. *The Chronic Fatigue Self Help Book* (Berkeley, CA: Celestial Arts, 1995).

2. McCarty, Daniel J., et al. "Treatment of Pain Due to Fibromyalgia With Topical Capsaicin: A Pilot." *Seminars in Arthritis and Rheumatism* 23:6 Suppl 3, 41–47.

3. Patient records of Dennis Zinner, D.C., of San Francisco, California.

4. Berne, Katrina, Ph.D. *Running on Empty: The Complete Guide to Chronic Fatigue Syndrome (CFIDS)* (Alameda, CA: Hunter House, 1995), 190.

5. Henry, C. J., and B. Emery. "Effect of Spiced Food on Metabolic Rate." *Human Nutrition Clinical Nutrition* 40:2 (March 1986), 165–168.

6. Glatzel, H. "Blood Circulation Effectiveness of Natural Spices." *Medizinische Klinik* 62:51 (December 1967), 1987–1989.

7. Buzzanca, G., and S. Laterza. "Clinical Trial with an Antirheumatic Ointment." *Clinica Terapeutica* 83:1 (October 1977), 71–83.

8. Mills, Simon Y., M.A. *The Dictionary of Modern Herbalism* (Rochester, VT: Healing Arts Press, 1988), 58–59.

9. ESCOP, European Scientific Cooperative for Phytotherapy. *Valerian Root.* (Meppel, The Netherlands: ESCOP, European Scientific Cooperative for Phytotherapy, 1990). Foster, S. *Chamomile.* Botanical Series 307 (Austin, TX: American Botanical Council, 1991).

10. Mills, Simon Y., M.A. *The Dictionary of Modern Herbalism* (Rochester, VT: Healing Arts Press, 1988), 75.

11. Puotinen, C. J. *Herbs for Detoxification* (New Canaan, CT: Keats, 1997), 67.

12. Foster, S. *Echinacea: The Purple Coneflowers. Botanical Series* 301 (Austin, TX: American Botanical Council, 1991).

13. German Ministry of Health. *Echinacea purpurea Leaf. Commission E Monographs for Phytomedicines* (Bonn, Germany: German Ministry of Health, 1989).

14. Foster, S. *Garlic. Botanical Series* 311 (Austin, TX: American Botanical Council, 1991).

15. Ibid.

16. Foster, S. *Garlic. Botanical Series* 311 (Austin, TX: American Botanical Council, 1991). Kleijnen, J., P. Knipschild, and G. Terriet. "Garlic, Onions and Cardiovascular Risk Factors. A Review of the Evidence from Human Experiments with Emphasis on Commercially Available Preparations." *British Journal of Clinical Pharmacology* 28:5 (November 1989), 535–544.

17. Berne, Katrina, Ph.D. *Running on Empty: The Complete Guide to Chronic Fatigue Syndrome (CFIDS)* (Alameda, CA: Hunter House, 1995), 191.

18. Braquet, P., ed. *Ginkgolides: Chemistry, Biology, Pharmacology and Clinical Perspectives*, Vol. 1 (Barcelona, Spain: J. Prous Science Publishers, 1988). Braquet, P., ed. *Ginkgolides: Chemistry, Biology, Pharmacology and Clinical Perspectives*, Vol. 2 (Barcelona, Spain: J. Prous Science Publishers, 1989). Fungfeld, E. W., ed. *Rokan: Ginkgo biloba* (New York: Springer Verlag, 1988).

19. Root, Jolie Martin. "16 Ways to Boost Your Brain Power." *Alternative Medicine Digest* 20 (November 1997), 17.

20. Shibata, S., et al. "Chemistry and Pharmacology of Panax." *Economic and Medicinal Plant Research* 1 (1985), 217–284.

21. Werbach, Melvyn R., M.D., and Michael T. Murray, N.D. *Botanical Influences on Illness: A Sourcebook of Clinical Research* (Tarzana, CA: Third Line Press, 1994).

22. Brekhman, I. I., and I. V. Dardymov. "Pharmacological Investigation of Glycosides From Ginseng and Eleutherococcus." *Lloydia* 32 (1969), 46–51.

23. Bombardelli, E., A. Cirstoni, and A. Lietti. "The Effect of Acute and Chronic (Panax) Ginseng Saponins Treatment on Adrenal Function; Biochemical and Pharmacological." *Proceedings of the 3rd International Ginseng Symposium* 1 (1980), 9–16. Fulder, S. J. "Ginseng and the Hypothalamic-Pituitary Control of Stress." *American Journal of Chinese Medicine* 9 (1981), 112–118.

24. Feng, L. M., H. Z. Pan, and W. W. Li. "Anti-Oxidant Action of Panax Ginseng." *Chung Hsi I Chieh Ho Tsa Chih* 7:5 (May 1987), 262, 288–290.

25. Hikino, H., et al. "Antihepatotoxic Actions of Ginsenosides From Panax Ginseng Roots." *Planta Medica* 52 (1985), 62–64.

26. Ng, T. B., and H. W. Yeung. "Hypoglycemic Constituents of Panax Ginseng." *General Pharmacology* 6 (1985), 549–552.

27. Huo, Y. S. "Anti-Senility Action of Saponin in Panax Ginseng Fruit in 327 Cases." *Chung Hsi I Chieh Ho Tsa Chih* 4:10 (October 1984), 578, 593–596.

28. Joo, C. N. "The Preventative Effect of Korean (P. Ginseng) Saponins on Aortic Atheroma Formation in Prolonged Cholesterol-Fed Rabbits." *Proceedings of the 3rd International Ginseng Symposium* (1980), 27–36.

29. Scaglione, F., et al. "Immunomodulatory Effects of Two Extracts of Panax Ginseng." *Drugs Under Experimental and Clinical Research* 16:10 (1990), 537–542.

30. Yamamoto, M., and T. Uemura. "Endocrinological and Metabolic Actions of P. Ginseng Principles." *Proceeding of the 3rd International Ginseng Symposium* (1980), 115–119.

31. Berdyshev, V. V. "Effect of the Long-Term Intake of Eleutherococcus on the Adaptation of Sailors in the Tropics." *Voenno-Meditsinskii Zhurnal* 5 (May 1981), 57–58.

32. Hoffmann, D. *The New Holistic Herbal* (Rockport, MA: Element, 1991), 204.

33. Hahn, F. E., and J. Ciak. "Berberine." *Antibiotics and Chemotherapy* 3 (1976), 577–588.

34. Choudhry, V. P., M. Sabir, and V. N. Bhide. "Berberine in Giardiasis." *Indian Pediatrics* 9:3 (March 1972), 143–146.

35. Kumazawa, Y., et al. "Activation of Peritoneal Macrophages by Berberine-Alkaloids in Terms of Induction of Cytostatic Activity." *International Journal of Immunopharmacology* 6 (1984), 587–592.

36. German Ministry of Health. *Hops. Commission E Monographs for Phytomedicines* (Bonn, Germany: German Ministry of Health, 1989).

37. Lehmann, E., et al. "Efficacy of a Special Kava Extract (Piper methysticum) in Patients with Anxiety, Tension, and Excitedness of Non-Mental Origin." *Phytomedicine* 3 (1996), 113–119.

38. Volz, H. P., and M. Kieser. "Kava-kava Extract WS 14490 Versus Placebo in Anxiety Disorders: A Randomized Placebo-Controlled 25-Week Outpatient Trial." *Pharmacopsychiatria* 30 (1997), 1–5.

39. Mills, Simon Y., M.A. *The Dictionary of Modern Herbalism* (Rochester, VT: Healing Arts Press, 1988), 138.

40. Armanini, D., et al. "Affinity of Liquorice Derivatives for Mineralo-corticoid and Glucocorticoid Receptors." *Clinical Endocrinology* 19 (November 1983), 609–612. Berne, Katrina, Ph.D. *Running on Empty: The Complete Guide to Chronic Fatigue Syndrome (CFIDS)* (Alameda, CA: Hunter House, 1995), 191.

41. Hikino, H., and Y. Kiso. "Natural Products for Liver Diseases." In: Wagner, H., H. Hikino, and N. R. Farnsworth. *Economic and Medicinal Plant Research*, 2nd ed. (London: Academic Press, 1988).

42. Pompei, R., et al. "Antiviral Activity of Glycrrhizic Acid." *Experientia* 36 (March 1980), 304–305.

43. Baschetti, Riccardo. "Chronic Fatigue Syndrome and Liquorice (Letter)." *New Zealand Medical Journal* 108 (April 26, 1995), 156–157.

44. Vogel, G. "Natural Substances with Effects on the Liver." In:

Wagner, H., and P. Wolff, eds. *New Natural Products and Plant Drugs with Pharmacological, Biological or Therapeutic Activity* (Heidelberg, Germany: Springer-Verlag, 1977).

45. Wagner, H., F. Willer, and B. Kreher. "Biologically Active Compounds From the Aqueous Extract of *Urtica dioica*." *Planta Medica* 55:5 (October 1989), 452–454.

46. Mittman, P. "Randomized, Double-Blind Study of Freeze-Dried *Urtica dioica* in the Treatment of Allergic Rhinitis." *Planta Medica* 56:1 (February 1990), 44–47.

47. Hoffmann, D. *The New Holistic Herbal* (Rockport, MA: Element, 1991), 218.

48. Hirazumi, A., E. Furusawa, S. C. Chou, and Y. Hokama. *Proceedings of the Western Pharmacology Society* 37 (1994), 145–146.

49. Mayell, Mark. "Increase Your Energy." *Off-the-Shelf Natural Health* (New York: Bantam Books, 1995), 123–124.

50. German Ministry of Health. *Passion Flower Leaves. Commission E Monographs for Phytomedicines* (Bonn, Germany: German Ministry of Health, 1985).

51. Mills, Simon Y., M.A. *The Dictionary of Modern Herbalism* (Rochester, VT: Healing Arts Press, 1988), 164.

52. Foster, S. *Passion Flower. Botanical Series* 314 (Austin, TX: American Botanical Council, 1993).

53. Foster, S. *Peppermint. Botanical Series* 306 (Austin, TX: American Botanical Council, 1991).

54. German Ministry of Health. *Peppermint Oil. Commission E Monographs for Phytomedicines* (Bonn, Germany: German Ministry of Health, 1989).

55. Suzuki, O., et al. "Inhibition of Monoamine Oxidase by Hypericin." *Planta Medica* 50 (1984), 272–274. Muldner, H., and M. Zoller. "Antidepressive Effect of a Hypericum Extract Standardized to an Active Hypericine Complex. Biochemical and Clinical Studies." *Arzneimittelforschung* 34:8 (1984), 918–920.

56. Meruelo, D., et al. "Therapeutic Agents with Dramatic Antiviral Activity and Little Toxicity at Effective Doses: Aromatic Polycyclicdiones Hypericin and Pseudohypericin." *Proceedings of the National Academy of Sciences* 85 (1988), 5230–5234.

57. De Smet, Peter, et al. "St. John's Wort as an Antidepressant." *British Medical Journal* 7052:313 (August 3, 1996), 241–242. Linde, Klaus, et al. "St. John's Wort for Depression—An Overview and Meta-Analysis of Randomized Clinical Trials." *British Medical Journal* 7052:313 (August 3, 1996), 253–258.

58. Hobbs, Christopher, L.Ac. *Stress and Natural Healing* (Loveland, CO: Interweave Press, 1997), 158–159.

59. German Ministry of Health. *Valerian. Commission E Monographs for Phytomedicines* (Bonn, Germany: German Ministry of Health, 1985).

60. ESCOP, European Scientific Cooperative for Phytotherapy. *Valerian Root* (Meppel, The Netherlands: European Scientific Cooperative for Phytotherapy, 1990).

61. Mills, Simon Y., M.A. *The Dictionary of Modern Herbalism* (Rochester, VT: Healing Arts Press, 1988), 211.

62. Hobbs, Christopher, L.Ac. "Valerian: A Literature Review." *Herbal-Gram* 21 (1989), 19–34.

## Chapter 13. Lipid Replacement Therapy

1. Seidman, M. "Polyunsaturated phosphatidylcholine in NT Factor improves mitochondrial function, auditory sensitivity and may slow some of the aging processes." *Anti-aging Medical News.* 2001; Winter (4): 5. Seidman, M., M. J. Khan , W. X. Tang, and W. S. Quirk. "Influence of lecithin on mitochondrial DNA and age-related hearing loss." *Otolaryngol Head Neck Surg* 2002; 127:138–144.

2. Block, J. B., and E. Stevens. "Clinical Evidence Supporting Cancer Risk Reduction with Antioxidants and Implications for Diet and Supplementation." *Journal of American Nutraceutical Association* 3:1 (Spring 2000), 6–16.

3. Block, J. B., and E. Stevens. "A Review of Recent Results Addressing the Potential Interactions of Antioxidants with Cancer Drug Therapy." *Journal of American Nutraceutical Association* 4:1 (Spring 2001), 11–20.

## Chapter 14. Additional Alternative Therapies

1. Fletcher, D. J. "Regaining the Ability to Heal." *Alternative Medicine* 35 (May 2000), 67.

2. "Chinese Display Qigong Energy for U.S. Doctors." *Brain/Mind Bulletin* 11:6 (March 3, 1986).

3. Dodd, G. H. "Receptor Events in Perfumery." In: Van toller, S., and G. H. Dodd, eds. *Perfumery: The Psychology and Biology of Fragrance* (London: Chapman and Hall, 1988).

## Chapter 15. Treating and Preventing Lyme Disease

1. Vanderhoof-Forschner, Karen. *Everything You Need to Know About Lyme Disease and Other Tick-Borne Disorders,* 2nd ed. (Hoboken, NJ: John Wiley & Sons, Inc., 2003), 39.

2. Ibid, 47.

3. Ibid.

4. Ibid.

5. Ibid, 58.

6. Ibid, 65.

7. Burrascano, Joseph. *Advanced Topics in Lyme Disease: Diagnostic Hints and Treatment Guidelines for Lyme and Other Tick Borne Illnesses*, 13th ed. (May 2000). Available from East End Medical Associates, P.C., 139 Springs Fireplace Road, East Hampton, NY 11937; tel: (631) 324-7337.

8. Vanderhoof-Forschner, Karen. *Everything You Need to Know About Lyme Disease and Other Tick-Borne Disorders*, 2nd ed. (Hoboken, NJ: John Wiley & Sons, Inc., 2003), 85.

9. Ibid, 89.

10. Ibid, 90.

11. Ibid, 90–91.

12. Ibid, 91–92.

13. Burrascano, Joseph. *Advanced Topics in Lyme Disease: Diagnostic Hints and Treatment Guidelines for Lyme and Other Tick Borne Illnesses*, 13th ed. (May 2000).

14. Ibid.

15. Ibid.

16. Ibid.

17. Ibid.

18. Ibid.

19. Ibid.

# Index

LECIPS, 246
Lecithin, 165
Lee, Lita, 17, 35, 55, 68, 91, 151, 161, 208–9, 213–14
Lee, Martin, 30
Lehmann, E., 314
LEM, 68
Leukocytes, 101, 336
Leukotrienes, 219
Levin, Norman, 274–78
Levy, Jay, 43
Lewis, Judith A., 288–91
Lichtenberg, H., 183
Licorice, 314, 315–16
Lieberman, Shari, 5, 68–71, 268, 279
Lifestyle choices/changes. *See also* Emotions; Psychological factors
CFS and, 250–51, 273, 278–81
depression and, 293
importance of, 127
Lyme disease and, 406–7
Ligaments, 368, 369
Light therapy, 104–5, 411–12
Linoleic acid, 270
Lipase, 55, 210–11
Lipid replacement therapy, 341–51
cellular energy and, 341–45
combining, with other therapies, 345–51
digestion and, 345–47
Lipotropic factors, 249–50
Liver
fatty infiltration of, 166
flushes, 136–38
importance of, 136
Lombard, Jay, 268
Long-chain fatty acids (LCFAs), 35
Loomis, Charles, 55
Loomis, Howard, 214, 215
Loomis urinalysis, 55
Lyme, Connecticut, 385, 391
Lyme carditis, 397
Lyme disease, 385–414
case study of, 408–13
future of, 413–14
heart problems and, 397

history of, 385, 391
incidence of, 389
misdiagnosis of, 22, 385–86, 389
preventing, 398–400
symptoms of, 386–89, 395–96
testing and diagnosing, 391–98
transmission of, 389–90
treating, 390–91, 400–414
yeast infections and, 403
Lyme Disease Foundation, 414
Lyme Disease Network, 414
Lymphatic system
draining, 138
improving function of, 374–75
Lymph nodes, 100, 139
Lymphocytes, 10, 11, 39, 41, 100, 101
Lymphokines, 39, 219
Lysine, 108–9

MacroForce, 110
Macrophages, 41, 101, 112, 256, 336
Magnesium, 250, 264–65, 274–75, 339, 349, 405–6
Magnet therapy, 221
*Ma-huang. See* Ephedra
Maitake mushrooms, 70, 406
Malic acid, 265, 349
Mandell, Marshall, 122, 224, 225
Manganese, 265–66
Martin, W. John, 76–77
Masking, 218
Massage
electrostatic, 221
essential oils for, 384
for fibromyalgia, 284
Mast cells, 219
*Matricaria recutita. See* Chamomile
Mattman, Lida, 392, 393, 394, 414
MCS (multiple chemical sensitivity), 334–35. *See also* Environmental illness

McTaggart, Lynne, 162
Meaning dimension, 166–67
Medications. *See* Drugs
Meditation, 291
Melatonin, 46
Meliae seeds, 94
Mellor, Judy M., 352–61
Membrane potential, 190
Mental symptoms, 246
*Mentha piperita. See* Peppermint
Mercury
detoxification programs for, 187–95
effects of, 151, 176, 180, 184, 185–87
safety standards for, 183
sources of, 151, 193
testing for, 53
Mercury amalgams (fillings)
ADA's position on, 195–96
bans or restrictions on, 179, 195
composition of, 175, 183
dangers of, 151, 175–76, 179–87
history of, 151, 195
removal of, 176–79, 181, 188, 189, 191
Mercury toxicity
domino effect of, 182–84
symptoms of, 151, 176, 181
Meridian Center, 234, 239
Meridians. *See* Acupuncture
Metabolism
anabolic vs. catabolic, 82, 213
definition of, 82, 213
process of, 212–13
Metals, heavy. *See also* Mercury
detoxification for, 133–34
exposure to, 53
testing for, 53–54
Metbal, 109–10
Methionine, 249–50, 267–68
Methylmercury, 185
Meyers, John, 222, 274
Meyers' Cocktail, 222, 274
Miasms, homeopathic, 289
Milk thistle, 165, 189, 314, 316, 406
Milliman, Bruce, 79

# About the Authors

**Burton Goldberg** (President) rose to national prominence in 1994 with the publication of the landmark volume *Alternative Medicine: The Definitive Guide*, produced by his own publishing company. As a result of the publication of the *Guide*, he has become a focal point and leading spokesperson for the entire field of alternative medicine. He has spent 25 years researching every aspect of holistic medicine, traveling worldwide to personally investigate innovative healing techniques. He is also the founder and publisher of *Alternative Medicine* magazine, which is critically acclaimed as a unique, consumer-oriented guide to all aspects of alternative medicine, and he has co-authored and published over a dozen other books on the same subject. Mr. Goldberg tirelessly promotes alternative medicine through media appearances each year and has rightly earned the reputation as "the voice of alternative medicine."

**Larry Trivieri, Jr.**, is a leading writer and editor in the field of holistic and alternative medicine, with over 30 years of personal experience in exploring techniques for optimal wellness and human transformation. From 1991 to 1994, he served as editor and principal writer of *Alternative Medicine: The Definitive Guide*, and between 2000 and 2002 he oversaw the *Guide*'s extensive revision. He is also the author of *Health on the Edge: Visionary Views of Healing in the New Millennium* (Tarcher/Putnam, Fall 2003), and *The American Holistic Medical Association Guide to Holistic Health* (John Wiley & Sons, Spring 2001), and co-author of *The Com-*

*plete Self-Care Guide to Holistic Medicine* (Tarcher/Putnam, Fall 1999). He has also written numerous articles for a variety of publications, including *Alternative Medicine* (for which he also served as contributing editor from 1999 through 2002), *Natural Health, Whole Life Times*, and *Yoga Journal*. In 2003, he founded www.1healthyworld.com, a comprehensive online resource dedicated to empowering personal health using holistic and alternative healing approaches. Mr. Trivieri resides in his hometown of Utica, New York.

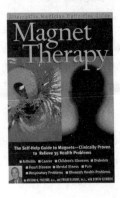

**T**hese titles are part of our Alternative Medicine Definitive Guide paperback series—offering practical proven advice that may mean the difference between sickness and robust health. We distill the work of hundreds of leading alternative physicians from all disciplines and put it into a reader-friendly format—medical knowledge without the jargon. Essential reading before your next doctor's visit. Because you need to know your medical alternatives.

# To order, call 800-333-2665
# or visit www.alternativemedicine.com

You can also find our books at your local health food store or bookstore

# Stay up-to-date...

## In each issue you will . . .

✻ **Learn** how alternative medicine can enhance the quality of your life.

✻ **Discover** secrets to a healthier lifestyle that will help protect you against disease.

✻ **Read** exciting news about new therapies, studies and emerging alternative treatments.

✻ **Find out** how to naturally boost your energy level and vitality.

✻ **Receive** delicious recipes for cooking and eating well.

✻ **Encounter** natural beauty products that go more than skin deep.

# Send for your FREE trial issue today!

For faster service, call **800-546-6707** or visit: www.alternativemedicine.com